INTERNATIONAL HAN POSITIVE AGING

As our global demographic shifts towards an increasingly aging population, we have an opportunity to transform how we experience and think about getting older and embrace the diversity and contribution that this population can bring to society. The *International Handbook of Positive Aging* showcases the latest research and theory into aging, examining the various challenges faced by older adults and the ways in which we can bring a much-needed positive focus towards dealing with these.

The handbook brings together disparate research from medical, academic, economic and social community fields, with contributions from NHS partners, service users, universities across the United Kingdom and collaborations with international research leaders in the field of aging. Divided into sections, the first part of the book focuses on introducing the concept of positive aging, then goes on to cover the body over the life course, well-being and care delivery. All contributors recognise it is the fact that we are living longer which is providing us with a tremendous opportunity to enjoy and flourish in healthy and fulfilling later lives, and this focus on the importance of patient empowerment is integral to the book.

This is a valuable reference source for those working in developmental psychology, clinical psychology, mental health, health sciences, medicine, neuropsychological rehabilitation, sociology, anthropology, social policy and social work. It will help encourage researchers, professionals and policymakers to make the most of opportunities and innovations to promote a person's sense of independence, dignity, well-being, good health and participation in society as they get older.

Dr Rachael E. Docking is Senior Evidence Manager at the Centre for Ageing Better and Senior Research Fellow at Anglia Ruskin University. Her research background is in the disciplines of psychology and epidemiology. Rachael's specific interests are in attitudes to aging, chronic and/or disabling pain in older adults, risk factors for pain onset and methods for self-management of pain. Additionally, she has an interest in dementia and pain, particularly in how accurately pain can be assessed in those with dementia. In her work at the Centre for Ageing Better, an independent charitable foundation working to help everybody enjoy a good later life, Rachael leads their programme on 'Homes and neighbourhoods'. As Senior Evidence Manager she works on their evidence work stream and on identifying evidence needs.

Dr Jennifer Stock was a Senior Research Fellow at Anglia Ruskin University at the time of submission. Jennifer's background is in psychology and she has been lead on a number of aging-related research projects. Jennifer's doctoral thesis investigated the role of psychosocial factors in the relationship between physical activity and cognitive ability in older adults. Jennifer's post-doctoral research interests have included psychological resilience with aging, improving attitudes towards aging amongst young people and healthcare staff, dementia, lifestyle interventions, innovative use of technology to improve the lives of older adults, psychosocial aspects to living with long-term conditions, and end-of-life care. Jennifer is currently undertaking her Doctorate in Clinical Psychology at the Institute of Psychiatry, Psychology and Neuroscience, King's College London.

THE ROUTLEDGE INTERNATIONAL HANDBOOK SERIES

THE ROUTLEDGE INTERNATIONAL HANDBOOK OF THE SOCIOLOGY OF EDUCATION
Edited by Michael W. Apple, Stephen J. Ball and Luis Armando Gandin

THE ROUTLEDGE INTERNATIONAL HANDBOOK OF CRITICAL EDUCATION
Edited by Michael W. Apple, Wayne Au, and Luis Armando Gandin

THE ROUTLEDGE INTERNATIONAL HANDBOOK OF LIFELONG LEARNING
Edited by Peter Jarvis

THE ROUTLEDGE INTERNATIONAL COMPANION TO MULTICULTURAL EDUCATION
Edited by James A. Banks

THE ROUTLEDGE INTERNATIONAL HANDBOOK OF ENGLISH, LANGUAGE AND LITERACY TEACHING
Edited by Dominic Wyse, Richard Andrews and James Hoffman

THE ROUTLEDGE INTERNATIONAL HANDBOOK OF HIGHER EDUCATION
Edited by Malcolm Tight, Ka Ho Mok, Jeroen Huisman and Christopher C. Morpew

THE ROUTLEDGE INTERNATIONAL HANDBOOK OF EARLY LITERACY EDUCATION
Edited by Natalia Kucirkova, Catherine E. Snow, Vibeke Grover and Catherine McBride

THE ROUTLEDGE INTERNATIONAL HANDBOOK OF EARLY CHILDHOOD PLAY
Edited by Tina Bruce, Pentti Hakkarainen and Milda Bredikyte

INTERNATIONAL HANDBOOK OF POSITIVE AGING
Edited by Rachael E. Docking and Jennifer Stock

INTERNATIONAL HANDBOOK OF POSITIVE AGING

Edited by Rachael E. Docking and Jennifer Stock

Routledge
Taylor & Francis Group
LONDON AND NEW YORK

First published 2017 by Routledge

2 Park Square, Milton Park, Abingdon, Oxfordshire OX14 4RN
52 Vanderbilt Avenue, New York, NY 10017

Routledge is an imprint of the Taylor & Francis Group, an informa business

First issued in paperback 2019

British Library Cataloguing-in-Publication Data
A catalogue record for this book is available from the British Library

Library of Congress Cataloguing-in-Publication Data
A catalog record for this book has been requested

ISBN: 978-1-138-93305-7 (hbk)
ISBN: 978-0-367-87349-3 (pbk)

Typeset in Bembo
by Apex CoVantage, LLC

CONTENTS

CONTRIBUTORS

Mustafa Al-Haboubi BDS, MSc, PhD, DDPH (RCS England) Policy Innovation Research Unit, Department of Health Services Research and Policy, Faculty of Public Health and Policy, London School of Hygiene & Tropical Medicine, London, UK. Formerly, Faculty of Education and Health, University of Greenwich, London, UK.

Geraldine Anthony, RN, RM, BSc, MSc, PhD School of Pharmacy & Life Sciences, Robert Gordon University, Aberdeen, Scotland, UK.

Koula Asimakopoulou, PhD Division of Population and Patient Health, King's College London, London, UK.

Liz Bacon, BSc, PhD, CEng, CSci, CITP, FBCS, PFHEA Faculty of Architecture, Computing and Humanities, University of Greenwich, London, UK.

Jane Banaszak-Holl, BA, MA, PhD School of Public Health, University of Michigan, Michigan, US; School of Medicine, University of Michigan, Michigan, US; Health Services Research, University of Greenwich, London, UK.

Sarah Barnes, BA (Hons), PgDip, PhD School of Health and Related Research (ScHARR), University of Sheffield, Sheffield, UK.

David Barron, BA, MA, PhD Saïd Business School, University of Oxford, Oxford, UK.

Gary Bellamy, BN (Hons), MA, PhD National Institute of Health Research, Clinical Research Network, North West London, UK.

Walter R. Boot, PhD Department of Psychology, Florida State University, Florida, US.

Tom Boterberg, MD, PhD Department of Radiation Oncology, Ghent University Hospital, Ghent, Belgium.

Etienne Brain, MD, PhD Hôpital René Huguenin – Institut Curie, Saint-Cloud, France & President of the International Society of Geriatric Oncology.

Joanne Brooke, BSc, MSc, PGCE HE, Professional Doctorate, RGN Oxford Institute of Nursing and Allied Health Research, Oxford Brookes University, UK.

Val Chandler, MBA Faculty of Education and Health, University of Greenwich, London, UK.

Tatiana Christides, BA, MSc, MD Faculty of Engineering and Science, University of Greenwich, Medway, UK.

Rachel Crockett, PhD School of Natural Sciences, University of Stirling, Stirling, UK.

Philip R. Debruyne, MD, PhD, MSc, FRCP (Glasg), FCP Department of Medical Oncology, Cancer Centre, General Hospital Groeninge, Kortrijk, Belgium; Faculty of Health, Social Care, & Education, Anglia Ruskin University, Chelmsford, UK.

Rachael E. Docking, MA (Hons), PhD Faculty of Health, Social Care, & Education, Anglia Ruskin University, Chelmsford, UK; Centre for Ageing Better, London, UK.

John Foster, BA (Hons), PGHCE, RMN, MSc, PhD Faculty of Education and Health, University of Greenwich, London, UK.

Leslie Gelling, BSc (Hons), MA, PhD, RN, FRSA Faculty of Health, Social Care, & Education, Anglia Ruskin University, Chelmsford, UK.

Eshtar Hamid, MD, MSc Faculty of Health, Social Care, & Education, Anglia Ruskin University, Chelmsford, UK.

Michelle Lycke, MSc Cancer Centre, General Hospital Groeninge, Kortrijk, Belgium.

Lachlan MacKinnon, FBCS, CITP, CEng, PhD, BSc, CQSW, CSS, RGN, RMN Faculty of Architecture, Computing and Humanities, University of Greenwich, London, UK.

Joanna Malone, BSc (Hons), MSc Faculty of Health, Social Care, & Education, Anglia Ruskin University, Chelmsford, UK.

Pauline McGovern, PhD Faculty of Business, University of Greenwich, London, UK.

M. Elena Mendoza, PhD Department of Rehabilitation Medicine, University of Washington, Seattle, Washington, US.

Supriya G. Mohile, MD, MS University of Rochester Medical Centre, Rochester, New York, US.

Carlos Moreno-Leguizamon, BA, PGCEHE, MA, PhD Faculty of Health and Education, University of Greenwich, London, UK.

Paul Newton, BA (Hons), MSc, PhD Faculty of Education and Health, University of Greenwich, London, UK.

Ann Pascoe, MSc Carer, Founder and Director of Dementia Friendly Communities Community Interest Company, Helmsdale, Scotland, UK.

Lies Pottel, MSc, PhD Cancer Centre, General Hospital Groeninge, Kortrijk, Belgium.

Nelson A. Roque, MS Department of Psychology, Florida State University, Florida, US.

Sasha Scambler, PhD Division of Population and Patient Health, King's College London, London, UK.

Pat Schofield, DipN, PGDip, PhD, RGN Faculty of Health, Social Care, & Education, Anglia Ruskin University, Chelmsford, UK.

David Smith, BA (Hons), TESOL Cert, PhD, PGCLT (HE) Faculty of Health and Education, University of Greenwich, London, UK.

Clarence Spigner, DrPH, MPH, AB School of Public Health, University of Washington, Seattle, Washington, US.

Jill Stewart, BSc (Hons), MCIEH, FRSPH, CMIH, FRGS, PGCE, MSc, PhD Faculty of Science and Technology, Middlesex University, London, UK.

Jennifer Stock, BSc (Hons) DPS, MRes, PhD Faculty of Health, Social Care, & Education, Anglia Ruskin University, Chelmsford, UK; Institute of Psychiatry, Psychology and Neuroscience, King's College London, London, UK.

Trevor Thompson, BSc, MSc, PhD Faculty of Education and Health, University of Greenwich, London, UK.

Hilde Verbeek, PhD Department of Health Services Research, Maastricht University, The Netherlands.

Elizabeth West, BSc, MSc, MA, PhD Faculty of Education and Health, University of Greenwich, London, UK; Faculty of Health, Social Care & Education, Anglia Ruskin University, Chelmsford, UK.

Katharine Whittingham, RGN, BSc (Hons), MPH, Fellow of HEA, M.I.H.P.E. School of Health Sciences, Queens Medical Centre, University of Nottingham, Nottingham, UK.

Elaine Wiersma, BRLS, MA, PhD Centre for Education and Research on Aging and Health, Lakehead University, Ontario, Canada.

PART I

Introduction to positive aging

1
INTRODUCTION

Rachael E. Docking and Jennifer Stock

Demographics

We are anticipating a major shift in the demographic in the United Kingdom over the next 20–30 years. Over the past century there has been a significant increase in life expectancy and it is estimated that by 2031 the proportion of people aged >65 years in the United Kingdom will have increased from 16 to 22 per cent, exceeding the population <25 years of age (Greengross et al., 1997). For the first time in history, people aged >60 years now outnumber those aged <16 years in developed countries (Office of National Statistics, 2010). The latest projections are for 5½ million additional older people in 20 years' time and the number will have nearly doubled to around 19 million by 2050. There are currently three million people aged more than 80 years and this is projected to almost double by 2030 and reach eight million by 2050. The pensioner population is expected to rise despite the increase in the women's state pension age to 65 between 2010 and 2020 and the increase for both men and women from 65 to 68 between 2024 and 2046. In 2008 there were 3.2 people of working age for every person of pensionable age. This ratio is projected to fall to 2.8 by 2033.

With the older population the fastest growing part of our society and with the majority of the population expecting to survive until their eighth and ninth decade, the implications of this are far reaching upon health and social care; with already stretched services being stretched even further, the impact on society will be considerable. However, while an aging population brings with it a range of challenges for society, it is also an emerging phenomenon that should be celebrated along with better healthcare and healthier lifestyles; living longer is potentially one of the greatest opportunities.

Concepts of aging

In the health and care sector, across media outlets, and within society generally, aging is often approached and described with negative language. Older people, and the aging population, are often labelled with words with negative connotations, such as bed blockers, aging tsunami, ticking time bomb, frail, and vulnerable, to name just a few. Even words such as mature, senior, or pensioner are used to diminish how we perceive the value of older adults.

It is time for society to move away from old fashioned, stereotypical views of aging, which focus on chronological age. While our society is changing, with older people active and valuable members within this, attitudes and language around aging are still lagging behind.

We have an opportunity to transform how we experience and think about getting older, and it is therefore time to leave behind labels and relish in the diversity and contribution that an aging population can bring to society.

Opportunity

The experience of aging varies hugely across the population. A recent report by the Centre for Ageing Better (Ipsos Mori, 'Later Life in 2015'), a not-for-profit organisation who aim to help people have a better later life by understanding what works and by making change happen, found that there are many ways in which people experience their later life. There are those who are 'struggling and alone' (12 per cent of those 50 years and over), who are characterised by having less money for their needs and are more likely to be in poverty. Many have a long-standing illness and suffer with frequent pain and most are socially isolated, which makes them feel dissatisfied with their life. However, the Centre for Ageing Better also found that three-quarters of people aged 50 and over report their general health as excellent or good, and report never or rarely feeling they have too little money to spend on their needs.

This research further found that the key dimensions to a good later life, as identified by older adults themselves, are health, financial security, and social connections. Within these, people have modest expectations, with their goals being to have 'good enough' health to maintain relationships and activities that they value, as well as enough money for essentials and to allow them to participate in activities socially and culturally, while also saving a little for the unexpected.

Society currently looks at older people as a burden; however, it is clear that the expectations and needs of this population are predominantly modest and it is essential for us to understand more about people's priorities as they age.

Provided with the right opportunities, this portion of the older population could be contributing to society and the economy, if provided with the right support.

Conclusion

Positive aging is not necessarily a life completely free of challenges, illness, or disabilities; people's expectations are not that they will live in perfect health. However it is about feeling a part of something, having a purpose, and being in control of one's life.

This book aims to provide an introduction to the national and international research and theory, both current and developing, that focuses on the various challenges faced by older adults and the ways in which we can shift towards a more positive focus within these. It brings together NHS partners, service users, universities across the United Kingdom, and collaborations with international research leaders in the field of aging. All contributors to this handbook recognise that the fact that we are living longer is providing us with a tremendous opportunity to enjoy and flourish in healthy and fulfilling later lives.

References

Greengross, S., Murphy, E., Quam, L., Rochon, P. & Smith, R. (1997). Aging: a subject that must be at the top world agendas. *British Medical Journal*, 315, 1029.

Office of National Statistics. (2010). www.statistics.gov.uk/default.asp (accessed March 2011).

2
WHAT IS POSITIVE AGING?

Jennifer Stock, Pat Schofield and Rachael E. Docking

This chapter discusses:

- A definition of positive aging
- The impact of negative attitudes towards aging
- The formation of attitudes towards aging
- What can be done to increase capacity for aging positively
- Interventions to improve attitudes towards aging
- Perspectives of positive aging
- Change at an organisational level
- Involvement of people with lived experience in research

A definition of positive aging

There are many terms that are used for aging-related initiatives including 'active aging' and 'healthy aging'. The Centre for Positive Ageing at the University of Greenwich was conceived, set up and led by Professor Pat Schofield, which brought together multidisciplinary academics from faculties across the University with expertise in aging-related topics to develop worthwhile research projects. As part of this work we sought to develop a term which emphasises that the process of aging is not necessarily associated with activity or good health, but that 'positive' steps may be taken to make the best of any scenario; so whilst one may not be completely healthy or active, that does not necessarily mean one is not aging positively or well. To reflect this belief, the following definition was constructed jointly by our academic team, collaborators of the Centre, and most importantly, our older adults advisory group:

> 'Positive Ageing' denotes the aspirations of individuals and communities to plan for, approach and live life's changes and challenges as they age and approach the end of their lives, in a productive, active and fulfilling manner. The focus embraces the idea of making the most of opportunities, innovations and research which promote a person's sense of independence, dignity, well-being, good health and enable their participation in society.
> *(2015)*

Attitudes towards aging

Previous studies have found that society has a generally negative perception of older people which in turn influences the behaviour of this population (Hale & Hewitt, 1998). Drennan et al. (2008) completed a review on public perceptions of older people and aging. Authors found that public perceptions of older adults can impact both positively and negatively on the lives of older people, in terms of access to health services and social/employment opportunities. Whilst there were some instances of positive attitudes towards aging, the majority of studies reviewed displayed some level of negative attitudes towards older people, from which the consequences are significant. A recent study found that attitudes towards aging held by young adults in the United Kingdom were significantly more negative compared to those held by young adults in China (Stock, 2014).

As our older population grows worldwide, it is essential we identify and target negative attitudes towards older adults in society. It is the public's perceptions of aging and older adults that impacts on the development of social policies (Arnold-Cathalifaud et al., 2008; Musaiger & D'Souza, 2009). Zhou (2007) stated that good-quality care service and healthy relationships with older adults are necessary, but are unlikely if people's views of older adults are negative. A 2009 Health Service Executive (HSE) report, "Open your eyes", detailed how the attitudes of others can significantly impact negatively on the lives of older adults due to ageist attitudes which create a culture of age discrimination, devaluing, and disempowering.

The impact of negative attitudes towards aging

There is evidence that young adults' attitudes towards aging affect how they engage with older adults. For example, negative attitudes from healthcare workers can also impact on quality of care provided (Levy, Slade & Kasl, 2002). Kemper (1994) found that nursing home caregivers with negative attitudes towards aging spoke to all older adults more slowly and used shorter words despite the varied cognitive abilities or physical health of the older adults they were addressing (Kemper, 1994). These interactions between young adults or caregivers and older adults provide social reinforcement for negative self-stereotypes of those older adults and there is evidence to suggest this has a priming and damaging effect on their physical and cognitive health (Meisner, 2012). This indicates that aging is not solely a biological process, but also a psychosocial process whereby attitudes, self-perceptions, and stereotypes of aging can affect cognitive and physical health outcomes (Levy, 2003). Negative priming of attitudes towards aging were found to elicit a three-times greater detrimental effect on health outcomes compared to the beneficial effect of positive age priming in older adults, either implicit or explicit. The detrimental effects of negative age priming on health outcomes included walking speed and gait (Hausdorff, Levy & Wei, 1999), cardiovascular responses (Levy et al., 2000), memory performance (Levy, 1996), and mental health (Levy, Pilver & Pietrzak, 2014). The aforementioned evidence suggests that ageism and negative attitudes towards aging impact negatively on cognitive and physical health outcomes and also the quality of care for older adults, thus it is essential that negative perceptions about aging across society are targeted.

Formation of attitudes towards aging

Young adults' attitudes towards aging become internalised when they reach older adulthood and manifest as self-perceptions of aging (Levy, 2003; Luborsky & McMullen, 1999; Sokolovsky, 1993). Young adults' stereotypes of older adults affect how they feel about aging and how they perceive their own future (Lowin, Knapp & Mccrone, 2001; Seefeldt et al., 1977). This could influence their perceived control of future health and the degree to which they believe age-related decline is inevitable. Longitudinal studies have demonstrated that negative self-perceptions of aging predict participation in preventative health behaviours (Levy & Myers, 2004) and functional health decline, even after controlling for baseline functional health (Levy, Slade & Kasl, 2002). Attitudes towards aging that are formed when younger have been found to predict health outcomes in later life, for example up to 38 years later for cardiovascular events (Levy et al., 2009). Positive attitudes towards aging were associated with living on average 7.5 years longer – measured up to 23 years earlier – (Levy et al., 2002) and a decline in self-perceptions of aging over time was related to an increased risk of mortality at 16-year follow-up (Sargent-Cox, Anstey & Luszcz, 2013) even after controlling for demographic characteristics and physical health. Negative attitudes towards aging also independently predicted poorer memory performance (Levy et al., 2011) and hearing loss after controlling for other established predictors (Levy, Slade & Gill, 2006).

What can be done to increase capacity for aging positively?

Interventions to improve attitudes towards aging

Drennan et al. (2008) suggested a number of recommendations following their review; one of these was that positive aging education programmes are needed and these should be targeted at all levels of society but specifically those who hold less favourable attitudes towards aging (e.g. young adults and men). The 'impressionable years' hypothesis proposes that individuals are highly susceptible to attitude change during late adolescence and early adulthood and that this susceptibility drops after this and remains low (Krosnick & Alwin, 1989). The 'increasing persistence' hypothesis proposes that individuals become increasingly resistant to change as they age. Evidence of the stability of political attitudes supports the impressionable years hypothesis but not the increasing persistence hypothesis. If these findings can be applied to attitudes towards aging then perhaps the young adults would be the most appropriate target for attitude change interventions.

There is currently limited evidence on the impact of aging education programmes to reduce ageist attitudes and increase positive attitudes towards aging. However the findings of those that have been carried out suggest that participating in such a programme can have a positive effect on attitudes to aging and older adults (e.g., Puentes & Cayer, 2001; Funderburk et al., 2006; Cottle & Glover, 2007; Gringart, Helmes & Speelman, 2008). For instance, Knapp & Stubblefield (2000) reported an improvement in the knowledge of aging in students who were enrolled on a gerontology course. There is evidence of successful intervention involving a fact sheet and inducing cognitive dissonance for improving attitudes towards older workers in a study aiming to reduce age-related employment discrimination (Gringart, Helmes & Speelman, 2008). Additionally, a creative-bonding intervention with Taiwanese nursing students was successful and resulted in significantly more positive attitudes towards older adults after the intervention compared to a 'friendly visit' control group (Chen & Walsh, 2009). Dooley & Frankel (1990) also implemented a friendly visitor type of program in which adolescents visited senior citizens; it was found that general attitudes toward older people improved following weekly contact with specific older adults. The perceived quality of the experience was found to have a significant impact on improving attitudes. The outcomes suggested that programs such as the one evaluated here can, therefore, have two outcomes: the provision of service to older individuals and the change of negative attitudes toward older people. However, an education intervention programme in secondary schools in Australia brought about little change in attitudes towards older people (Scott, Minichiello & Browning, 1998). This education intervention was designed to increase the knowledge of students about the aging process, in terms of biological and psychological changes associated with growing older and the social determinants of aging. This unsuccessful intervention highlights the importance of developing well-thought through and evaluated interventions which are relevant to the target populations. Future research needs to develop interventions for specific populations which can lead to long-term meaningful changes in attitudes towards aging.

Peer education

A recently completed project involved the development of a self-management training programme on positive aging for older adults and was delivered by older adults (Stock, Docking & Schofield, 2016). The rationale of utilising peer education in this context is based on a number of established theories. There is a common belief that advice is more readily accepted from contemporaries who are of a similar age and level of experience to the recipients (Allen, 2004; Buonocore & Sussman-Skalka, 2002). Whilst adult learning theory demonstrates the benefits of cooperative learning environments (Clemson & Swann, 2008). Furthermore social identity theory supports the notion of peer education in that people have multiple social identities and the ability to identify with a group contributes to the decision-making process. Thus, people are more influenced by others who share similar characteristics. So older adults can foster a more positive attitude to growing older, which challenges negative ageist stereotyping. Finally, according to the innovation theory, new information is more likely to be taken on board from those who are well integrated and practicing. Success of peer education models is based upon a number of key factors. For example, older people have a high level of rapport with people of the same age and hold the belief that information from peers is more credible and less biased than that from others not of a similar age (Beckingham & Watt, 1995; Shiner, 1999). It moves away from the model that healthcare professionals are the 'experts', it is seen as less 'threatening', and older peer educators have similar problems as the recipients and are therefore seen as more credible. Finally peer education amongst older adults is less socially isolating and more likely to reach 'hard-to-reach' groups such as BME populations (Quine, 1998; Bratter & Freeman, 1990).

As part of this project we recruited older adults from local community groups and pensioner forums and a University older adult research advisory group. We also involved healthcare professionals across London and South East England. Workshops were facilitated to capture insights and perceptions of what positive aging means to older adults and healthcare professionals. Insight gathered from these workshops was collated, synthesised, and used as part of discussions, within the research team, to develop curriculum and teaching materials. Discussions topics included the following, which are presented in this chapter as word cloud summaries: What does aging mean to you? (see Figure 2.1); What does positive aging mean to you? (see Figure 2.2); What are barriers to positive aging? (see Figure 2.3); What are the facilitators to positive aging? (see Figure 2.4). This study enabled us to understand our own pre-conceptions regarding aging and positive aging. Again, as healthcare professionals, researchers, and generally younger adults, we are guilty of having our own opinions regarding aging and what is positive or negative aging. The views and opinions held by us are often reflected amongst many others in the population and these are not the views and opinions of the older population with whom we worked on this project. A caveat of course is that the views and opinions of the participants may be different to those of the general older population, as we are fully aware that the older population is not a homogenous group and we should also acknowledge that this group is changing constantly.

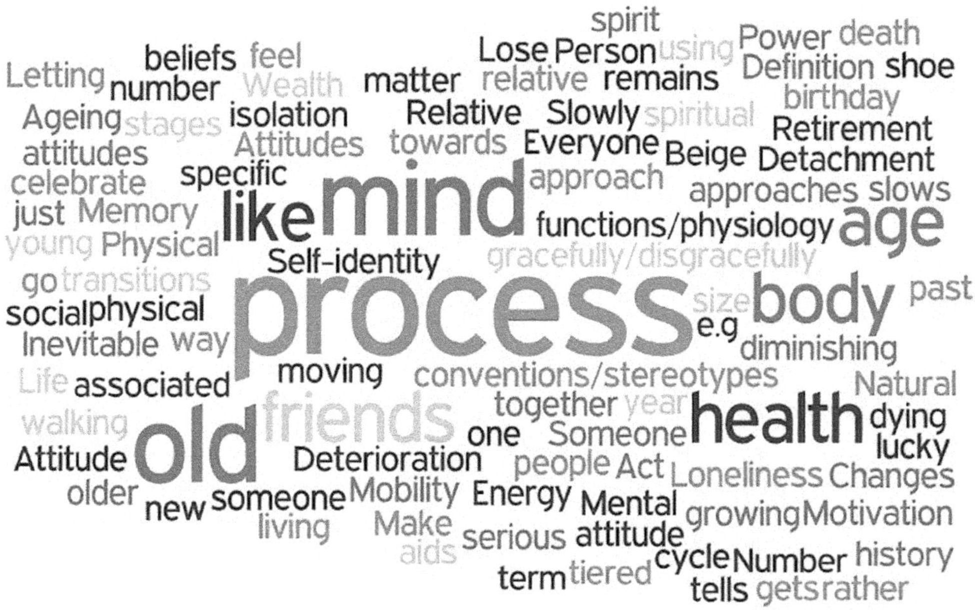

Figure 2.1 What does aging mean to you?

(Stock, Docking & Schofield, 2016).

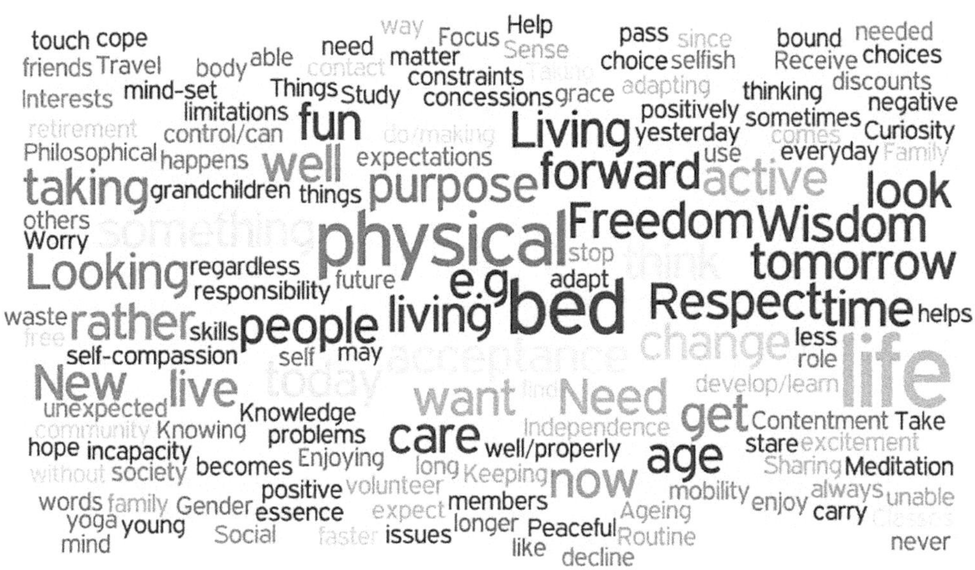

Figure 2.2 What does positive aging mean to you?

(Stock, Docking & Schofield, 2016).

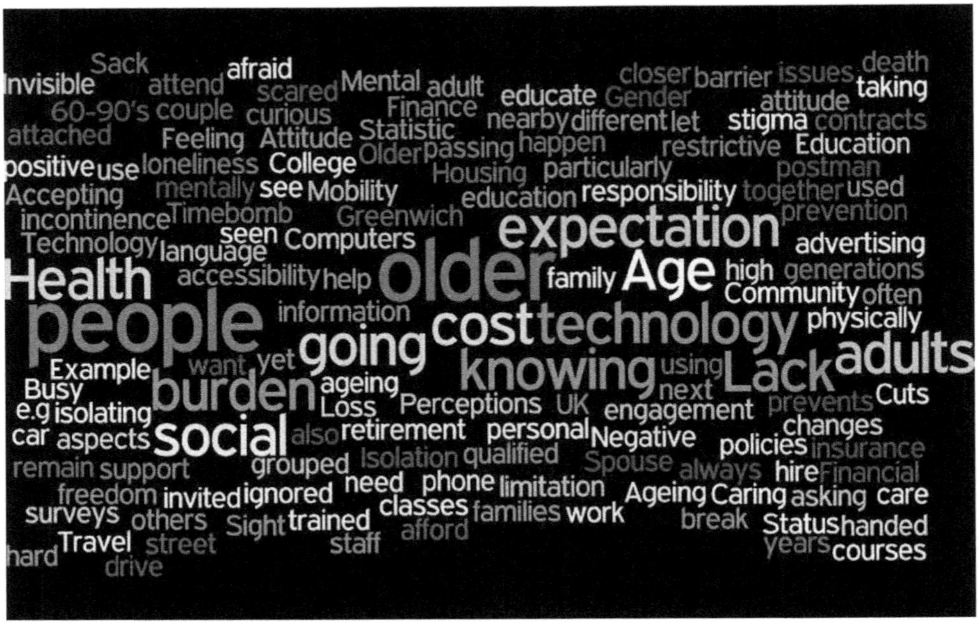

Figure 2.3 What are barriers to positive aging?

(Stock, Docking & Schofield, 2016).

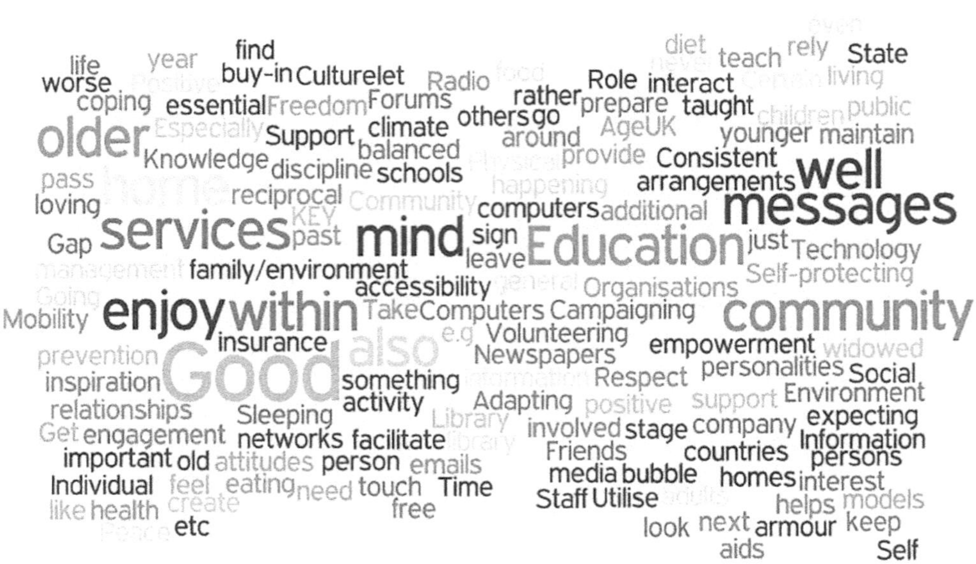

Figure 2.4 What are the facilitators to positive aging?

(Stock, Docking & Schofield, 2016).

Change at an organisational level

Typically, in the United Kingdom, adults have a working lifespan of 18–65/7 years. At this point, it is accepted that the older population are expected to retire from full-time work and take up their pension. At this point many older adults are viewed as no longer contributing to society and, in some areas, they are even considered to be a 'drain'. Whilst for some occupations, this may be the only option, such as where good vision or physical fitness is considered an essential part of the role, it is often a glaring generalisation, as there are many older adults who are still active, physically fit, and have good eyesight. Furthermore, the skills and expertise gained over many years are lost to society. Perhaps, new ways of thinking could enable use of this growing population to share their life stories and experiences to children in schools and colleges. Or maybe a network of retired electricians, carpenters, and plumbers could be established to provide services to their peers. There are many unused opportunities which could be explored rather than using the blanket approach or compulsory retirement for all which results in a huge skill loss to society. In the academic world, for example, older scholars are considered beneficial to the organisation.

Organisations should be encouraged to support the positive aging agenda; perhaps they could promote positive aging in the years before retirement. So for example, the electrician or plumber, as they are approaching retirement, could be trained in teaching skills to enable them to move into a role whereby they can pass on their skills and expertise. At the same time programmes could be offered which empower individuals to view aging in a more positive way, thus becoming more proactive in their health and well-being.

Involvement of people with lived experience in research

As researchers we need to listen to the experiences of older adults as they are people with lived experience. Their input is valuable because researchers often have pre-conceived ideas regarding what the general population 'need' or 'think'. This approach uses a co-action strategy, whereby users and researchers learn together (Seng, 1988). It may not always be the information that we are expecting or that we are hoping to hear. Thus, this requires a high degree of flexibility and excellent communication skills to enable those with whom we are working to feel 'safe' in airing their opinions. We also need to be able to 'listen' to the views of our research participants. The involvement of people with lived experience also ensures that the work we carry out has real-world relevance and is therefore important and meaningful to those we are aiming to help.

Conclusion

Socio-demographic changes are occurring in the United Kingdom and the rest of the world. With these changes come pressures upon the delivery of health and social care services. We also know that our aging population numbers are rapidly overtaking our younger population numbers. So the key question is to ask who will care for our older adults in the future? New models of care will need to be considered which address these increasing demands and pressures. However, we will also need to consider ways of viewing our older population and enabling them to view themselves more as being in control of their 'own destiny'. Rather than viewing aging as a negative consequence, we should promote it positively and say instead "what older adults can contribute to society".

This seed change will require new thinking about aging, health, and well-being which must come from employers, health services, and older adults themselves. Amongst all of this, we have to remember that older adults are not a homogenous group. We already know that the definition of aging varies between nations (50 or 65 years) and between philosophical perspectives (for example, sociological, psychological, or biological). Furthermore, strategies put into place today may not be appropriate for the older population of tomorrow. The only way that this can happen is to empower individuals to take control and influence the socio-political agenda which in turn will shape the health and social care agenda and provide services that can be fit for purpose and reactive to the changing needs of society.

References

Allen, T. (2004). Preventing falls in older people: Evaluating a peer education approach. *British Journal of Community Nursing*, 9(5), 195–200.

Arnold-Cathalifaud, M., Thumala, D., Urquiza, A., & Ojeda, A. (2008). Young people's images of old age in Chile: Exploratory research. *Educational Gerontology*, 34(2), 105–123.

Beckingham, A. C., & Watt, S. (1995). Daring to grow old: Lessons in healthy aging and empowerment. *Educational Gerontology*, 21, 479–495.

Bratter, B., & Freeman, E. (1990). The maturing of peer counseling. *Generations*, 14, 49.

Buonocore, S., & Sussman-Skalka, C. (2002). Project InSights: An evaluation of a community vision education project for older adults. *Educational Gerontology*, 28(4), 289–299.

Chen, S., & Walsh, S. (2009). Effect of a creative-bonding intervention on Taiwanese nursing students' self-transcendence and attitudes toward elders. *Research in Nursing & Health*, 32(2), 204–216.

Clemson, L., & Swann, M. (2008). *Stepping on: Building confidence and reducing falls: A community-based program for older people*. Sydney: Sydney University Press.

Cottle, N. R., & Glover, R. J. (2007). Combating ageism: Change in student knowledge and attitudes regarding aging. *Educational Gerontology*, 33(6), 501–512.

Dooley, S., & Frankel, G. (1990). Improving attitudes toward elderly people: Evaluation of an intervention program for adolescents. *Canadian Journal on Aging*, 9, 400–409.

Drennan, J., Treacy, M., Butler, M., Byrne, A., Fealy, G., Frazer, K., & Irving, K. (2008). The experience of social and emotional loneliness of older people in Ireland. *Ageing & Society*, 28, 1113–1132.

Funderburk, B., Damron-Rodriguez, J., Storms, L. L., & Solomon, D. H. (2006). Endurance of undergraduate attitudes toward older adults. *Educational Gerontology*, 32(6), 447–462.

Gringart, E., Helmes, E., & Speelman, C. (2008). Harnessing cognitive dissonance to promote positive attitudes toward older workers in Australia. *Journal of Applied Social Psychology*, 38(3), 751–778.

Hale, N., & Hewitt, J. (1998). Negative aging stereotypes and the agentic – communal dichotomy. *Perceptual and Motor Skills*, 87(3), 915–918.

Hausdorff, J., Levy, B., & Wei, J. (1999). The power of ageism on physical function of older persons: Reversibility of age-related gait changes. *Journal of the American Geriatrics Society*, 47(11), 1346–1349.

Kemper, S. (1994). Elderspeak: Speech accommodations to older adults. *Aging, Neuropsychology, and Cognition*, 1(1), 17–28.

Knapp, J. L., & Stubblefield, P. (2000). Changing students' perceptions of aging: The impact of an intergenerational service learning course. *Educational Gerontology*, 26(7), 611–621.

Krosnick, J., & Alwin, D. (1989). Aging and susceptibility to attitude change. *Journal of Personality and Social Psychology*, 57(3), 416–425.

Levy, B. R. (1996). Improving memory in old age through implicit self-stereotyping. *Journal of Personality and Social Psychology*, 71(6), 1092–1107.

Levy, B. R. (2003). Mind matters: Cognitive and physical effects of aging self-stereotypes. *The Journals of Gerontology. Series B, Psychological Sciences and Social Sciences*, 58(4), 203–211.

Levy, B. R., Hausdorff, J. M., Hencke, R., & Wei, J. Y. (2000). Reducing cardiovascular stress with positive self-stereotypes of aging. *The Journals Gerontology: Psychological Sciences*, 55B(4), 205–213.

Levy, B. R., and Myers, L. (2004). Preventive health behaviors influenced by self-perceptions of aging. *Preventive Medicine*, 39(3), 625–629.

Levy, B. R., Pilver, C. E., & Pietrzak, R. H. (2014). Lower prevalence of psychiatric conditions when negative age stereotypes are resisted. *Social Science & Medicine*, 119, 170–174.

Levy, B. R., Slade, M. D., & Gill, T. M. (2006). Hearing decline predicted by elders' stereotypes, *Journal of Gerontology: Psychological Sciences*, 61(2), 82–87.

Levy, B. R., Slade, M. D., & Kasl, S. V. (2002). Longitudinal benefit of positive self-perceptions of aging on functional health. *The Journals of Gerontology Series B: Psychological Sciences and Social Sciences*, 57(5), P409–P417.

Levy, B. R., Slade, M. D., Kunkel, S. R., & Kasl, S.V. (2002). Longevity increased by positive self-perceptions of aging. *Journal of Personality and Social Psychology*, 83(2), 261–270. doi:10.1037//0022-3514.83.2.261

Levy, B. R., Zonderman, A. B., Slade, M. D., & Ferrucci, L. (2009). Age stereotypes held earlier in life predict cardiovascular events in later life. *Psychological Science*, 20(3), 296–298.

Levy, B. R., Zonderman, A. B., Slade, M. D., & Ferrucci, L. (2011). Memory shaped by age stereotypes over time. *The Journals of Gerontology: Series B*, 67(4), 432–436.

Lowin, A., Knapp, M., & Mccrone, P. (2001). Alzheimer's disease in the UK: Comparative evidence on cost of illness and volume of health services research funding. *International Journal of Geriatric Psychiatry*, 16(12), 1143–1148.

Luborsky, M., & McMullen, C. (1999). Culture and aging. In J. C. Cavanaugh & S. K. Whitbourne (Eds.), *Gerontology: An interdisciplinary perspective* (pp. 65–90). New York: Oxford University Press.

Meisner, B. A. (2012). A meta-analysis of positive and negative age stereotype priming effects on behavior among older adults. *The Journals of Gerontology: Series B*, 67(1), 13–17.

Musaiger, A. O., & D'Souza, R. (2009). Role of age and gender in the perception of aging: A community-based survey in Kuwait. *Archives of Gerontology & Geriatrics*, 48(1), 50–57.

Puentes, W. J., & Cayer, C. A. (2001). Effects of a Modified Version of Feeley's Campus liveliness Vacation on Baccalaureate Registered Nurse Students' Knowledge of and Attitudes Toward Older Adults. Journal *of Nursing Education*, 40(2), 86–89.

Quine, S. (1998). Evaluation of a medicine information training program for older people. *Educational Gerontology*, 24(7), 661–673.

Sargent-Cox, K. A., Anstey, K. J., & Luszcz, M. A. (2013). Longitudinal change of self-perceptions of aging and mortality. *The Journals of Gerontology. Series B, Psychological Sciences and Social Sciences*, 69(2), 168–173.

Scott, T., Minichiello, V., & Browning, C. (1998). Secondary school students' knowledge of and attitudes towards older people: does an education intervention programme make a difference? *Ageing and Society*, 18(02), 167–183.

Seefeldt, C., Jantz, R., Galper, A., & Serock, K. (1977). Using pictures to explore children's attitudes toward the elderly. *The Gerontologist*, 17(6), 506–512.

Seng, J. (1988). Praxis as a conceptual framework for participatory research in Nursing. *Advanced Journal of Nursing Science*, 14(4), 37–48.

Shiner, M. (1999). Defining peer education. *Journal of Adolescence*, 22(4), 555–566.

Sokolovsky, J. (1993). Images of aging: A cross-cultural perspective. In D. Shenk & W. A. Achenbaum (Eds.), *Changing perceptions of aging and the aged* (pp. 85–94). New York: Springer.

Stock, J. (2014). *Physical activity and cognitive ability in older adults: The role of psychosocial factors*. A Doctoral Thesis, Loughborough University.

Stock, J., Docking, R. E., & Schofield, P. (June 2016). *Developing a positive self-management training programme on positive ageing for older adults & by older adults*. World Congress on Active Ageing. Melbourne, Australia.

Zhou, L.Y. (2007). What college students know about older adults: A crosscultural qualitative study. *Educational Gerontology*, 33(10), 811–831.

3
EPIDEMIOLOGY AND AGING

John Foster

This chapter discusses:

- Basic epidemiological data concerning older people
- The first section will consider some of the wider international trends both in the developed and developing world
- Part two considers some of the international trends concerning four issues particularly pertinent for older people: a) cardiovascular diabetes, b) diabetes, c) dementia and d) falls
- Part three considers two long-standing longitudinal general population studies; firstly the US Health and Retirement Study and secondly the English Longitudinal Study of Ageing (ELSA)
- Part four will summarise findings from the last ELSA report

Part one

General international epidemiological trends

The age structure of the population in many developed countries is shifting towards a greater proportion of people in older age categories (United Nations, 2002). It has been estimated that there will be a 50 per cent increase in the number of older people (65 or more) in the United Kingdom between 2001 and 2031(Office for National Statistics, 2004). Historically the main causes of death and illness have been as a result of infectious diseases, under-nutrition and inadequate hygiene. The past century has seen this shift to "diseases of wealth" (Caldwell, 1993) and this is especially so in the developed world. As individuals are living longer, the question is whether they are living better (Manton, Corder and Stallard, 1997) as the incidence of chronic diseases such as diabetes and dementia increases in older people. In the United Kingdom and many other parts of the developed world the trend is towards less use of secondary care services (such as general hospitals) to greater use of community services. This is also linked to an emphasis upon public health and health promotion and a policy shift of expecting individuals taking greater responsibility for their own health as some of the "diseases of wealth" become more commonplace. These diseases of wealth include obesity and diabetes linked to greater consumption of sugar and fats in many Western diets and liver disease links to greater alcohol consumption compared to previous generations (Royal College of Psychiatrists, 2011).

The emergence of "diseases of wealth" and more chronic diseases is now a trend in the developed world. In this context one of the major challenges is improving access to diagnostic services (both primary and secondary care) especially in rural areas. Other challenges include increasing awareness of diseases in older people. The developed world are prone to attributing diseases to being part of the aging process rather than being disease-related (Lloyd-Sherlock, 2005).

The World Health Organization (1998) has made a number of predictions about the impact of aging upon global health. One of these is by 2020 three-quarters of all deaths in developing countries will be related to old age. The main diseases implicated are related to the circulatory system, cancers, hypertension and diabetes. The current projection is that from 2000–2030 the incidence of diabetes in Africa and South East Asia will increase by 160 per cent. In India alone the prediction is that, by 2030, 80 million people will be living with diabetes.

Another important area is mental health. Older people can be prone to isolation as result of bereavement, retirement and loss of contact with family and friends both in the developed and developing world (Van Der Geest, 2004.) Depression and anxiety disorders account for 20–30 per cent of all worldwide primary care visits (Desjarlais et al., 1995). This is likely to be an underestimate of the true incidence of mental health problems.

Most studies suggest that the prevalence of dementia doubles in every five-year age band from 60–90 and it is estimated that in the United Kingdom the dementia prevalence is 6.5 per cent for the population over 65 (Desjarlais et al., 1995). WHO projections estimate that by 2020 more than 55 million people in Africa, Asia and Latin America will have senile dementia (World Health Organization, 1998). These WHO projections have led to greater emphasis being placed on the importance of encouraging lifestyle changes and health promotion (World Health Organization, 2004).

Part two

Data relating to specific conditions

Other chapters will look at these conditions in much greater depth but the author will now introduce some of the international epidemiological data concerning four diseases.

a) Cardiovascular diseases (CVD)

Cardiovascular disease (CVD) is the leading cause of mortality worldwide. It is estimated that in 2010 the worldwide burden for CVD-related deaths was 29.6 per cent (15.6 billion). In Europe there are 4 million deaths per year (2014) attributable to CVD, nearly half of all European deaths (Nichols et al., 2014). Across Europe women are more likely to die from CVD (51 per cent) and the equivalent figure for men is 42 per cent. Coronary heart disease alone accounts for 1.8 million (20 per cent) of European deaths annually. However across Europe mortality rates are falling (Nichols et al., 2014), but the fall is not uniform. Hospital discharge data (notwithstanding the difficulties of comparing uniform reporting methodologies across different countries) can be used to track morbidity rates for CVD. Whilst the trend is towards a fall in mortality there has been a rise in CVD morbidity rates. Thirty-four European countries have seen an increase in CVD hospital discharge rates. Most countries (32) have again seen an increase in equivalent stroke rates but these have fallen in 18 countries. The overall message is that more people are living longer across Europe with underlying cardiovascular diseases and this presents challenges for secondary and primary care health and social support services.

b) Dementia

Desjarlais et al. (1995) suggest that dementia rates double with every five-year age band beyond 60 and dementia has received increased attention from policymakers, healthcare services and the press. However a recently published study assessing data during the past 20–30 years conducted in Sweden, the Netherlands, England and Spain (Wu et al., 2015) presents a more optimistic picture than commonly portrayed. The Wu et al. study showed very few significant changes in dementia rates over the study period. The only study centre that experienced a significant fall in dementia was the United Kingdom (22 per cent reduction, $p=0.003$). The authors suggest that the main explanation for the non-significant trends have been the rises in life expectancy, improved health and living conditions. Furthermore the explanation for the non-significant Scandinavian and Dutch findings may be health service configurations that have targeted prevention and treatment of vascular and other chronic conditions. Other chapters in this book will explore this in greater depth; however there is an emerging body of evidence that one of the keys to positive aging is a healthy diet, stopping smoking and measures to improve cognitive function and the extension of services that pick up signs of cognitive decline at an early stage so that support services can be put in place.

c) Diabetes

Whilst the picture for dementia is possibly not as pessimistic as commonly supposed, the opposite is true for diabetes, which is a disease whereby the pancreas produces insufficient insulin and as a result there is a significant rise in blood glucose levels. This causes damage to blood vessels, nerves and other body tissues. Serious complications can be cardiovascular disease, impaired vision and sometimes blindness and kidney disease. Wild et al. (2004) have projected the likely prevalence of diabetes in 2030. (Type 1 and Type 2 Diabetes are not differentiated in most international data sets.) In 2000 the worldwide estimate for diabetes was 2.8 per cent (171 million) and the projection is that by 2030 this will be 4.4 per cent (366 million). The rise in diabetes prevalence is related to increased worldwide obesity rates and an increasingly aging population. In consequence it is possible the projections of Wild et al. may be underestimates. The group where the largest increase is expected is over 65 and in order to reduce the likely burden of diabetes (and indeed dementia and CVD), interventions will need to target changes in diet and promote an increase in physical activities.

d) Falls

Falls have an impact on individuals, carers and secondary and primary healthcare services. They can result in prolonged hospital admissions and it is estimated that fracture management (mainly hips) cost the NHS £1.7 billion annually (Lawrence et al., 2005). They are the most common form of accidental injury in older people and the most common cause of accidental death in individuals over 75 (British Geriatrics Society, 2005). Also, frequent falling can be linked with anxiety and depression as an individual develops a fear of falling. US data indicates that 30 per cent of all "community-dwelling adults" fall annually and this figure rises to 40 per cent for those individuals over 75 and half of individuals who fall do so at least twice annually (Hauer et al., 2006). Six per cent of falls in individuals over 65 result in a fracture and 1 per cent of these are hip fractures. Falls are the most common reason older people are admitted to accident and emergency services and, for those over 75, hip fractures, resulting in hospital admissions, present a significant burden for healthcare services (Lawrence et al., 2005).

Part three

Collecting epidemiological data

As the previous section indicates, the main variables of interest for epidemiologists are trends relating to disease morbidity (prevalence) and mortality rates. However another way of collecting epidemiological data is general population surveys. This section will briefly consider two international longitudinal surveys.

a) The US Health and Retirement Study (HRS)

This is a study administered by the University of Michigan. It is supported by the US National Institute of Aging and Social Security Administration and the first wave was conducted in 1992. The main aim is to explore changes in employment and health trends and the data collected includes income, work, assets, pension plans, health insurance, disability, physical health and functioning, cognitive functioning and healthcare utilisation. The participants are a representative sample of approximately 20,000 Americans over the age of 50 who are given an in-depth interview every two years. Thus it "provides an invaluable and growing body of multidisciplinary data that researchers can use to address important questions about the challenges and opportunities of aging" (Hodes and Suzman, 2015). A website (National Institute of Aging, 2015) provides further details about the study and details about how to access the study data once a researcher has been registered on the system.

b) English Longitudinal Study of Ageing (ELSA)

The English Longitudinal Study of Ageing (ELSA) (ELSA, 2011) is an epidemiological study covering health, employment and financial status, access to support services and participation in wider society, amongst other issues. There is an interview by a trained researcher and a subsequent visit by a nurse where data such as height, weight, blood pressure and prescription drug use is collected. Participants for ELSA were recruited from a representative sample of the population aged 50 and older. Wave 1 consisted of a sample of 11,050 respondents and commenced in March 2002. The participants were originally drawn from the Health Survey of England (HSE) (UK Data Service, 2014). However the HSE concentrates on individuals living in private households and from Wave 3 onwards participants were recruited from residential care homes or similar institutions. The latest data collection (Wave 6) took place from June 2012 to June 2013.

Part four

Diseases of prosperity/consumption: case study on alcohol and cigarettes

There is now evidence (Royal College of Psychiatrists, 2011) that older people are drinking more than previous generations. There are a number of possible reasons for this but the reason often postulated is the fact that alcohol is cheap and increasingly convenient to buy. This links to one of the challenges that will face policymakers and service designers, and this is how to lessen the health burden presented by "diseases of wealth", most notably food, alcohol and tobacco. A recent report (Matthews et al., 2014) was able to track data from Wave 0 (2002–2003) to Wave 6 (2012–2013) and consider some health-related behaviours over time. These included cigarette smoking and alcohol consumption. The trajectory for smoking-related behaviours was uniformly in a healthy direction and this was particularly marked in the higher social classes and better-educated groups.

The main trends for alcohol were less clear cut and will be outlined in brief. Heavy drinking in this analysis (Matthews et al., 2014) was defined as daily or almost daily drinking. Almost a fifth of individuals were drinking daily. It is worth noting that this may not be a proxy for heavy drinking in the elderly, as aging is associated with a greater likelihood of daily or almost daily drinking (Burns Murdoch, 2012). The general trend was that there was little change in heavy drinking rates from Wave 0 to Wave 6. There was a small increase (non-significant) in heavy drinking rates and men were most likely to be heavy drinkers but marital status had no relationship to heavy drinking. The relationship between greater wealth, higher educational level and increased likelihood of heavy drinking was confirmed. Better health was associated with increased drinking and those individuals with impaired health were less likely to drink daily and almost twice as many individuals reduced their drinking as increased it.

Alcohol presents a conundrum because drinking in older people is associated with positive outcomes and there are some commentators (Iparraguire, 2015) who suggest that alcohol consumption is a proxy for "successful aging". It is unlikely this is connected to the chemical make-up of alcohol; rather alcohol is likely to be a proxy for having a greater social contact and integration, which is related to positive health and social outcomes. Older people, like their younger counterparts, only tend to reduce their drinking if they become unwell and frail. This belief that alcohol may be integral to successful aging now has to be put into the context of recent NICE guidelines (NICE, 2015) that suggest there is a link between excessive drinking, cognitive decline and, most notably, dementia. Some media commentators have mistakenly interpreted this as a direction to drink no alcohol if an individual wishes to avoid dementia (Donnelly, 2015).

Part five

Concluding thoughts

As this chapter has shown the trend is that due to improvement in health services, environment and overall prosperity, individuals are living longer and probably "living better". However it is questionable whether these trends can and will continue. The most prevalent diseases – cardiovascular diseases and diabetes – are at least in part diseases of consumption and prosperity and the key to reducing these burdens is education and lifestyle changes. Many governments have become increasingly neoliberal with policies that will result in less health and social care provision by the state and possibly diminished pension provision. Neoliberal regimes also tend to emphasise encouraging personal responsibility and diabetes, cardiovascular disease and even possibly dementia may be seen as diseases which can be lessened if individuals can be encouraged to make lifestyle changes that will lessen the health and social care burden for the state. It is possible that, in days of scarce resource, in future years the promotion of "positive aging" will not be seen as the responsibility of the state but the individual.

References

British Geriatrics Society. (2005). *Falls*. www.bgs.org.uk/index.php/topresources/publicationfind/goodpractice/365-falls2 (accessed October 28, 2015).

Burns Murdoch, J. (2012). Over-45s more likely to drink almost every day, survey reveals. *The Guardian*, Thursday March 8, 2012.

Caldwell, J. (1993). Health transition: The cultural, social and behavioural determinants of health in the third world. *Social Science and Medicine*, 36, 125–135.

Desjarlais, R., Eisenberg, L., Good, B., and Klienmann, A. (1995). *World mental health problems and priorities in low income countries*. New York: Oxford University Press.

Donnelly, L. (2015). Go teetotal to reduce dementia risks, NHS says: Official NHS advice on prevention of dementia warns "there is no safe level of alcohol consumption" which does not increase risk of the condition. *Daily Telegraph*, October 21, 2015.

ELSA. (2011). *English longitudinal study of aging*. www.ifs.org.uk/ELSA (accessed October 28, 2015).

Hodes, R., and Suzman, R. (2015). *Health and aging: Growing old in America*. Bethesda, MD: National Institute of Aging.

Iparraguire, J. (2015). Socioeconomic determinants of risk of harmful alcohol drinking among people aged 50 or over in England. *BMJ Open*, 5, e007684. doi:10.1136/bmjopen-2015-007684

Lawrence, T., White, C., Wrenn, R., and Moran, C. (2005). The current hospital costs of treating hip-fractures. *Injury*, 36, 88–91.

Lloyd-Sherlock, P. (2005). Epidemiological change and health policy for older people in developing countries: Some preliminary thoughts. *Ageing Horizons*, 2, 21–24.

Manton, K., Corder, L., and Stallard, E. (1997). Chronic disability trends in elderly United States populations 1982–1994. *Proceedings of the National Academy of Sciences*, 94, 2593–2598.

Matthews, K., Panayotes, D., Nazroo, J., and Shankar, A. (2014). The evolution of lifestyles in older age in England. In J. Banks, J. Nazroo, and A. Steptoe (Eds.), *The dynamics of ageing-evidence from the English longitudinal study of ageing 2002–2012 (wave 6)* (pp. 51–94). London: Institute of Fiscal Studies.

National Institute of Ageing. (2015). *Health and aging: Growing old in America: The health and retirement study*. www.nia.nih.gov/health/publication/growing-older-america-health-and-retirement-study/references (accessed October 28, 2015).

NICE. (2015). *Dementia, disability and frailty in later life-mid-life approaches to delay or prevent onset*. www.nice.org.uk/guidance/ng16 (accessed October 28, 2015).

Nichols, M., Townsend, N., Scarborough, P., and Rayner, M. (2014). Cardiovascular disease in Europe 2014: Epidemiological update. *European Heart Journal*. 35(42), 2950–2959.

Office for National Statistics. (2004). *National population projections: 2002-based*. London: TSO (The Stationery Office).

Royal College of Psychiatrists. (2011). *"Our invisible addicts": First report of the older persons' substance misuse working group of the Royal College of Psychiatrists*. London: Royal College of Psychiatrists.

UK Data Service. (2014). *Health survey for England*. http://discover.ukdataservice.ac.uk/series/?sn=2000021 (accessed October 28, 2015).

United Nations. (2002). *World population ageing 1950–2050*. New York: United Nations Publications.

Van Der Geest, S. (2004). "They don't come to listen": The experience of loneliness among older people in Kwahu, Ghana. *Journal of Cross Cultural Gerontology*, 19, 77–96.

Wild, S., Roglic, G., Green, A., Sicree, R., and King, H. (2004). Global prevalence of diabetes: Estimates for the year 2000 and projections for 2030. *Diabetes Care*, 27, 1047–1053.

World Health Organization. (1998). *Population ageing-a public health challenge*. Fact Sheet No. 135. Geneva: WHO.

World Health Organization. (2004). *Preventing chronic diseases- a vital investment*. Geneva: WHO. www.who.int/chp/chronic_disease_report/full_report.pdf (accessed October 28, 2015).

Wu, T.Y., Fratiglioni, L., Matthews, F., Lobo, A., Breteler, M., Skoog, I., and Brayne, C. (2015). Dementia in western Europe: Epidemiological evidence and implications for policy making. *The Lancet: Neurology*, Online edition. http://dx.doi.org/10.1016/S1474-4422(15)00092-7

4

POSITIVE AGING, POSITIVE DYING

Intersectional and daily communicational issues surrounding palliative and end-of-life care services in minority groups in the United Kingdom and the United States

Carlos Moreno-Leguizamon, David Smith and Clarence Spigner

This chapter discusses:

- Palliative and end-of-life care services
- The UK and the USA ethnic classification and a further need for intersectionality
- Death and dying main concerns for ethnic minorities in the UK and the USA as per the literature

Introduction

The journey through life has an end and an ending process: physical death and physical dying. As Kakar (2014) states, objectively speaking, our physical death – when our heart stops working, our kidneys fail, brain dies and we cease breathing – are actions that should not carry mystery because these are not more than the processes of a body deteriorating and ceasing to exist. However, we humans insist on constructing death and dying as mysteries and, if not, as deniable practices: why? Probably because physical death is the only experience that we do not survive to tell. In the case of dying, societies are increasingly reluctant to reflect seriously about this life event and the social, economic, political and cultural consequences it entails. As some literature already demonstrates, services for the elderly and aging are a low priority for government agendas, health and medical services (Tinker, 2014a, 2014b). However, social policy and healthcare provision for aging populations is being contested from political, economic and social policy angles by the inter-generational equity debate. According to this debate, which focuses mainly on industrialised countries, as elderly groups are growing as a proportion of the population and are more likely to vote than younger voters, they have increasing political power. Similarly it is argued that these elderly populations are in a more advantageous position than their younger cohorts through occupational and final salary pensions that are now largely closed to younger people, higher state pensions (with the triple lock guarantee in the UK) paid for by working age tax payers, rising property prices benefiting older home owners when many youngsters cannot get on the property ladder, and, of course, disproportionate use of health services.

Throughout history, human societies, cultures and groups have responded in different, complex, nuanced and imaginative ways to death and, to a lesser extent, to the dying process. From mummifying, cremating and burying the body to planning to send the bodies' ashes into space, humans have always crafted diverse ways to deal with death. However, this is not so true with regards to the dying process. Historically most people have died at "home", connoting[1] a familiar place and under the care of family, community, friends or, more recently, by health professionals. Gawande (2014) notes that it is only since the mid-twentieth century with the rapid progress and consolidation of both "scientific" biomedicine and the hospital as a site synonymous with cure and the extension of life that the move from dying at home to dying in sites such as the hospital and other institutions has occurred. As a medical doctor, Gawande (2014) states, "the experience of making mortality a medical experience is just decades old. It is young. And the evidence is failing" (p. 9). So is the focus on the physical death a contributing factor in sanitising death and removing it from our daily and familiar landscape, "home"?

Contemporary societies are being challenged to rethink death and dying mainly due to the fact that humans are living longer and, secondly, national populations are becoming increasingly diverse racially, ethnically and religiously at the same time as they are aging. This means that practices and customs surrounding death and dying are increasingly heterogeneous, posing significant challenges for healthcare providers who deal with death and dying on a daily basis. Thus, keeping in the background this new emerging and controversial global question on how our physical death and dying processes are taking shape, this chapter aims to contribute to the debate over what a "good" or "positive" death and dying process might mean. Specifically in the context of palliative and end-of-life (EoL) care services in the United Kingdom (UK) and the United States of America (USA) the article seeks to i) discuss what the main themes about death and dying are according to the literature for both minorities and palliative and EoL services and ii) bring to the forefront what intersectional and communicational issues could affect individuals and the respective services they receive at the EoL who, in either society, are defined or self-identified as members of ethnic minorities.

The justification for contrasting the UK and the USA is centred on various reasons but the quintessential one is that the authors annually conduct a seminar series (Dark Empire: Health and Race) with undergraduate students from the universities of Washington (USA) and Greenwich (UK). The main objectives are to invite the students to reflect on healthcare issues such as i) why the USA has a market-oriented healthcare system compared to the UK's national health system; ii) the USA's entire 237-year history (since independence) is of multiculturalism, while the UK's much longer history is roughly only 60 years of multiculturalism; iii) the USA is 40 times the size of the UK with 321 million persons compared to just over 64 million in the whole of the UK; and, finally, and a very significant issue in 2015, iv) the UK was ranked number 1 on the Quality of Death Index compared to the USA, which ranked number 9 along with Canada (Economist Intelligence Unit, 2010).

The chapter is structured around four components: i) a definition and characterisation of palliative and EoL care services; ii) how ethnic minorities are classified in both countries; iii) how more culturally sensitive communicational and intersectional approaches could capture the complexities of identity markers in minorities around physical death and the process of dying; and iv) what the literature in both countries, supported by some empirical data from a one-year study in the UK[2] illustrate are common themes in both countries for minorities in general and for some country-specific groups.

Palliative and EoL care services

Gawande (2014) notes that the medicalisation of physical death is a relatively recent biomedical phenomena taking place mostly in hospitals, nursing homes and care homes. The process of dying has been removed from what most patients denote and connote as "home", and this trend is apparently not satisfying populations, particularly the elderly. Why is this the case? Recent historical developments in the management of death and dying in the past 60 years and the definition and characterisation of palliative and EoL care may contain the clues to why this is the case.

Firstly, like any other social movement, the consolidation and mainstreaming of palliative care medicine within mainstream biomedicine – a process still very much in progress – has been the result of creative and innovative health professionals advocating for a change on what, based on anecdotal evidence and individual cases, some saw as failing to maximise quality of life for those near death. In the UK, Cicely Saunders was central in developing hospice and palliative care. She – herself an intersectional case: woman, nurse, social worker and medical doctor – collected 1100 individual experiences of patients in the final stages of life between 1960 and 1967. According to Clark (2007):

> [a] striking feature of her papers was her articulation of the relation between physical and mental suffering, seen in almost dialectical terms, each capable of affecting the other. Her description of this relation reached full expression in her idea of total pain, which was taken to include physical symptoms, mental distress, social problems, and emotional difficulties – captured so comprehensively by the patient who told her: "all of me is wrong".
>
> *(p. 431)*

The work of Saunders was significant in advancing the view that death and dying were more than merely biomedical or physical processes. They were also social, emotional, psychological and cultural processes involving various intersectional identity markers such as gender, ethnicity, class, sexual orientation, disability, age and religion.

Secondly, Saunders's work on the concept of total pain challenged the historical body-mind dichotomy so pervasively used in biomedicine in the last three hundred years in which the physical or material has been prioritised over the mental (Moreno-Leguizamon, 2005, 2012). The failing evidence of medicalising death and dying that Gawande (2014) observes is reflected in Saunders's concepts of total pain and the modern hospice as the site for providing a different type of care. The biomedical emphasis that all physical processes of the body including its death are material processes has disregarded the complementary role that the mind or the psyche plays and the corresponding influence of this in the behaviour of health services. Even today in palliative inter-disciplinary teams, the professions that are less present are psychology and psychotherapy. Heubber and Sellschopp (2014) observe that, in Germany,

> [t]he membership statistics of the German Association for Palliative Medicine confirm the impression that psychological competences are still a project in progress: Less than 10 percent of the members are psychologists or psychotherapists by profession, and the statistics do not offer any information about the quality of their psychotherapeutic and psycho-oncological training.
>
> *(p. 216)*

The fact that the modern hospice is increasingly considered as a friendlier site for death and dying compared to the hospital or nursing home is in many ways due to the total pain approach in which the physical, mental and social is taken into account. As Heubber and Sellschopp (2014) note, Saunders herself stated that the "Hospice is not a place to go to die, but rather a concept of care based on the promise that when medical science can no longer add days to life, more life will be added to each day" (p. 215).

Thirdly, although palliative care and EoL care services are offered to all cases in which patients' diseases are malignant and non-malignant (Keeley and Noble, 2011), the origin of palliative care is rooted in cancer as the disease and the modern hospice as the site. Clark (2007) notes that palliative care has contributed to a considerable shift in attitude: from a "casual" attitude in the 1970s when doctors would send patients to die at home because they could not offer anything else, to the continuous effort of expanding palliative care and EoL services globally for malignant and non-malignant diseases today. Clark also mentions that in the USA Elisabeth Kübler-Ross's work at the end of the 1960s – another woman and a psychiatrist – at the Billings Hospital in Chicago initiated a ground-breaking work on death and dying in that country. However, despite the pioneering work of these women in the 1970s it was only towards the end of the 1980s (1987) in the UK and near the end of the first decade of the twenty-first century (2008) in the USA that palliative care became recognised as a specialty of biomedicine.

The first definition of palliative care by the World Health Organization (WHO) was in 1986 and from then onwards re-definitions have taken place. Accordingly the definition today states:

> Palliative care is an approach that improves the quality of life of patients and their families facing the problems associated with life-threatening illness, through the prevention and relief of suffering by means of early identification and impeccable assessment and treatment of pain and other problems, physical, psychosocial and spiritual.
>
> *(WHO, 2015)*

Additional underpinning characteristics of the WHO's definition of palliative care include those suggested by Saunders and Kübler-Ross, such as a more ample conceptualisation of pain, the affirmation of life, a better attempt to integrate body and mind, an ordinary and reflexive acceptance of death as an inevitable process and care rather than treatment at the moment of dying.

In fact, care at the moment of dying or near the moment of dying is what EoL care services comprise as a more focused and specialised activity within palliative care. Incorporating the philosophy, concept and approach from palliative care, EoL care addresses issues such as: i) death with dignity and autonomy; and ii) identification of wishes and preferences of the dying individual (part of patient centred care), and decisions on the preferred site of death. On the side of the service providers, EoL care services address the ethics and responsibility of the multidisciplinary team to provide high-quality care that involves, as early as possible, a death without too much total pain. In the National Health Service (NHS) in the UK this gets summarised in a compassionate, competent and respectful EoL care service (NHS, 2015). Similarly, after having scrapped the Liverpool Care Pathway in the UK for being perceived as a speedy pathway to get rid of dying people, the NHS is now talking in terms of the EoL care pathway in which six key activities are deemed noteworthy: i) frank and honest discussion as the EoL approaches; ii) assessment and agreement of care planning and its review; iii) coordination amongst all parties involved; iv) delivery of quality care as per site chosen; v) specific care for the last days, and vi) care after death for the ones in mourning and bereavement (NHS, 2015).

Many of the above characteristics of both palliative and EoL care are amongst the ones that have led to the UK recently being rated as the best place to die amongst 80 countries according to "Quality of Death: Ranking End-of-Life Care Across the World" report from the (Economist Intelligence Unit, 2010). In the same ranking, the USA was ranked 9. However, a challenging issue for both palliative and EoL care is the emerging global discussion on the right to die as one of the maximum expressions of autonomy by patients. So far the global picture in this discussion does not involve many countries, as few countries have approved it. Assisted dying is legal in the Netherlands, Switzerland, Belgium, Luxembourg and Colombia while assisted dying laws exist in California, Washington, Oregon, Vermont and Montana in the USA.

The UK and the USA ethnic classification and a further need for intersectionality

Marking ethnicity or race chiefly amongst a range of other possible identity markers is one way that societies such as the UK and the USA have governmentally decided to classify and count the non-white and white populations. As Moreno-Leguizamon et al. (2015) point out, ethnic recognition has not been an acknowledged and given political right in either society but a right that carries a political history of struggle that in the UK was closely related to the struggle for gender equality and in the USA to the civil rights movement. Obviously a common denominator in both struggles has been issues of racism, discrimination and inequalities in social, educational, political and economic life, including health issues, as is the case in this chapter with palliative care and EoL. When discussing the literature from both countries, minorities experience inequalities in life and inequalities even when dying. Table 4.1 displays the main ethnic categories used in the two countries. In the case of the UK data is drawn from the national Census of 2011 (Office for National Statistics, Census, 2011) and in the USA from the 2010 Population Census (United States Census Bureau, 2015).

As shown in Table 4.1 the UK and the USA are both different and yet alike in certain respects. At 321 million residents, the USA has more than five times the population of the UK at 56 billion for England and Wales. Racial and ethnic diversity has been integral to the USA population even before it won independence as a colony from the UK more than 240 years ago. The UK has only dealt with large-scale multi-racialism since around 1950. The definitions "race" and "ethnicity" can differ across the two nations. "Race" is generally defined as superficial physical characteristics between people or according to biology. "Ethnicity" is defined as people identified by a shared history, nationality, language or religion. In the UK, the Irish have been defined as a group distinct from the English group whereas, in the USA, Irish Americans are part of the white population. The UK's white population is 86 per cent (England and Wales) compared to 79.9 per cent of the USA's population. Racial and ethnic distinctions, critical for assessing the epidemiology of the public's health can however be deceiving. In the UK, the all-encompassing "Asian/Asian Britain" population include South Asians with ancestry in the Indian sub-continent. Those with origins in the Far East are excluded and are placed under the "Other" category. In the USA however, the Asian designation comprises 4.4 per cent of the population and includes those with ancestry in South Asia, India and the Far East. The USA's Hispanic designation is an ethnic classification, assessed by surname, and includes those who are "white". The USA white population includes therefore approximately 15 per cent Hispanics. However, Hispanics are not singled out in the UK population and would be classified under "white other" with a diverse range of other national and ethnic groups. The all-encompassing "Black" designation in both nations includes people who are descendants of black people from the African continent. The UK has a registered 3 per cent Black population and the USA has a 12.8 per cent Black population.

Examining the role of ethnicity without acknowledging how ethnic experiences intersect with wider identity markers or categories and other socioeconomic processes would give a very partial view of the dynamics influencing their engagement with palliative and EoL services. Social class status is closely related to race and ethnicity in both the UK and the USA

Table 4.1 Ethnic/race categories in the UK and the USA

UK ethnic categories (England and Wales)	*Demographics*	*US race categories*	*Demographics*
White	48.2 million (86%)	One race	
White British	45.1 million (80.5%)	White	223,553,265 (72.4)
White Irish	531.1 (0.9%)	Black or African	38,929,319 (12.6)
Gypsy or Irish traveller	57.7 (0.1%)	American	2,932,248 (0.9)
Other White	2,485 (4.4%)	American Indian and	
		Alaska Native	14,674,252 (4.8)
		Asian	540,013 (0.2)
		Native Hawaiian and	
		other Pacific Islander	47,435,002 (15.4)
		Hispanic or Latino race	
Mixed/multiple ethnic groups			
White and Black Caribbean	426.7 (0.8)	In the US census there are all types of consideration to combinations of two and three races amongst all the above categories; either they have been specified or not. Since our interest in this chapter is the ethnic categories, we do not list the combinations. For details see the figures for the 2010 census.	
White and Asian	341.7. (0.6)		
White and Black African	166.0 (0.3)		
Other mixed	290.0 (0.5)		
Asian/Asian British			
Indian	1,413 (2.5)		
Pakistani	1,124 (2.0)		
Bangladeshi	447.2 (0.8)		
Chinese	393.1 (0.7)		
Other Asian	835.7 (1.5)		
Black/African/Caribbean/Black British			
African	989.6 (1.8)		
Caribbean	594.8 (1.1)		
Other Black	280.4 (0.5)		
Other ethnic group			
Arab	230.6 (0.4)		
Any other ethnic group	333.1 (0.6)		

and impacts hugely on life chances and health status. In the UK, 40 per cent of ethnic minority households live in low-income households, twice the rate of White British households. Significant differences exist between groups, with 70 per cent of Bangladeshi and 60 per cent of Pakistani households classified as low income compared to 30 per cent for Indians and Black Caribbeans and 20 per cent for white households (Poverty.org.uk, 2015). In the USA, in 2010 whites and Asians have median household incomes that are higher than the median income of all races combined ($54,620 and $64,308, respectively) while Hispanics ($37,759) and blacks ($32,068) have median incomes significantly lower. Kessler et al. (2005) identified no social class differences in attitudes and beliefs surrounding death and dying in the UK, but found that patients from social class V were less likely to die in a hospice.

In both countries ethnic minorities are more likely to live in deprived areas, which impacts on the accessibility and quality of services they receive. In the UK, over one in three Bangladeshi and Pakistani households live in a deprived neighbourhood compared to one in five Black, African and Caribbean and one in twelve White British households. In the USA residents of predominately black or Hispanic neighbourhoods have access to roughly half as many social services as those in white neighbourhoods (National Poverty Centre, 2015). When ethnicity intersects with social class and geographical inequalities, Evans et al. (2011) identified an inverse relation between areas of high poverty and provision of palliative care services with poorer areas being less well provided than more affluent areas. Ethnic minorities therefore face a 'dual disadvantage' of being over-represented in areas of deprivation and, even within those areas, having lower levels of service use than deprived White British residents. In the USA, even after controlling for socioeconomic variables, there were differences in the use of palliative care services between whites, blacks and Hispanics (Hanchate et al., 2009). However, in the UK Karim, Bailey and Tunna (2000) noted higher referral rates to palliative services in areas with a higher percentage of ethnic minority patients.

Uncritically examining the role of ethnicity without acknowledging how ethnic experiences intersect with other identity and socioeconomic markers (something currently missing in the literature and research in palliative care) therefore gives a very partial view of the dynamics influencing the engagement of different groups, ethnic and otherwise, with palliative and EoL services. It is in this specific context that the need for considering an intersectional approach is briefly raised.

As an approach developed by a Black feminist (Crenshaw, 1989) to address the limitation of identifying only a singular category (ethnicity or gender) when capturing an act of discrimination or inequality, but not both (gender and ethnicity), this approach brings to the forefront a set of arguments needed to be included in contemporary research and policy in health services. Defined as a promising research paradigm to improve the understanding of and response to diversity in health and illness (Hankivsky and De Leeuw, 2011), intersectionality in broad terms focuses on critically examining the "intersections of life stages with selected identity markers and with axes of power, privilege and oppression" (Hankivsky and De Leeuw, 2011, p. 6). Further characteristics are a reflection on the dynamic relationship of simultaneity and mutuality of the identity markers or categories rather than their conceptualisation in isolation or as an additive operation. Similarly, as Hankivsky and De Leeuw (2011) suggest, the approach "provides a way to address the complexity of othering – namely the ways in which difference is produced so as to (re)assert standards of normalcy" (p. 13). Intersectionality also challenges the homogenisation of any group by including differences within differences in specific contexts. Power as another significant element of this approach is not always an oppressive force but can be a productive one with its corresponding resistances. Finally, the approach considers identity as a necessary element in people's lives.

With the unfolding equality regimes all over the world, but particularly in the developed world (for example the UK and the USA), the need for implementing and documenting inclusive research and policy experiences is important. The intersectionality approach aiming at social justice and equality as its goals can help here enormously. Palliative care and EoL services are not the exception from either its research or policy angle. As Krizsan, Skjeie and Squires (2012) state, researchers and academics are increasingly noting "that legal frameworks tend to compartmentalize people's experiences into 'prefabricated' legal categories failing to reflect the complexity of social identifications" (p. 19). Within intersectionality debates, identity rather than a discrete and permanent force is seen as a fluid, imagined, constructed and reconstructed element in people's daily life from the self and from relational and structural angles.

Death and dying main concerns for ethnic minorities in the UK and the USA as per the literature

In both the UK and the USA, ethnic minority groups access palliative and EoL services less than the majority population. Ethnicity has been recognised as a 'tracer' for measuring the success of palliative services, and it is within this context that healthcare providers have been trying to increase the quality and uptake of such services for minority groups (Calanzani et al., 2013). As indicated, some common themes were identified based on a research project in the UK, which explored experiences of and attitudes towards palliative care from the perspective of minority service users and a literature review covering both countries. From the minority perspectives there were differences both between and within groups. However the main overarching concerns were around knowledge of palliative and EoL care services; the levels of trust towards healthcare professionals; and how ethnicity intersects with class, gender, generation and other markers of identity when accessing these services. From the health provider's perspective, the themes related to their own understanding of minorities' cultural beliefs and practices around death and dying; how to communicate effectively and compassionately, given this diversity, at what is a traumatic and highly emotional period both for the patient and their family and friends; and policy frameworks that govern service delivery and the way those services are organised and delivered.

Minorities' lack of knowledge and awareness surrounding palliative and EoL care services

Lack of knowledge and awareness of available services is an important factor shaping differential access. Palliative services are often unavailable or minimal in under-developed or medium-developed countries compared to in Europe and in English-speaking countries, meaning immigrants may have had little or no prior exposure to palliative care services and may be unaware of available palliative services in their new countries (Koffman, 2014). Likewise focus groups conducted as part of the study conducted by the authors with gypsies and travellers and South Asians in the UK (see endnote 1) indicated relatively low levels of knowledge about available services. In the USA, Latinos, Chinese and Koreans all demonstrated low familiarity and a lack of knowledge about palliative services but a high level of interest in learning about them (Pan et al., 2015). The issue of knowledge and increased likelihood of accessing services, however, varies according to first-, second- and third-generation migrants. Diver, Molassiotis and Les Weeks (2003) note that social scientists and health professionals often neglect the process of acculturation and change in the minority individual's orientation to the majority culture. An apparent acculturation factor in the USA was revealed in Park et al.'s (2015) survey of the willingness of older Floridians – comprised of 504 non-Hispanic whites, 360 African Americans, 328 Cuban Americans and 241 non-Cuban Americans – to use hospice services. They found a greater willingness amongst younger non-Hispanics whites and African Americans who had less functional disabilities. Interestingly, amongst non-Cuban Hispanics, they also found English proficiency increased propensity to access hospice care.

Randhawa et al. (2003) observed how communication was a significant problem in the delivery of palliative care to South Asians in the UK. Similarly in the USA, Johnson, Kuchibhatla and Tulsky's (2009) survey of 200 community-dwelling people aged 65 years or older (comprised of 95 whites and 105 African Americans) found African Americans reported less exposure to information about hospice compared to whites. Reynolds et al. (2008), in their study of nursing home residents in the USA, recommend that in-depth discussions on the values and goals of care can upgrade palliative care and lessen racial disparities in EoL care. Cintron and Morrison (2006) recommended educational interventions to improve patient–provider communication regarding pain treatment. In the UK, Jack, Penny and Nazar (2001) recommend a strategy to promote racial and ethnic sensitivities in palliative care services. However, better promotion of palliative care services is insufficient in encouraging uptake by itself, according to Phillips and Taylor (2012). Their study found that an intervention to increase use of palliative care by using translated leaflets made little difference to access rates, as it failed to address why some individuals and groups view palliative care as inappropriate, as discussed further below.

Lack of trust due to relational prejudice

A lack of trust between minority groups and providers of health services has been identified as a barrier to access. Focusing on mistrust, however, frames the problem as rooted in the attitudes of ethnic minority group members. The historical context of prejudice and discrimination can result in minority mistrust of the medical profession as well as the wider society. Vulnerability or the threat of being subjected to harm due to ethnicity is an issue in both countries which can make palliative care an arduous task (Waisel, 2013). Koffman et al.'s (2009) secondary analysis of qualitative data found vulnerability in healthcare settings more prominent amongst Black Caribbean patients than White British patients. Such views concerning accessing healthcare and treatment in healthcare settings have also been prominent in studies of gypsies and travellers in the UK and contribute to their reluctance to use such services, as the authors found in their UK study (Parry et al., 2007; Smith and Ruston, 2013). The USA, with its longer history of racial dynamics, reveal similar concerns of vulnerability, especially regarding African Americans who often cited previous racial discrimination and medical mistreatment as influencing their willingness to access healthcare in the present (Duffy et al., 2006).

EoL care preferences for minority groups

As already discussed, increased referrals, improved information and more accessible palliative care services will not necessarily increase use of those services by minority groups, as they fail to address why some groups may reject this form of care. Koffman and Higginson's (2004) survey of 50 first-generation Black Caribbean and 50 native-born White British patients with terminal illnesses found no significant differences in preferred place of death between the two groups. Thirty-four per cent of Caribbean compared to 27 per cent of white patients expressed a preference for place of death. Eighty per cent of all patients wished to die at home and of these similar levels of Caribbean patients (53 per cent) and white patients (56 per cent) who wished to die at home did so. Coupland et al.'s (2011) database examination of over 68,000 patients who died from cancer between 1998 and 2006 in South East England however indicated significant differences in place of death by ethnicity. Pakistani Indian and Bangladeshi patients were significantly less likely to die in a hospice. Black African, Black Caribbean and Chinese patients were more likely to die at home and all groups had a higher likelihood of dying in hospital than white patients. Johnson et al. (2005) found that in the USA elderly minorities are more likely to die in inpatient settings than white people, while older African Americans were more likely than older whites of dying in an inpatient hospice setting than a nursing home. However, these studies were unable to determine the extent to which these patterns indicate the ethnic/cultural preferences of different groups, knowledge of available services or institutional and practice based factors discussed above.

Studies indicate differences in the role of the family in relation to individual decision-making at the EoL. Amongst frail elderly people in the USA, whites were more likely to express their healthcare preferences than Hispanic, Asian and Black patients and were less likely than the other groups to have an alternative decision-maker (Hornung et al., 1998). This is consistent with more recent research from the USA which indicates a higher preference for family-centred decision-making at the EoL amongst Asians and Hispanics than amongst other groups (Kwak and Haley, 2005). A study of elderly South Asians in London highlighted two themes relevant to understanding perceptions of EoL discussions and their role within those discussions. The first was 'avoidance as a cultural norm' – referring to a lack of discussions around death and dying within the family and a reluctance to play a role in decision-making. The second was 'avoidance as protection' and referred to beliefs about delegating such decisions to family members (Venkatasalu, Arthur and Seymour, 2013). Amongst Korean Americans a lower percentage (73 per cent) reported that they were willing to consider hospice care than white Americans (94 per cent) and African Americans (90 per cent). Younger and more educated Korean Americans, those with more chronic conditions, those with health insurance and those with a higher level of acculturation indicated a greater preference for hospice care (Jang et al., 2010).

In the study conducted by the authors (see endnote 1) most of the African women interviewed expressed a strong aversion to ending their lives in an institutional setting (whether hospital, hospice or nursing home) and was based in three factors: firstly, a high proportion had worked in the health and social care sector and they had perceptions of low standards of care towards the elderly and of experiencing racism and discrimination from other staff, making them reluctant to enter such environments themselves when they became old and vulnerable. Secondly, they had the strongly engrained belief that it is the responsibility of the family and particularly the (adult) offspring to provide appropriate care. Thirdly, they had a preference for either returning to their land of birth to die or if this is not possible having their bodies buried 'at home'. The theme of family (primarily female) based care and a desire to die in their home country or be buried there was also prominent in focus groups with South Asian participants particularly amongst first-generation migrants though there was a feeling amongst the focus group participants (mainly second generation South Asian women) that this preference would decline in subsequent generations supporting the acculturation arguments discussed above.

Health professionals and use of palliative and EoL services

Studies have identified how the practices of health professionals may lead to lower use of palliative and EoL services amongst minority groups. The main reasons include a lack of knowledge of different groups' customs and practices surrounding the EoL amongst health professionals and practitioners and an assumption that minority groups prefer family based to 'formal' care. Another factor was language and communication difficulties, which can contribute to a lower level of referrals (Ahmed et al., 2004). Family members may be asked to interpret between the patient and healthcare professionals increasing the risk of misinterpretation and non-disclosure (Firth, 2001). Problems may continue after services have been accessed with poor communication between patients and staff, a common theme in the literature (Evans et al., 2011). Bereaved Caribbean relatives in the UK were more likely than bereaved white relatives to feel that the deceased relative was not given sufficient choice regarding place of death (Koffman and Higginson, 2004).

The age and gender of the healthcare professional can also affect what type of care is provided with older male physicians more likely to end life support and life sustaining methods than younger female physicians (Hinkka, 2002). Mebane et al. (1999) found that in the USA, the racial and ethnic background of the physician was significant with white American physicians more likely to promote advance directives and to support early discussion of EoL options with their patients than their black counterparts. Moreover a diversity of cultural beliefs and practices surrounding death and dying means that the potential for conflict when considering EoL care for patients from minority ethnic groups in a Western medical system 'dominated by the principles of patient autonomy, beneficence, non-maleficence and avoiding futile care' (Brown, 2014, p. 3). Difficulties arise from often implicit values around disclosure, care and responsibility; the desire to carry burden collectively; resistance to talking explicitly about death and dying in healthcare settings; preferences over place of death and the use of traditional methods as an element of supportive care (Broom et al., 2013).

Conclusion

The way the physical process of death and dying is handled by most Western societies is showing signs of exhaustion due to some basic phenomena that this chapter has addressed. Firstly, the biomedicalisation of dying insists on treating, curing and extending life at any cost rather than ensuring a high-quality standard of life during the last days of life. Secondly, the dying process has been removed from familiar sites ("home") to hospitals and other such sites where many dying people do not want to be in their final days. Thirdly, this perspective persists in emphasising the material side of the dying process at the expense of the integration of psyche/mind and body. Even careful and novel palliative care services do not give the same level of importance to the professionals of the mind when forming interprofessional or inter-disciplinary teams. Fourthly, the biomedicalisation of death is a phenomenon of the last 60 years and there is still time to correct the excesses.

The brief history of both palliative and EoL care in as much as a social and a research movement has been linked to two interesting and intersectional cases of women doctors in the UK and the USA. It is due to these two figures that palliative care has been acknowledged as a branch of medicine with the corresponding global adoption by the WHO. With the innovative concept of total pain as something not only physical but also social, emotional, psychological and cultural, Saunders opened the ground for thinking about the relationship between body and mind, which gave birth to the hospice movement. Historically her work has contributed to the fact that the UK is ranked as the best place to die.

In multicultural societies such as the UK and the USA there is a need for government authorities, including health service planners, to be more sensitive culturally. Ethnicity, gender, age, disability, class and religion, amongst others, are categories or identity markers that help to capture when acts of inequality and discrimination occur. One advantage of the intersectional approach is that it helps to capture, simultaneously and mutually, when discrimination and inequity take place in more than one category rather than to each one in an isolated and discrete way. Identity and power as two of the underpinning concepts of the intersectional approach bring innovative light to how health professionals can think of these concepts in their daily interaction with service users. Palliative and EoL care services will benefit from using the intersectional approach. Examining the role of ethnicity without acknowledging how ethnic experiences intersect with wider identity markers or categories and other socioeconomic processes would give a very partial view of the dynamics influencing their engagement with palliative and EoL services.

Research and literature on palliative and EoL services regarding ethnic minorities in the UK and the USA demonstrate that these groups access these services less than the majority population. The main overarching concerns found from the perspective of minority service users were around knowledge of palliative and EoL care services; levels of trust towards healthcare professionals and how ethnicity intersects with class, gender, generation, religion, disability, age, sexual orientation and immigration status when accessing these services. The concerns found from the health provider's perspective are related to their understanding of minority cultural beliefs and practices around death and dying, how to communicate effectively and compassionately with the patient and their family and friends, and the organisation and delivery of those services.

Racial/ethnic commonalities about palliative and hospice care cut across social, economic and cultural dimensions in both nations. In the UK and the USA, dying with care must be communicated to patients and caregivers as a medical intervention that is well within the framework of healthcare. With expressions of pain still falling within frameworks of ethnicity and determining a patient's discomfort risk being an arbitrary and capricious judgement by health providers, relieving patients' pain, mental anguish and physical stress should be conveyed as improving the patients' quality of life as they face the inevitability of death.

Dying occurs at home more frequently in the USA, Canada and Britain, though, in the USA, some research found that racial/ethnic minorities would rather die in a hospital than at home. In the UK, the need for high-quality palliative and EoL services for minorities is because the majority of deaths still occur in hospitals. The UK, compared to the USA, ranks better in the provision of palliative care. However, inadequate care can be compounded by feelings of vulnerability that many minorities in both nations might experience due to being defined (and treated) as racial/ethnic minorities. Communication does not necessarily mean speaking the same language but the ability to convey compassionate care in a diverse population. Identities are not static and permanent forces but are fluid, imagined, constructed and reconstructed forces and it is to these identities that health services in palliative and EoL care need to respond ethically on a daily basis.

Acknowledgements

This chapter is dedicated to Dipti Shome, who made it home late, and Allan McNaught, who would like to have made it home!

Notes

1 In anthropological research when it comes to meaning, there are two notions: denoting and connoting. The denotation of a word is its explicit definition as listed in a dictionary. Home for example is a place where one lives; a residence. Meanwhile connoting refers to the set of associations that a word usually brings to mind. The connotative meaning of "home" is a place of safety, comfort, and above all

a familiar site. It is the connotation of the meaning of home when it comes to service users of palliative and EoL care that this chapter wants to use.

2 Smith, D., Moreno-Leguizamon, C., and Grohman, S. (2015). *EoL practices and palliative care among Black and Minority Ethnic Groups (BME).* The one-year feasibility study was supported by Health Education Kent Surrey and Sussex (UK).

References

Ahmed, N., et al. (2004). Systematic review of the problems and issues of accessing specialist palliative care by patients, carers and health and social care professionals. *Palliative Medicine*, 18(6), 525.

Broom, A., et al. (2013). Negotiating palliative care in the context of culturally and linguistically diverse patients. *Internal Medicine Journal*, 43, 1043–1046.

Brown, E. A. (2014). Ethnic and cultural challenges at the end-of-life: Setting the scene. *Journal of Renal Care*, 40(Suppl. 1), 2–5.

Calanzani, N., et al. (2013). *Palliative and EoL care for black and minority ethnic groups in the UK.* London: Public Health England.

Cintron, A., and Morrison, R. S. (2006). Pain and ethnicity in the USA: A systematic review. *Journal of Palliative Medicine*, 9(6), 1454–1473.

Clark, D. (2007). From margins to centre: A review of the history of palliative care in cancer. *The Lancet Oncology*, 8(5), 430–438.

Coupland, V. H., Madden, P., Jack, R. H., Møller, H., and Davies, E. A. (2011). Does place of death from cancer vary between ethnic groups in South East England? *Palliative Medicine*, 25(4), 314–322.

Crenshaw, K. (1989). Demarginalizing the intersection of race and sex: A black feminist critique of anti-discrimination doctrine, feminist theory and antiracist politics. *University of Chicago Legal Forum*, 1989, 139–167.

Diver, F., Molassiotis, A., and Les Weeks, L. (2003). The palliative care needs of ethnic minority patients attending a day-care centre: A qualitative study. *International Journal of Palliative Nursing*, 9(9), 389–396.

Duffy, S., Jackson, F., Schim, S., Ronis, D., and Fowler, K. (2006). Racial/ethnic preferences, sex preferences, and perceived discrimination related to end-of-life care. *Journal of the American Geriatrics Society*, 54(1), 150–157.

Economist Intelligence Unit. (2010). *The quality of death: ranking end-of-life care across the world.* A report from the Economist Intelligence Unit commissioned by Lien Foundation. http://graphics.eiu.com/upload/QOD_main_final_edition_Jul12_toprint.pdf (accessed May 5, 2017).

Evans, N., Menaca, A., Andrew, E. V., Koffman, J., Harding, J., Higginson, I. J., Pool, R., and Gysels, M. (2011). Systematic review of the primary research on minority ethnic groups and end-of-life care from the United Kingdom. *Journal of Pain Symptom Management*, 43(2), 261–286.

Firth, S. (2001). *Wider horizons: Care of the dying in a multicultural society.* London: NCHSPC.

Gawande, A. (2014). *Being mortal.* New York: Picador.

Hanchate, A., et al. (2009). Racial and ethnic differences in end-of-life costs: Why do minorities cost more than Whites? *Archives of Internal Medicine*, 169(5), 493–501.

Hankivsky, O., and De Leeuw, S. (2011). *Health inequities in Canada.* Vancouver: UBC Press.

Heubber, S., and Sellschopp, A. (2014). Adding life to the dying: Palliative care and psycho-oncology. In S. Kakar (Ed.), *Death and dying* (1st ed.) (pp. 213–222). New Delhi: Penguin India.

Hinkka, H., et al. (2002). Factors affecting physicians' decisions to forgo life-sustaining treatments in terminal care. *Journal of Medical Ethics*, 28(2), 109–114.

Hornung, C. A., Eleazer, G. P., Strothers, H. S., Wieland, G. D., Eng, C., McCann, R., and Sapir, M. (1998). Ethnicity and decision-makers in a group of frail older people. *Journal of the American Geriatric Society*, 46(3), 280–286.

Jack, C. M., Penny, L., and Nazar, W. (2001). Effective palliative care for minority ethnic groups: The role of a liaison worker. *International Journal of Palliative Nursing*, 7(8), 375–380.

Jang, Y., Chiriboga, D., Allen, J., Kwak, J., and Haley, W. (2010). Willingness of older Korean-American adults to use hospice. *Journal of the American Geriatrics Society*, 58(2), 352–356.

Johnson, K. S., Kuchibhatala, M., Sloane, R. J., Tanis, D., Galanos, A. N., and Tulsky, J. A. (2005). Ethnic differences in the place of death of elderly hospice enrollees. *Journal of the American Geriatrics Society*, 53(12), 2209–2215.

Johnson, K. S., Kuchibhatla, M., and Tulsky, J. A. (2009). Racial differences in self-reported exposure to information about hospice care. *Journal of Palliative Medicine*, 12(10), 921–927.

Kakar, S. (2014). *Death and dying*. New Delhi: Penguin Books.

Karim, K., Bailey, M., and Tunna, K. (2000). Nonwhite ethnicity and the provision of specialist palliative care services: Factors affecting doctors' referral patterns. *Palliative Medicine*, 14(6), 471–478.

Keeley, P., and Noble, S. (2011). Palliative care: Introduction. *Medicine*, 39(11), 635.

Kessler, D., Peters, T. J., Lee, L., and Parr, S. (2005). Social class and access to specialist palliative care services. *Palliative Medicine*, 19(2), 105–110.

Koffman, J. (2014). Servicing multi-cultural needs at the EoL. *Journal of Renal Care*, 40(Suppl. 1), 6–15.

Koffman, J., and Higginson, I. J. (2004). Dying to be home? Preferred locations of death of first generation black Caribbean and native-born white patients in the United Kingdom. *Journal of Palliative Medicine*, 7, 628–636.

Koffman, J., Morgan, M., Edmonds, P., Speck, P., & Higginson, I. J. (2009). Vulnerability in palliative care research: findings from a qualitative study of black Caribbean and white British patients with advanced cancer. *Journal of Medical Ethics*, 35(7), 440–444.

Krizsan, A., Skjeie, H., and Squires, J. (2012). *Institutionalizing intersectionality*. London: Palgrave Macmillan.

Kwak, J., and Haley, W. E. (2005). Current research findings on end-of-life decision making among racially or ethnically diverse groups. *Gerontologist*, 45(5), 634–641.

Mebane, E. W., et al. (1999). The influence of physicians' race, age and gender on physician attitudes towards advance care directives and preferences for end-of-life decision making. *Journal of the American Geriatrics Society*, 47(5), 579–591.

Moreno-Leguizamon, C. J. (2005). Dichotomies in western biomedicine and ayurveda, health-illness and body-mind. *Economic and Political Weekly*, XL(30), July, India, 3302–3310.

Moreno-Leguizamon, C. J. (2012). *Ayurveda, biomedicine, and indigenous medicine: Three medical discourses, one critical discourse analysis (CDA)*. Germany: Lambert Academic Publishing. ISBN 978-3-659-22912-1.

Moreno-Leguizamon, C. J., Tovar-Restrepo, M., Irazábal, C., and Locke, C. (2015). Learning alliance methodology: Contributions and challenges for multicultural planning in health service provision: A case study in Kent, UK. *Planning Theory & Practice*, 16(1), 79–96.

National Health Service (NHS). (2015). *End of life care – NHS choices*. [online] www.nhs.uk/planners/end-of-life-care/Pages/End-of-life-care.aspx (accessed December 23, 2015).

National Poverty Centre. (2015). *National poverty center | University of Michigan*. [online] www.npc.umich.edu/ (accessed December 23, 2015).

Office for National Statistics. (2015). 2011 Census – ONS. [online]. *ONS.gov.uk*. www.ons.gov.uk/ons/guidemethod/census/2011/index.html?utm_source=twitterfeed&utm_medium=twitter (accessed December 23, 2015).

Pan, C. X., et al. (2015). Just ask: Hospice familiarity in Asian and Hispanic adults. *Journal of Pain and Symptom Management*, 49(5), 928–933.

Park, N., Jang, Y., Ko, J., and Chiriboga, D. (2015). Factors affecting willingness to use hospice in racially/ethnically diverse older men and women. *American Journal of Hospice and Palliative Medicine*, 33(8), 770–776.

Parry, G., Van Cleemput, P., Peters, J., Walters, S., Thomas, K., and Cooper, C. (2007). Health status of gypsies and travellers in England. *Journal of Epidemiology & Community Health*, 61(3), 198–204.

Phillips, L., and Taylor, V. (2012). Addressing the palliative care needs of minority groups. *Primary Health Care*, 22(1), 26–30.

Poverty.org.uk. (2015). *Poverty indicators – The poverty site*. [online] www.poverty.org.uk/ (accessed December 23, 2015).

Randhawa, G., Owens, A., Fitches, R., and Khan, Z. (2003). The role of communication In developing culturally competent palliative care services In the UK: A Luton case study. *International Journal of Palliative Nursing*, 9, 24–31.
Reynolds, K. S., Hanson, L. C., Henderson, M., and Steinhauser, K. E. (2008). End-of-life care in nursing home settings: Do race or age matter? *Palliative Support Care*, 6(1), 21–27.
Smith, D., and Ruston, A. M. (2013). If you feel that nobody wants you you'll withdraw into your own Gypsy/Travellers, networks and health care utilisation. *Sociology of Health and Illness*, 35(8), 1196–1210.
Tinker, A. (2014a). *Review of transforming your care and older people*. Committee for Health, Social Services and Public Safety. Northern Ireland Assembly.
Tinker, A. (2014b). *Older people in modern society* (4th ed.). London: Routledge.
United States Census Bureau. (2015). Population. [online] *Census.gov*. www.census.gov/topics/population.html (accessed December 23, 2015).
Venkatasalu, M. R., Arthur, A., and Seymour, J. (2013). Talking about end-of-life care: The perspectives of older South Asians living in East London. *Journal of Research in Nursing*, 18(5), 394–406.
Waisel, D. B. (2013). Vulnerable populations in health care. *Curr Opin Anaesthesiol*, 26(2), 186–192.
World Health Organization (WHO). (2015). *WHO definition of palliative care*. www.who.int/cancer/palliative/definition/en/ (accessed December 23, 2015).

PART II

The body over the life course

5
CANCER

Michelle Lycke, Lies Pottel, Tom Boterberg, Supriya G. Mohile, Etienne Brain and Philip R. Debruyne

This chapter discusses:

- Current evidence in the field of aging and cancer
- The integration of geriatric principles in oncology
- The content of a Comprehensive Geriatric Assessment
- Comprehensive Geriatric Assessment in routine practice
- Discussion of work performed by the authors
- International perspective

Introduction

Due to growth of the aging population and a prolonged exposure to carcinogens, cancer has become an important disease in older people (Yancik, 1997; Siegel et al., 2012). As represented in Figure 5.1, between 2009 and 2011, more than a third of cancers were diagnosed in people aged 75 and over in the United Kingdom (UK) (Cancer Research, 2015). Looking at these data, it is no surprise that individuals aged 65 or older have an 11-fold higher risk of developing cancer compared to their younger counterparts. Further, they have a 15 per cent greater cancer-related mortality rate (Yancik, 1997). In the European Union, an approximate 14 per cent increase of the total projected cancer incidence is estimated to occur from 2009 to 2020 (Davey et al., 1983; Mistry et al., 2011).

Cancer is a very serious health problem at any age; however, combined with increasing age, it creates even more challenging situations for healthcare providers. Decreasing physiologic reserves, leading to distinct variations in functional status, cognition and co-morbidity may affect life expectancy in an individualized manner. As a consequence, their chronological and functional age may not correspond (Hoffe and Balducci, 2012). The spectrum of impairment ranges from more independent individuals, to those who are at moderate risk of health deterioration, to patients who have a high risk of functional decline or mortality (Mohile et al., 2007). Therefore, proper patient selection is an important step to administering a safe and effective cancer treatment (Hurria et al., 2011).

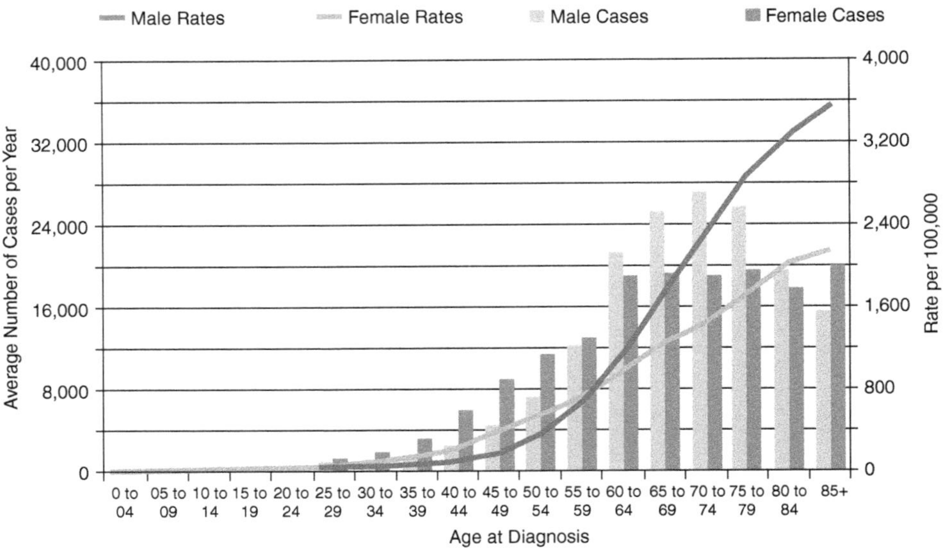

Figure 5.1 Cancer incidence UK: 2009–2011.

The darker grey line indicates the average number of new cases per year and age-specific incidence rates per 100,000 people in the United Kingdom. The lighter grey line represents all cancers, excluding non-melanoma skin cancer.

(Reproduced with permission from Cancer Research UK (Cancer Research, 2015).)

Medical and radiation oncologists are faced with another challenge since evidence-based data of the risks and benefits of cancer treatments in older patients are lacking. Currently applied tools, such as the Eastern Cooperative Oncology Group (ECOG) performance status (PS) and Karnofsky (K) PS, have proven to be insensitive in estimating the functional capabilities of an older patient (Pal, Katheria and Hurria, 2010). Consequently, as a result of doubts concerning the patients' fitness and their ability to tolerate treatment, physicians are less likely to provide appropriate and curative life-saving therapies to older patients when compared to their younger counterparts (Rocco et al., 2013; Camilon et al., 2014). For this reason, a Comprehensive Geriatric Assessment (CGA) has become the cornerstone in modern geriatric oncology care (Hoppe et al., 2013; Lycke et al., 2015).

Current evidence in the field

The integration of geriatric principles in oncology

The initial geriatric assessment was developed in 1930 by Marjory Warren. She established the first geriatric care unit in the United Kingdom in which ill older patients were more adequately managed through assessment of a CGA. A CGA can be defined as:

> a multidisciplinary evaluation in which the multiple problems of older persons are uncovered, described and explained, if possible, and in which the resources and strengths of the person are catalogued, need for services assessed, and a coordinated care plan developed to focus interventions on the person's problems.
>
> *(Solomon et al., 1988; Brunello, Sandri and Extermann, 2009)*

Table 5.1 Overview of the advantages of performing a CGA in oncology

Advantage	*Reference*
Guides treatment decision	(Aliamus et al., 2011; Caillet et al., 2011; Kenis et al., 2013)
Predicts and improves survival	(Extermann et al., 2004; Clough-Gorr et al., 2012)
Prevention of functional decline	(Maas et al., 2007; Vande Walle et al., 2014)
Predicts and improves quality of life	(Wedding, Pientka and Hoffken, 2007; Pottel et al., 2014)
Prediction of the risk on chemotherapy toxicity	(Chen et al., 2003; Hurria et al., 2011)

Since those first steps of Marjory Warren, a CGA has been the advised approach in the evaluation and treatment of general geriatric patients and has been applied all over the world, as it is known to have multiple advantages (Table 5.1) (Matthews, 1984; Hurria and Balducci, 2009).

These geriatric principles have found their way into oncology practice since the 1990s, when Monfardini and colleagues made a first attempt to adapt the CGA for use in cancer patients (Monfardini et al., 1996). Their adapted CGA has later been prospectively validated by the Italian Group of Geriatric Oncology (Repetto et al., 2002). Around the year 2000, several research groups indicated the value of using a CGA in routine oncology practice (Monfardini and Balducci, 1999; Extermann and Hurria, 2007). In an ideal situation, a CGA should be performed by a multidisciplinary geriatric team, which includes a geriatrician, nurse, social worker, pharmacist, dietician and occupational therapist (Chapman et al., 2014). However, other approaches (including for example a geriatric oncology nurse) have also been proposed, as they are more feasible in ambulatory oncology practice (Kenis et al., 2015).

Extermann and Terret were the first to report that a CGA could detect multiple problems in older breast and prostate cancer patients, respectively (Extermann et al., 2004; Terret, Albrand and Droz, 2004). Many papers followed which described different health problems in distinct cancer populations (Mohile et al., 2007; Kellen et al., 2010; Molina-Garrido and Guillen-Ponce, 2011; Bellera et al., 2012; Puts et al., 2012; Kenis et al., 2013). Further, Repetto et al. suggested that a CGA has an added value to ECOG PS and KPS (Repetto et al., 2002; Wedding, Pientkas and Hoffken, 2007).

The content of a CGA

In oncology, a CGA is described as a multidisciplinary, in-depth evaluation to assess the risk of morbidity and mortality (Extermann and Hurria, 2007; Hurria et al., 2014). It aims at identifying vulnerabilities in different age-related domains such as functional status, physical performance, cognition, nutrition, social state, emotional status, co-morbidity and polypharmacy. Though only a limited number of oncology trials could be found that examined the psychometric properties of CGA as a whole, researchers generally agreed about the CGA's feasibility, reliability and validity (Reuben et al., 1996; Hurria et al., 2005; Diachun et al., 2012; Puts et al., 2012). Hamaker reported a median number of seven examined domains within CGA and consequently resulting in a different estimation of vulnerability prevalence (range 28 per cent to 94 per cent) (Hamaker et al., 2012). Moreover, for each health domain, a plethora of validated tools are in use and no consensus exists as to which one is most suited. International oncology societies such as the National Comprehensive Cancer Network (www.nccn.org), the International Society for Geriatric Oncology (www.siog.org) and the European Organization for

Research and Treatment of Cancer (EORTC) (www.eortc.org) have published guidelines suggesting those core domains that should be incorporated within CGA and that could be assessed by the oncologist or a geriatric oncology nurse (Table 5.2) (Extermann et al., 2005; Hurria et al., 2005; Rodin and Mohile, 2007; Pottel, 2014).

Assessing the functional and physical status are cardinal components of geriatric care. Cancer is considered to be life changing in all its aspects because it induces major changes in the living patterns of older adults (Chen et al., 2004). Further, there is evidence that the level of dependence in daily activities influences survival in older patients (Rockwood et al., 1999). The most commonly used instruments to screen for functional dependence are the Activities of Daily Living (ADL) and the Instrumental Activities of Daily Living (IADL) (Katz et al., 1963; Lawton and Brody, 1969). The ADL rates the patient's ability to fulfil basic activities of daily living including bathing, dressing, toileting, transferring, continence and feeding. The IADL looks at activities that require a higher level of cognition and judgement such as cooking, shopping,

Table 5.2 Overview of the principle domains within CGA (Adapted with permission from Pottel, 2014)

Principal domains	*Description*	*Most commonly applied validated tools*
Functional status	Assessment to estimate patient's self-sufficiency, as well as their ability to live independently and function in the community	Katz's Activities of daily living (ADL)(Katz et al., 1963), Barthel-index(Mahoney and Barthel, 1965), Lawtons's instrumental activities of daily living (IADL)(Lawton and Brody, 1969)
Physical performance	Mobility, gait, balance, muscle strength	Tinetti Balance and Gait test (Tinetti, 1986), Timed up and go (TUG) (Podsiadlo and Richardson, 1991), Grip strength (Matsui et al., 2014), specific questions
Cognition	Assessment of patient's cognitive performance	Mini-Mental State Examination (MMSE) (Folstein, Folstein and McHugh, 1975), Clock Drawing Test (CDT) (Lycke et al., 2014), Montreal Cognitive Assessment (MoCA) (Nasreddine et al., 2005)
Nutrition	Assessment of patient's nourishment, weight changes	Mini-Nutritional Assessment (MNA) (Vellas et al., 1999)
Social state	Patient's social network, available social support resources	Specific questions
Emotional state	Assessment of the patient's emotional status	Geriatric depression scale (GDS) (Yesavage, 1988)
Co-morbidities	Rating of the number and severity of co-existing morbidities	Charlson Comorbidity Index (CCI) (Charlson et al., 1987), Cumulative Illness Rating Scale for Geriatrics (CIRS-G) (Miller and Tower, 1991), Adult Comorbidity Evaluation (ACE-27) (Paleri and Wight, 2002)
Polypharmacy	Assessment of the number of medications, possible drug–drug and drug–disease interactions, medications contraindicated in older patients (principles of geriatric pharmacology)	Online drug interaction tool (Hammann and Drewe, 2014), Drug burden index (DBI) (Hilmer et al., 2009), Beers criteria(2012)

transportation and others (Droz et al., 2014). Ideally, grip strength and an evaluation of gait, balance and risk of falls should also be included as a direct measure of the patient's physical status (Hurria et al., 2005).

Another essential domain within a CGA is the assessment of the patient's cognitive function. Studies have shown that up to 50 per cent of patients can present with cognitive abnormalities that need further attention. It is further shown that a cognitive disorder can impact the ability to weigh the risk and benefits of the suggested treatment plan and that it may cause difficulties in recognizing signs of adverse effects that warrant closer observation (Extermann and Hurria, 2007). Cognitive functioning within a CGA is mostly evaluated with the well-known Folstein Mini-Mental State Examination (MMSE) (Folstein, Folstein and McHugh, 1975). Although validated in multiple populations, others have encountered difficulties when having to perform the MMSE in older cancer patients. Therefore, recent studies have suggested that the Freund Clock Drawing Test may be more favourable as an initial screening instrument in this population since it reduces the assessment time, is well accepted by the patient and uses a quick and easy scoring system (Freund et al., 2005; Ketelaars et al., 2013; Lycke et al., 2014).

Nutrition is another crucial element included in a CGA. Several studies have demonstrated the importance of weight loss as a prognostic factor for survival in patients with cancer (Extermann and Hurria, 2007). Up to 40 per cent of general geriatric patients are found to be at risk for malnutrition, and without proper nutritional support, an intensive cancer treatment could induce cachexia. Nutrition can be assessed through the Mini-Nutritional Assessment (MNA), which is frequently used to identify geriatric patients at risk of malnutrition (Vellas et al., 1999).

An important aspect to consider when approaching older cancer patients is the social state of the patient. Social isolation in older adults leads to psychological distress and the absence of social support is a predictor of mortality, independent of the age of the patient (Seeman et al., 1993; Extermann and Hurria, 2007). To examine the social state of the patients, specific questions can be asked regarding their marital status, living situation, number of children, etc.

The emotional status cannot be un-assessed within a CGA, as up to 50 per cent of older patients have been found to show signs of depression (Repetto et al., 2002; Brunello, Sandri and Extermann, 2009). Depression in older adults has been associated with increased risk for resource requirements and informal caregiving needs. An assessment of the older patient's psychological state is becoming increasingly important as the care of oncology patients is primarily moving to the outpatients settings, with an increased reliance on caregivers to assist with symptom management and daily activities (Extermann and Hurria, 2007). The Geriatric Depression Scale (GDS) is a commonly used tool to screen for depression in older patients (Extermann et al., 2004). The GDS was originally developed including 30 questions, although shorter versions exist (Yesavage, 1988; Burke, Roccaforte and Wengel, 1991).

The relative incidence of co-morbidities increases with age. Research has shown an association between the presence of co-morbidities and the older cancer patient's prognosis (Mohile and Magnuson, 2013). Further, it is stated that concomitant diseases not only impact survival but that they also may impact the behaviour of the cancer itself. Therefore, screening for co-morbidities forms an essential part of the CGA (Extermann and Hurria, 2007). Co-morbidities can be assessed through the Charlson Comorbidity Index which includes 19 diseases weighted from one to six points (Charlson et al., 1987) or through the Cumulative Illness Rating Scale for Geriatrics (Miller and Tower, 1991).

The final element included in the older cancer patient's assessment is polypharmacy. The reported prevalence of concomitant drug use in the elderly ranges widely and is dependent on the population under study (Mohile and Magnuson, 2013). However, changes in physiology, associated with aging, can induce differences in the pharmacokinetics and pharmacodynamics of cancer treatments and can result – in combination with polypharmacy – in drug–drug or drug–disease interactions, causing adverse clinical events (Extermann and Hurria, 2007; Pottel et al., 2012b; Nightingale et al., 2015).

CGA in routine practice

When the CGA was first introduced into oncology, the assessment could take up to two hours, without incorporating the time needed to review the data, score the patient's health status and develop an individualized care plan. To overcome this limitation, researchers have focused on a two-step approach in which older patients are first assessed with a brief screening tool, followed by a more comprehensive geriatric assessment for those who screen positive (see Figure 5.2) (Extermann, 2010).

Hamaker and his colleagues provided an overview of the screening tools that have been mostly investigated for use in oncogeriatric patients. All of the screening tools assess functional status and most of those also address psychosocial functioning. However, the inclusion of other geriatric domains was observed to vary widely amongst the different screening methods. Further, the use of different contents and cut-off scores leads to a large discrepancy in sensitivity and specificity to identify vulnerability. Nevertheless, the G8-questionnaire (G-8) remains the most favourable screening tool for use as it has a strong prognostic value for functional decline and overall survival (Hamaker, Mitrovi and Stauder, 2014; Kenis et al., 2014; Pottel et al., 2014).

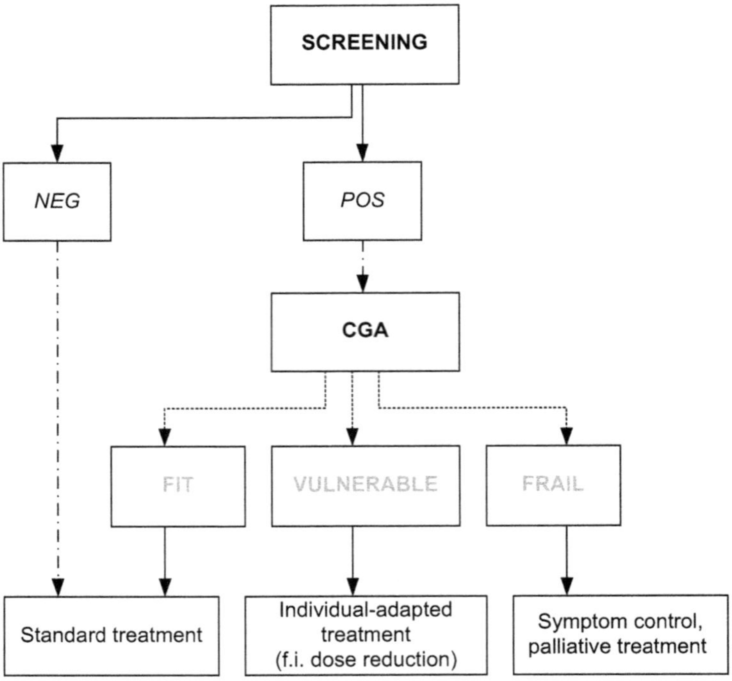

Figure 5.2 Schematic overview of CGA approach in oncology.

(Adapted with permission from Pottel, 2014).

Abbreviations: NEG: negative, POS: positive, CGA: comprehensive geriatric assessment

In addition, since there is not one precise definition of frailty, classification of patients' fitness for treatment into 'fit', 'vulnerable' or 'frail' based on CGA also differs according to the criteria applied. Balducci was the first to publish three classes of fitness in the older patient, based on the presence of co-morbidities, geriatric syndromes (e.g. incontinence, distress, delirium) or functional dependence (Balducci and Extermann, 2001). Further, some have included parameters such as muscle weakness, weight loss and other (Fried et al., 2001; Ensrud et al., 2008). At present, an impairment on a CGA is defined as meeting the cut-off scores for impairment in at least one (Bellera et al., 2012) or at least two (Mohile et al., 2007; Kellen et al., 2010; Luciani et al., 2010; Molina-Garrido and Guillen-Ponce, 2011) domains within CGA, based on the finding that deficits in two or more of the CGA scales indicate an increased risk of disability or death (Extermann et al., 1998; Inouye et al., 1998). Moreover, one single numerical scale to address frailty, based on CGA, has also been proposed (Teymoori et al. 2009; Jones et al., 2005; Pilotto et al., 2008). A more disease-specific definition of 'frailty' might be more adequate, in which more weight is attributed to specific CGA domains, considering the different health problems that might be associated with a specific cancer diagnosis. Recently, such a treatment decision-tree was established based on expert opinion, specifically for prostate cancer patients with respectively localized or metastatic disease, based on CGA. In this scenario, Droz et al. classified patients into four categories ('fit', 'vulnerable', 'frail' and 'too sick') based on impairments in co-morbidity, ADL, IADL and nutritional status, and suggested respectively standard or adaptive treatment according to declining order of fitness (Droz et al., 2010).

Presentation of the work performed by the authors

We started to focus on aging and cancer in 2009. In a first trial (OMGIANT-trial), which was a prospective multi-centric study, we examined the prevalence of vulnerability, assessed through (serial) CGA, in elderly head and neck cancer (HNCA) patients undergoing curative radio(chemo)therapy. Initial results showed that the G-8 is the most optimal tool to screen for fit-vulnerable HNCA patients, but suggested that a combination of both tools could lead to better performance scores (Pottel et al., 2012a). Dr Debruyne and his team tried to validate their new screening tool; however, data suggested that the G-8 remained favourable. Secondary endpoints also showed that CGA evaluation halfway through treatment is feasible and that it can be valuable considering the high impact of the treatment on the health status, both in fit and vulnerable patients. Moreover, serial CGA classification was found to be indicative of the health-related quality-of-life scores and can therefore provide useful information on the changing patient needs (Pottel et al., 2014).

We also studied the potential for optimization of the CGA and looked into the following domains: polypharmacy, cognition and hearing disorders. Firstly, we studied the applicability of Lexicomp®, an online drug information database, for adequate identification of drug–drug interactions (DDIs) within a CGA. Results indicated that Lexicomp® could reduce the administration of inappropriate drugs, resulting in an improved quality of patient-individualized treatment (Pottel et al., 2012b). In the PROACTIVE trial, we aimed at validating the user-friendly Freund Clock Drawing Test, with its retrospectively determined cut-off score of ≤4, as a screening tool to detect cognitive dysfunctions in older cancer patients within a CGA. It was compared against the time-consuming Folstein MMSE as gold standard. Results showed that the Freund CDT is well accepted by patients, time efficient and easy to score, and that it can be used as a stand-alone screening tool within a CGA in this population (Ketelaars et al., 2013; Lycke et al., 2014). During our most recent work, we looked at a screening tool to detect hearing disorders in older cancer patients. The NCCN Guidelines in Older Adult Oncology recommend an assessment of the sensory functions such as vision and hearing. We examined the efficacy of an iPod-based application, uHear™, to screen for hearing loss in older cancer patients as part of a CGA. uHear™ indeed showed promising results with good diagnostic performance scores. However, the application was not validated with its most optimal cut-off. We aim at validating uHear™ with its best cut-off in a future trial.

International perspective

Prof Dr Supriya Mohile

The incidence of cancer, particularly gynaecologic malignancy, increases with advanced age. The geriatric population is a heterogeneous group and a patient's chronologic age does not always reflect their overall health status. Therefore, oncologists need to be adept at assessing physiologic and functional capacity in older patients. A dedicated group of researchers and clinicians in the United States has formed the Cancer and Aging Research Group (CARG) with the mission of supporting research to improve the care of the older adult with cancer (Hurria et al., 2008). The CGA is supported by CARG as the gold standard for evaluation of the older patient with cancer. The various components of the CGA have been shown to influence cancer-related therapy in a multitude of ways. The combined data from the CGA can be used to stratify patients into risk categories to better predict their tolerance to treatment and risk for chemotherapy toxicity. It has been shown that in geriatric patients with malignancy, performance status evaluation is not a sensitive tool to detect risk factors in this population. For example, Extermann and Hurria demonstrated that although only 20 per cent of geriatric oncology patients present with a performance status of two or greater, more than half of this population needs assistance with IADLs, which measure the ability of a person to perform tasks that allow for living independently in the community (Extermann and Hurria, 2007).

Patients who have good functional and nutritional status, low level of co-morbidity and strong social support are classified as 'fit' for treatment. Patients with multiple CGA deficits are considered 'frail' and would have high risk for toxicity with treatments. Those patients in-between may have modifiable risk factors and are considered 'vulnerable'. These patients are at increased risk of treatment related toxicity as compared to 'fit' patients and should be evaluated for potential modification or dose-reduction of their treatment (with escalation as tolerated) to facilitate completion of therapy with minimum toxicity.

A CARG study sought to identify baseline characteristics of the geriatric oncology population, which would predict increased risk toxicity (Hurria et al., 2011). The investigators collected pre-chemotherapy clinical data and CGA results on 500 patients and followed them throughout their treatment course, monitoring for toxicity events. Characteristics predicting increased risk for toxicity included age ≥72, cancer type (gastro-intestinal or genitourinary malignancy), standard dosing of chemotherapy, polychemotherapy regimen, decreased hemoglobin (males <11, females <10), creatinine clearance <34, hearing impairment, one or more falls in the past six months, limited ability to walk one block, need for assistance with taking medications and decreased social activities. Authors were able to develop a risk-stratification schema by assigning a risk score for each of these factors. They demonstrated that the total risk score for a patient correlated with the incidence of treatment-related toxicity events. Extermann et al. developed and validated the CRASH score in 500 older patients which also included GA factors that predicted risk of toxicity (Extermann et al., 2012).

While CGA has been shown to identify impairments in older patients and to help identify those at most risk for chemotherapy toxicity and mortality, less is known about how CGA can guide interventions to improve outcomes of older cancer patients. The development of structured care processes can provide a framework for how oncologists can incorporate GA into clinical practice and improve outcomes of vulnerable older adults with cancer. Firstly, CGA is used to identify specific evidence-based geriatric interventions to be implemented, such as social work referral for patients who live alone and require assistance with planning for a higher level of care. Secondly, CGA is used to guide cancer treatment decisions, such as not using a neuro-toxic chemotherapy in an older patient with balance issues who is at risk for falls. A US-based study surveyed geriatric oncology experts who provided a consensus using Delphi methodology on assessment tools and interventions that could be provided to older patients with cancer with impairments on GA (Mohile et al., 2015). These types of approaches require further validation in large randomized studies.

Prof Dr Etienne Brain (SIOG President)

The pioneers and landmark actions led around CGA by Silvio Monfardini, Lodovico Balducci, Matti Aapro, Jean Pierre Droz and many others (Monfardini et al., 1996; Monfardini and Balducci, 1999; Repetto et al., 2002; Terret, Albrand and Droz, 2004; Extermann et al., 2005) were a real dawning eye-opener for the community of healthcare givers. However, around the twenty-first century, despite growing evidence that geriatric oncology would become a key component in the daily oncology practice, interest in geriatric oncology within the oncology world remained arduous. As a result, for those who were already involved in the management of elderly cancer patients and who underlined its importance, the International Society of Geriatric Oncology or Société Internationale d'Onco Gériatrie (SIOG) was launched in 2000. Since then, SIOG has deeply committed to supporting research linking aging and cancer, developing education and expanding international outreach and dimension, as summarized in its ten priorities (www.siog.org).

In research, SIOG has been a constant supporter to brainstorm and disseminate the great strides to predict treatment toxicity in elderly, either with chemotherapy (CRASH and Cancer and Aging Research Group programs) (Hurria et al., 2011; Extermann et al., 2012) or after surgery (PACE and PREOP studies) (Audisio et al., 2008; Huisman et al., 2015). It has progressively engaged in developing and disseminating specific high-standard guidelines that advocate fine-tuned strategies in elderly cancer patients (see SIOG Guidelines on www.siog.org). It still appreciates the need to demonstrate that CGA may result in corrective measures (or geriatric interventions) improving cancer prognosis and overall outcome, as in the large French randomized clinical trial PREPARE that will be launched in early 2016 (Pierre Soubeyran, personal communication). Indeed, this seems to be the only way we can convince others of the CGA's added value and to decrease the still too-often-blinded oncology practice in the elderly population.

Geriatric oncology also needs to spread internationally: one may have to adapt geriatric tools according to culture and countries, prioritizing some domains according to local conditions and resources. The SIOG has created bridges between (inter)national and cooperative groups: GERICO/Unicancer in France, CARG in US, the Cancer in the Elderly Task Force of the EORTC, the Gruppo Italiano di Oncologia Geriatrica (GIOGER) in Italy, etc. It has allowed launching oncology policy acts through the development of a solid, visible and international expertise, making the voice of elderly cancer patients more and more heard. Beside its annual conference, SIOG has also decided to launch alternating and rotating events to move to regions of the world which are less covered, such as Asia Pacific (APAC) or Latin America (LATAM) (www.siog.org).

This all would never have happened without education. In our aging society, education is the most important cornerstone dedicated to build the future and to get a tangible change now! The society therefore launched its first SIOG Treviso Advanced Post Graduate Course in 2014, with the support of the Università Cattolica del Sacro Cuore and European School of Oncology, and under the auspices of American Society of Clinical Oncology (ASCO), resurrecting a long-standing Italian tradition of cenacoli as during the Rinascimento. There is no doubt that young oncologists and geriatricians from all around the world learning how to work together more efficiently is the way to make things happen!

Conclusion

Due to the aging of the population, researchers' attention towards the management of older cancer patients has increased. At present, CGA has established its added value in the geriatric oncology population since it can predict the risk on morbidity and mortality that is associated with a cancer treatment. Despite extensive documentation of its efficacy, and suggestions for its incorporation by international guidelines for geriatric oncology, not all physicians have started to implement geriatric assessments into their oncology practice. Therefore, in the coming years, the efficient and widespread implementation of CGA in daily geriatric oncology care programs will be of utmost importance.

References

Aliamus, V., Adam, C., Druet-Cabanac, M., Dantoine, T., and Vergnenegre, A. (2011). Geriatric assessment contribution to treatment decision-making in thoracic oncology. *Revue Des Maladies Respiratoires*, 28, 1124–1130.

Audisio, R. A., Pope, D., Ramesh, H. S., Gennari, R., Van Leeuwen, B. L., West, C., Corsini, G., Maffezzini, M., Hoekstra, H. J., Mobarak, D., Bozzetti, F., Colledan, M., Wildiers, H., Stotter, A., Capewell, A., and Marshall, E. (2008). Shall we operate? Preoperative assessment in elderly cancer patients (PACE) can help. A SIOG surgical task force prospective study. *Critical Reviews in Oncology/Hematology*, 65, 156–163.

Balducci, L., and Extermann, M. (2001). A practical approach to the older patient with cancer. *Current Problems in Cancer*, 25, 6–76.

Bellera, C. A., Rainfray, M., Mathoulin-Pelissier, S., Mertens, C., Delva, F., Fonck, M., and Soubeyran, P. L. (2012). Screening older cancer patients: First evaluation of the G-8 geriatric screening tool. *Annals of Oncology*, 23, 2166–2172.

Brunello, A., Sandri, R., and Extermann, M. (2009). Multidimensional geriatric evaluation for older cancer patients as a clinical and research tool. *Cancer Treatment Reviews*, 35, 487–492.

Burke, W. J., Roccaforte, W. H., and Wengel, S. P. (1991). The short form of the Geriatric Depression Scale: A comparison with the 30-item form. *Journal of Geriatric Psychiatry and Neurology*, 4, 173–178.

Caillet, P., Canoui-Poitrine, F., Vouriot, J., Berle, M., Reinald, N., Krypciak, S., Bastuji-Garin, S., Culine, S., and Paillaud, E. (2011). Comprehensive geriatric assessment in the decision-making process in elderly patients with cancer: ELCAPA study. *Journal of Clinical Oncology*, 29, 3636–3642.

Camilon, P. R., Stokes, W. A., Nguyen, S. A., and Lentsch, E. J. (2014). Are the elderly with oropharyngeal carcinoma undertreated? *Laryngoscope*. 124(9), 2057–2063.

Campanelli, C. M. (2012). American geriatrics society updated beers criteria for potentially inappropriate medication use in older adults. *Journal of the American Geriatrics Society*, 60, 616–631.

Cancer Research, U. K. (2015). www.cancerresearchuk.org/health-professional/cancer-statistics/incidence/age#heading-Zero (accessed August, 2015).

Chapman, A. E., Swartz, K., Schoppe, J., and Arenson, C. (2014). Development of a comprehensive multidisciplinary geriatric oncology center, the Thomas Jefferson University Experience. *Journal of Geriatric Oncology*, 5, 164–170.

Charlson, M. E., Pompei, P., Ales, K. L., and Mackenzie, C. R. (1987). A new method of classifying prognostic comorbidity in longitudinal studies: Development and validation. *Journal of Chronic Disease*, 40, 373–383.

Chen, C. C., Kenefick, A. L., Tang, S. T., and McCorkle, R. (2004). Utilization of comprehensive geriatric assessment in cancer patients. *Critical Reviews in Oncology/Hematology*, 49, 53–67.

Chen, H., Cantor, A., Meyer, J., Beth Corcoran, M., Grendys, E., Cavanaugh, D., Antonek, S., Camarata, A., Haley, W., Balducci, L., and Extermann, M. (2003). Can older cancer patients tolerate chemotherapy? A prospective pilot study. *Cancer*, 97, 1107–1114.

Clough-Gorr, K. M., Thwin, S. S., Stuck, A. E., and Silliman, R. A. (2012). Examining five- and ten-year survival in older women with breast cancer using cancer-specific geriatric assessment. *European Journal of Cancer*, 48, 805–812.

Davey, P. G., Jabeen, F. J., Harpur, E. S., Shenoi, P. M., and Geddes, A. M. (1983). A controlled study of the reliability of pure tone audiometry for the detection of gentamicin auditory toxicity. *Journal of Laryngology & Otology*, 97, 27–36.

Diachun, L. L., Klages, K. B., Hansen, K. T., Blake, K., and Gordon, J. (2012). The comprehensive geriatric assessment guide: An exploratory analysis of a medical trainee performance evaluation tool. *Academic Medicine*, 87, 1679–1684.

Droz, J. P., Aapro, M., Balducci, L., Boyle, H., Van den Broeck, T., Cathcart, P., Dickinson, L., Efstathiou, E., Emberton, M., Fitzpatrick, J. M., Heidenreich, A., Hughes, S., Joniau, S., Kattan, M., Mottet, N., Oudard, S., Payne, H., Saad, F., and Sugihara, T. (2014). Management of prostate cancer in older patients: Updated recommendations of a working group of the International Society of Geriatric Oncology. *The Lancet Oncology*, 15, e404–e414.

Droz, J. P., Balducci, L., Bolla, M., Emberton, M., Fitzpatrick, J. M., Joniau, S., Kattan, M. W., Monfardini, S., Moul, J. W., Naeim, A., Van Poppel, H., Saad, F., and Sternberg, C. N. (2010). Management of prostate cancer in older men: Recommendations of a working group of the International Society of Geriatric Oncology. *BJU Int*, 106, 462–469.

Ensrud, K. E., Ewing, S. K., Taylor, B. C., Fink, H. A., Cawthon, P. M., Stone, K. L., Hillier, T. A., Cauley, J. A., Hochberg, M. C., Rodondi, N., Tracy, J. K., and Cummings, S. R. (2008). Comparison of 2 frailty indexes for prediction of falls, disability, fractures, and death in older women. *Archives of Internal Medicine*, 168, 382–389.

Extermann, M. (2010). Geriatric oncology: An overview of progresses and challenges. *Cancer Research and Treatment*, 42, 61–68.

Extermann, M., Aapro, M., Bernabei, R., Cohen, H. J., Droz, J. P., Lichtman, S., Mor, V., Monfardini, S., Repetto, L., Sorbye, L., Topinkova, E., and Task Force on CGA of the International Society of Geriatric Oncology. (2005). Use of comprehensive geriatric assessment in older cancer patients: Recommendations from the task force on CGA of the International Society of Geriatric Oncology (SIOG). *Critical Reviews in Oncology/Hematology*, 55, 241–252.

Extermann, M., Boler, I., Reich, R. R., Lyman, G. H., Brown, R. H., Defelice, J., Levine, R. M., Lubiner, E. T., Reyes, P., Schreiber, F. J., 3rd, and Balducci, L. (2012). Predicting the risk of chemotherapy toxicity in older patients: The Chemotherapy Risk Assessment Scale for High-Age Patients (CRASH) score. *Cancer*, 118, 3377–3386.

Extermann, M., and Hurria, A. (2007). Comprehensive geriatric assessment for older patients with cancer. *Journal of Clinical Oncology*, 25, 1824–1831.

Extermann, M., Meyer, J., Mcginnis, M., Crocker, T. T., Corcoran, M. B., Yoder, J., Haley, W. E., Chen, H., Boulware, D., and Balducci, L. (2004). A comprehensive geriatric intervention detects multiple problems in older breast cancer patients. *Critical Reviews in Oncology/Hematology*, 49, 69–75.

Extermann, M., Overcash, J., Lyman, G. H., Parr, J., and Balducci, L. (1998). Comorbidity and functional status are independent in older cancer patients. *Journal of Clinical Oncology*, 16, 1582–1587.

Folstein, M. F., Folstein, S. E., and Mchugh, P. R. (1975). "Mini-mental state": A practical method for grading the cognitive state of patients for the clinician. *Journal of Psychiatric Research*, 12, 189–198.

Freund, B., Gravenstein, S., Ferris, R., Burke, B. L., and Shaheen, E. (2005). Drawing clocks and driving cars. *Journal of General Internal Medicine*, 20, 240–244.

Fried, L. P., Tangen, C. M., Walston, J., Newman, A. B., Hirsch, C., Gottdiener, J., Seeman, T., Tracy, R., Kop, W. J., Burke, G., and Mcburnie, M. A. (2001). Frailty in older adults: Evidence for a phenotype. *Journal of Gerontology Series A: Biological Sciences and Medical Science*, 56, M146–M156.

Hamaker, M. E., Jonker, J. M., De Rooij, S. E., Vos, A. G., Smorenburg, C. H., and Van Munster, B. C. (2012). Frailty screening methods for predicting outcome of a comprehensive geriatric assessment in elderly patients with cancer: A systematic review. *Lancet Oncol*, 13, e437–e444.

Hamaker, M. E., Mitrovic, M., and Stauder, R. (2014). The G8 screening tool detects relevant geriatric impairments and predicts survival in elderly patients with a haematological malignancy. *Ann Hematol*, 93, 1031–1040.

Hammann, F., and Drewe, J. (2014). Data mining for potential adverse drug-drug interactions. *Expert Opinion on Drug Metabolism & Toxicology*, 10, 665–671.

Hilmer, S. N., Mager, D. E., Simonsick, E. M., Ling, S. M., Windham, B. G., Harris, T. B., Shorr, R. I., Bauer, D. C., and Abernethy, D. R. (2009). Drug burden index score and functional decline in older people. *American Journal of Medicine*, 122, 1142–1149, e1–e2.

Hoffe, S., and Balducci, L. (2012). Cancer and age: General considerations. *Clinics in Geriatric Medicine*, 28, 1–18.

Hoppe, S., Rainfray, M., Fonck, M., Hoppenreys, L., Blanc, J. F., Ceccaldi, J., Mertens, C., Blanc-Bisson, C., Imbert, Y., Cany, L., Vogt, L., Dauba, J., Houede, N., Bellera, C. A., Floquet, A., Fabry, M. N., Ravaud, A., Chakiba, C., Mathoulin-Pelissier, S., and Soubeyran, P. (2013). Functional decline in older patients with cancer receiving first-line chemotherapy. *Journal of Clinical Oncology*, 31, 3877–3882.

Huisman, M. G., Audisio, R. A., Ugolini, G., Montroni, I., Vigano, A., Spiliotis, J., Stabilini, C., De Liguori Carino, N., Farinella, E., Stanojevic, G., Veering, B. T., Reed, M. W., Somasundar, P. S., De Bock, G. H., and Van Leeuwen, B. L. (2015). Screening for predictors of adverse outcome in onco-geriatric surgical patients: A multicenter prospective cohort study. *European Journal of Surgical Oncology*, 41, 844–851.

Hurria, A., and Balducci, L. (2009). *Geriatric oncology: Treatment, assessment and management*. New York: Springer.

Hurria, A., Balducci, L., Naeim, A., Gross, C., Mohile, S., Klepin, H., Tew, W., Downey, L., Gajra, A., Owusu, C., Sanati, H., Suh, T., and Figlin, R. (2008). Mentoring junior faculty in geriatric oncology: Report from the Cancer and Aging Research Group. *Journal of Clinical Oncology*, 26, 3125–3127.

Hurria, A., Gupta, S., Zauderer, M., Zuckerman, E. L., Cohen, H. J., Muss, H., Rodin, M., Panageas, K. S., Holland, J. C., Saltz, L., Kris, M. G., Noy, A., Gomez, J., Jakubowski, A., Hudis, C., and Kornblith, A. B. (2005). Developing a cancer-specific geriatric assessment: A feasibility study. *Cancer*, 104, 1998–2005.

Hurria, A., Togawa, K., Mohile, S. G., Owusu, C., Klepin, H. D., Gross, C. P., Lichtman, S. M., Gajra, A., Bhatia, S., Katheria, V., Klapper, S., Hansen, K., Ramani, R., Lachs, M., Wong, F. L., and Tew, W. P. (2011). Predicting chemotherapy toxicity in older adults with cancer: A prospective multicenter study. *Journal of Clinical Oncology*, 29, 3457–3465.

Hurria, A., Wildes, T., Blair, S. L., Browner, I. S., Cohen, H. J., Deshazo, M., Dotan, E., Edil, B. H., Extermann, M., Ganti, A. K., Holmes, H. M., Jagsi, R., Karlekar, M. B., Keating, N. L., Korc-Grodzicki, B., Mckoy, J. M., Medeiros, B. C., Mrozek, E., O'Connor, T., Rugo, H. S., Rupper, R. W., Silliman, R. A., Stirewalt, D. L., Tew, W. P., Walter, L. C., Weir, A. B., 3rd, Bergman, M. A., and Sundar, H. (2014). Senior adult oncology, version 2.2014: Clinical practice guidelines in oncology. *Journal of National Comprehensive Cancer Network*, 12, 82–126.

Inouye, S. K., Peduzzi, P. N., Robison, J. T., Hughes, J. S., Horwitz, R. I., and Concato, J. (1998). Importance of functional measures in predicting mortality among older hospitalized patients. *JAMA*, 279, 1187–1193.

Jones, D., Song, X., Mitnitski, A., and Rockwood, K. (2005). Evaluation of a frailty index based on a comprehensive geriatric assessment in a population based study of elderly Canadians. *Aging Clinical and Experimental Research*, 17, 465–471.

Katz, S., Ford, A. B., Moskowitz, R. W., Jackson, B. A., and Jaffe, M. W. (1963). Studies of illness in the aged. The index of ADL: A Standardized measure of biological and psychosocial function. *JAMA*, 185, 914–919.

Kellen, E., Bulens, P., Deckx, L., Schouten, H., Van Dijk, M., Verdonck, I., and Buntinx, F. (2010). Identifying an accurate pre-screening tool in geriatric oncology. *Critical Reviews in Oncology/Hematology*, 75, 243–248.

Kenis, C., Bron, D., Libert, Y., Decoster, L., Van Puyvelde, K., Scalliet, P., Cornette, P., Pepersack, T., Luce, S., Langenaeken, C., Rasschaert, M., Allepaerts, S., Van Rijswijk, R., Milisen, K., Flamaing, J., Lobelle, J. P., and Wildiers, H. (2013). Relevance of a systematic geriatric screening and assessment in older patients with cancer: Results of a prospective multicentric study. *Annals of Oncology*, 24, 1306–1312.

Kenis, C., Decoster, L., Van Puyvelde, K., De Greve, J., Conings, G., Milisen, K., Flamaing, J., Lobelle, J. P., and Wildiers, H. (2014). Performance of two geriatric screening tools in older patients with cancer. *Journal of Clinical Oncology*, 32, 19–26.

Kenis, C., Flamaing, J., Debruyne, P. R., Rasschaert, M., Focan, C., Cornelis, F., Verschaeve, V., Vanoverbeke, K., Libert, Y., Luce, S., Decoster, L., Nols, N., Van den Bulck, H., Goeminne, J.-C., Baitar, A., Geboers, K., Petit, B., Langenaeken, C., Van Rijswijk, R., Specenier, P., Jerusalem, G., Praet, J.-P., Vandenborre, K., Lobelle, J. P., Lycke, M., Milisen, K., and Wildiers, H. (2015). A nationwide implementation of a multidisciplinary geriatric assessment and intervention program in Belgian older patients with cancer. In *SIOG 2015*, Prague, Czech Republic.

Ketelaars, L., Pottel, L., Lycke, M., Goethals, L., Ghekiere, V., Santy, L., Boterberg, T., Van Den Noortgate, N., Pottel, H., and Debruyne, P. R. (2013). Use of the Freund clock drawing test within the Mini-Cog as a screening tool for cognitive impairment in elderly patients with or without cancer. *Journal of Geriatric Oncology*, 4, 174–182.

Lawton, M. P., and Brody, E. M. (1969). Assessment of older people: Self-maintaining and instrumental activities of daily living. *Gerontologist*, 9, 179–186.

Luciani, A., Ascione, G., Bertuzzi, C., Marussi, D., Codeca, C., Di Maria, G., Caldiera, S. E., Floriani, I., Zonato, S., Ferrari, D., and Foa, P. (2010). Detecting disabilities in older patients with cancer: Comparison between comprehensive geriatric assessment and vulnerable elders survey-13. *Journal of Clinical Oncology*, 28, 2046–2050.

Lycke, M., Ketelaars, L., Boterberg, T., Pottel, L., Pottel, H., Vergauwe, P., Goethals, L., Van Eygen, K., Werbrouck, P., Debruyne, D., Derijcke, S., Borms, M., Ghekiere, V., Wildiers, H., and Debruyne, P. R. (2014). Validation of the Freund clock drawing test as a screening tool to detect cognitive dysfunction in elderly cancer patients undergoing comprehensive geriatric assessment. *Psycho-Oncology*, 23, 1172–1177.

Lycke, M., Pottel, L., Boterberg, T., Ketelaars, L., Wildiers, H., Schofield, P., Weller, D., and Debruyne, P. R. (2015). Integration of geriatric oncology in daily multidisciplinary cancer care: The time is now. *European Journal of Cancer Care (Engl)*, 24, 143–146.

Maas, H. A., Janssen-Heijnen, M. L., Olde Rikkert, M. G., and Machteld Wymenga, A. N. (2007). Comprehensive geriatric assessment and its clinical impact in oncology. *European Journal of Cancer*, 43, 2161–2169.

Mahoney, F. I., and Barthel, D. W. (1965). Functional evaluation: The Barthel index. *Maryland State Medical Journal*, 14, 61–65.

Matsui, Y., Fujita, R., Harada, A., Sakurai, T., Nemoto, T., Noda, N., and Toba, K. (2014). Association of grip strength and related indices with independence of activities of daily living in older adults, investigated by a newly-developed grip strength measuring device. *Geriatrics & Gerontology International*, 14(Suppl. 2), 77–86.

Matthews, D. A. (1984). Dr. Marjory Warren and the origin of British geriatrics. *Journal of American Geriatrics Society*, 32, 253–258.

Miller, M., and Tower, A. (1991). *A manual of guidelines for scoring the cumulative illness rating scale for geriatrics (CIRS-G)*. Pittsburgh: University of Pittsburgh.

Mistry, M., Parkin, D. M., Ahmad, A. S., and Sasieni, P. (2011). Cancer incidence in the United Kingdom: Projections to the year 2030. *British Journal of Cancer*, 105, 1795–1803.

Mohile, S. G., Bylow, K., Dale, W., Dignam, J., Martin, K., Petrylak, D. P., Stadler, W. M., and Rodin, M. (2007). A pilot study of the vulnerable elders survey-13 compared with the comprehensive geriatric assessment for identifying disability in older patients with prostate cancer who receive androgen ablation. *Cancer*, 109, 802–810.

Mohile, S. G., and Magnuson, A. (2013). Comprehensive geriatric assessment in oncology. *Interdisciplinary Top in Gerontology*, 38, 85–103.

Mohile, S. G., Velarde, C., Hurria, A., Magnuson, A., Lowenstein, L., Pandya, C., O'Donovan, A., Gorawara-Bhat, R., and Dale, W. (2015). Geriatric assessment-guided care processes for older adults: A Delphi consensus of geriatric oncology experts. *Journal of the National Comprehensive Cancer Network*, 13, 1120–1130.

Molina-Garrido, M. J., and Guillen-Ponce, C. (2011). Comparison of two frailty screening tools in older women with early breast cancer. *Critical Reviews in Oncology/Hematology*, 79, 51–64.

Monfardini, S., and Balducci, L. (1999). A comprehensive geriatric assessment (CGA) is necessary for the study and the management of cancer in the elderly. *European Journal of Cancer*, 35, 1771–1772.

Monfardini, S., Ferrucci, L., Fratino, L., Del Lungo, I., Serraino, D., and Zagonel, V. (1996). Validation of a multidimensional evaluation scale for use in elderly cancer patients. *Cancer*, 77, 395–401.

Nasreddine, Z. S., Phillips, N. A., Bedirian, V., Charbonneau, S., Whitehead, V., Collin, I., Cummings, J. L., and Chertkow, H. (2005). The Montreal Cognitive Assessment, MoCA: A brief screening tool for mild cognitive impairment. *Journal of the American Geriatrics Society*, 53, 695–699.

Nightingale, G., Hajjar, E., Swartz, K., Andrel-Sendecki, J., and Chapman, A. (2015). Evaluation of a pharmacist-led medication assessment used to identify prevalence of and associations with polypharmacy and potentially inappropriate medication use among ambulatory senior adults with cancer. *Journal of Clinical Oncology*, 33, 1453–1459.

Pal, S. K., Katheria, V., and Hurria, A. (2010). Evaluating the older patient with cancer: Understanding frailty and the geriatric assessment. *CA: A Cancer Journal for Clinicians*, 60, 120–132.

Paleri, V., and Wight, R. G. (2002). Applicability of the adult comorbidity evaluation – 27 and the Charlson indexes to assess comorbidity by notes extraction in a cohort of United Kingdom patients with head and neck cancer: A retrospective study. *The Journal of Laryngology & Otology*, 116, 200–205.

Pilotto, A., Ferrucci, L., Franceschi, M., D'ambrosio, L. P., Scarcelli, C., Cascavilla, L., Paris, F., Placentino, G., Seripa, D., Dallapiccola, B., and Leandro, G. (2008). Development and validation of a multidimensional prognostic index for one-year mortality from comprehensive geriatric assessment in hospitalized older patients. *Rejuvenation Research*, 11, 151–161.

Podsiadlo, D., and Richardson, S. (1991). The timed "Up & Go": A test of basic functional mobility for frail elderly persons. *Journal of the American Geriatric Society*, 39, 142–148.

Pottel, L. (2014). *Towards individualised care for (older) head and neck cancer patients treated with curative radio-chemotherapy*. Ph.D., Ghent University.

Pottel, L., Boterberg, T., Pottel, H., Goethals, L., Van Den Noortgate, N., Duprez, F., De Neve, W., Rottey, S., Geldhof, K., Van Eygen, K., Kargar-Samani, K., Ghekiere, V., Cornelis, F., Mohile, S., and Debruyne, P. R. (2012a). Determination of an adequate screening tool for identification of vulnerable elderly head and neck cancer patients treated with radio(chemo)therapy. *Journal of Geriatric Oncology*, 3, 24–32.

Pottel, L., Lycke, M., Boterberg, T., Ketelaars, L., Pottel, H., Goethals, L., Van Den Noortgate, N., Duprez, F., De Neve, W., Rottey, S., Geldhof, K., Van Eygen, K., Kargar-Samani, K., Ghekiere, V., Verhaeghe, A., and Debruyne, P. (2012b). Experience with Lexicomp® Online Drug Database for medication review and drug-drug interaction analysis within a comprehensive geriatric assessment in elderly cancer patients. *Journal of Analytical Oncology*, 1, 32–41.

Pottel, L., Lycke, M., Boterberg, T., Pottel, H., Goethals, L., Duprez, F., Van Den Noortgate, N., De Neve, W., Rottey, S., Geldhof, K., Buyse, V., Kargar-Samani, K., Ghekiere, V., and Debruyne, P. R. (2014). Serial comprehensive geriatric assessment in elderly head and neck cancer patients undergoing curative radiotherapy identifies evolution of multidimensional health problems and is indicative of quality of life. *European Journal of Cancer Care*, 23, 401–412.

Puts, M. T., Hardt, J., Monette, J., Girre, V., Springall, E., and Alibhai, S. M. (2012). Use of geriatric assessment for older adults in the oncology setting: A systematic review. *Journal of the National Cancer Institute*, 104, 1133–1163.

Repetto, L., Fratino, L., Audisio, R. A., Venturino, A., Gianni, W., Vercelli, M., Parodi, S., Dal Logo, D., Gioia, F., Monfardini, S., Aapro, M. S., Serraino, D., and Zagonel, V. (2002). Comprehensive geriatric assessment adds information to Eastern Cooperative Oncology Group performance status in elderly cancer patients: An Italian group for geriatric oncology study. *Journal of Clinical Oncology*, 20, 494–502.

Reuben, D. B., Fishman, L. K., Mcnabney, M., and Wolde-Tsadik, G. (1996). Looking inside the black box of comprehensive geriatric assessment: A classification system for problems, recommendations, and implementation strategies. *Journal of the American Geriatric Society*, 44, 835–838.

Rocco, N., Rispoli, C., Pagano, G., Ascione, S., Compagna, R., Danzi, M., Accurso, A., and Amato, B. (2013). Undertreatment of breast cancer in the elderly. *BMC Surgery*, 13(Suppl. 2), S26.

Rockwood, K., Stadnyk, K., Macknight, C., Mcdowell, I., Hebert, R., and Hogan, D. B. (1999). A brief clinical instrument to classify frailty in elderly people. *Lancet*, 353, 205–206.

Rodin, M. B., and Mohile, S. G. (2007). A practical approach to geriatric assessment in oncology. *Journal of Clinical Oncology*, 25, 1936–1944.

Seeman, T. E., Berkman, L. F., Kohout, F., Lacroix, A., Glynn, R., and Blazer, D. (1993). Intercommunity variations in the association between social ties and mortality in the elderly: A comparative analysis of three communities. *Annals of Epidemiology*, 3, 325–335.

Siegel, R., Desantis, C., Virgo, K., Stein, K., Mariotto, A., Smith, T., Cooper, D., Gansler, T., Lerro, C., Fedewa, S., Lin, C., Leach, C., Cannady, R. S., Cho, H., Scoppa, S., Hachey, M., Kirch, R., Jemal, A., and Ward, E. (2012). Cancer treatment and survivorship statistics, 2012. *CA: A Cancer Journal for Clinicians*, 62, 220–241.

Solomon, D. H., Judd, H. L., Sier, H. C., Rubenstein, L. Z., and Morley, J. E. (1988). New issues in geriatric care. *Annals of Internal Medicine*, 108, 718–732.

Terret, C., Albrand, G., and Droz, J. P. (2004). Geriatric assessment in elderly patients with prostate cancer. *Clinical Prostate Cancer*, 2, 236–240.

Teymoori, F., Mousavi, M. T., Shirazikhah, M., Abharilaleh, B., Biglarian, R., Franco, A., and Demongeot, J. (2009). FI-CGA score of old people by community based information system. In *Proceedings of the International Conference on Complex, Intelligent and Software Intensive Systems (CISIS)*, Fukuoka, Japan (pp. 949–954).

Tinetti, M. E. (1986). Performance-oriented assessment of mobility problems in elderly patients. *Journal of the American Geriatric Society*, 34, 119–126.

Vande Walle, N., Kenis, C., Heeren, P., Van Puyvelde, K., Decoster, L., Beyer, I., Conings, G., Flamaing, J., Lobelle, J. P., Wildiers, H., and Milisen, K. (2014). Fall predictors in older cancer patients: A multicenter prospective study. *BMC Geriatric*, 14, 135.

Vellas, B., Guigoz, Y., Garry, P. J., Nourhashemi, F., Bennahum, D., Lauque, S., and Albarede, J. L. (1999). The Mini Nutritional Assessment (MNA) and its use in grading the nutritional state of elderly patients. *Nutrition*, 15, 116–122.

Wedding, U., Pientka, L., and Hoffken, K. (2007). Quality-of-life in elderly patients with cancer: A short review. *European Journal of Cancer*, 43, 2203–2210.

Yancik, R. (1997). Cancer burden in the aged: An epidemiologic and demographic overview. *Cancer*, 80, 1273–1283.

Yesavage, J. A. (1988). Geriatric Depression Scale. *Psychopharmacol Bull*, 24, 709–711.

6
HEART FAILURE

Sarah Barnes and Katharine Whittingham

This chapter discusses:

- Heart failure as a condition including prevalence, symptoms and provision of heart failure services in community settings
- The role of communication in heart failure between patients, their informal carers and the healthcare professionals who are responsible for their case management
- The role of informal carers in supporting heart failure patients in the community, including positive aspects of providing care to people with heart failure

Learning outcomes

In this chapter you will learn how to:

- Identify the physiology, prevalence and symptoms of heart failure
- Understand the barriers to patient–professional communication in heart failure
- Identify some strategies to improve communication between healthcare providers and patients
- Gain an understanding of some challenges of providing informal care to heart failure patients
- Identify some positive aspects of caring for patients with heart failure living in community settings

Introduction to heart failure

Physiology

Heart failure is a condition caused by the heart failing to pump enough blood around the body at the right pressure and usually occurs because the heart muscle has become too weak to work properly.

There are three main types of heart failure: left ventricular systolic dysfunction (LVSD), heart failure with preserved ejection fraction (HFPEF) and heart failure caused by diseased or damaged heart valves. In most cases, heart failure does not have a single cause; rather, there are a number of other conditions that increase the chances of developing heart failure. These can include: high blood pressure (hypertension); coronary heart disease (CHD), which may cause angina or a heart attack; heart muscle weakness (cardiomyopathy); heart rhythm disturbance (atrial fibrillation); anaemia; or an overactive thyroid gland (National Institute for Health and Care Excellence (NICE), (2010).

Prevalence

Heart failure is often referred to as a 'disease of older people'. It has a poor prognosis, with a survival rate worse than that of breast or prostate cancer, and presents a major challenge for healthcare delivery in an aging population. Figures for the United Kingdom indicate that around 900,000 people are living with heart failure and, globally, it is estimated that 23 million people are living with the disease (NICE, 2010; Bui, Horwich and Fonarow, 2011). The prevalence of heart failure is increasing due to improved diagnosis, with the average age at diagnosis being 76 years. This prevalence in an aging population presents not only the challenge of managing the condition, but also the need to address the complexities associated with existing co-morbidities and psychosocial issues in this patient cohort. A resulting factor of these complexities is that the condition is associated with frequent readmission to hospital. In the United Kingdom, heart failure is the most common cause of medical admission to hospital in patients and readmission rates are high when post-discharge care in the community is limited (Cowie, 2010). However, the introduction of more effective interventions in acute cardiac care means that more people are surviving with heart failure.

Disease trajectory

Heart failure is a life-limiting condition with a poor prognosis and is associated with debilitating symptoms resulting in poor quality of life. Dying from heart failure is unpredictable; for example, in up to 50 per cent of patients, death can be sudden and at any stage of the disease trajectory, whilst for the remaining patients the disease process is progressive with debilitating symptoms that can result in episodic and prolonged hospitalisation (Connolly et al., 2010). It is this variability in the disease trajectory (see Figure 6.1) that brings additional challenges both physically and emotionally for both the patient and carer (O'Leary et al., 2009; Gott et al., 2007).

Symptoms

The main signs and symptoms associated with heart failure are breathlessness (dyspnoea), fatigue, and swelling in the lower limbs (oedema). Other common symptoms include palpitations, chest pain, memory loss, and sleeplessness. Symptoms such as breathlessness and fatigue can limit the extent of daily physical activities, requiring careful planning to allow for slow performance and frequent stops. Depressive symptoms also predict greater mortality in heart failure patients and negative mood is associated with exacerbated physical symptoms (Woltz et al., 2012). Older people are more likely to attribute symptoms such as fatigue and sleeplessness to normal aging rather than heart failure, so seeking treatment can be delayed until symptoms become acute and distressing.

The New York Heart Association (NYHA) classification, devised by the Criteria Committee of the American Heart Association (1994), is widely recognized as a measure of how the condition impacts on the patients' day-to-day life and is categorized as shown in Table 6.1 (NICE, 2010).

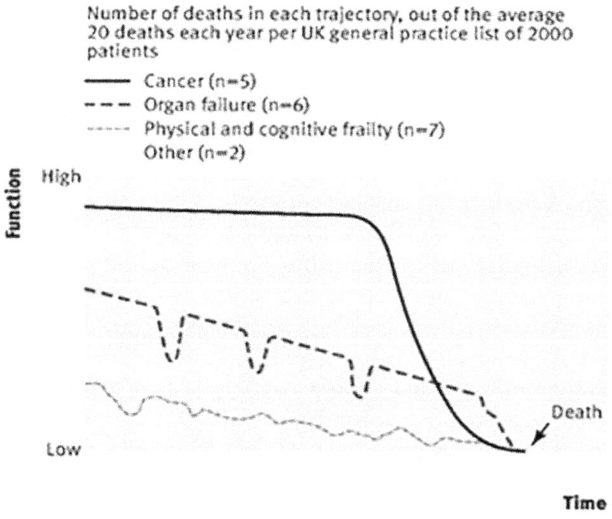

Figure 6.1 The three main trajectories of decline at the end of life.
(Murray and Sheikh, 2008).

Community-based health services for heart failure

Recent UK policies (British Heart Foundation, 2008) mean that people living with heart failure are increasingly cared for at home in the community. Services are provided by general practitioners (GPs), community matrons and, depending on support referral criteria, heart failure nurse specialists (HFNS). The primary goals of heart failure management include reducing disease progression, minimizing symptom burden and improving quality of life.

In the United Kingdom, the National Institute for Health and Care Excellence (NICE) guidance (2010) recommends that a systematic detailed history and clinical assessment is undertaken when a patient presents with symptoms of heart failure. If, following the assessment, heart failure is suspected, the patient should then be referred for an echocardiogram to confirm the diagnosis within two weeks. Echocardiograms are traditionally carried out in hospitals, although they are increasingly becoming available in community settings.

In response to increasing numbers of patients living with heart failure, community-based Heart Failure Nurse Services have been established with the aim, in partnership with GPs

Table 6.1 New York Heart Classification table (Criteria Committee of the American Heart Association, 1994)

Class I	No limitation of physical activity. Ordinary physical activity does not cause undue fatigue, palpitation or dyspnoea.
Class II	Slight limitation of physical activity. Comfortable at rest but ordinary physical activity results in fatigue, palpitation or dyspnoea.
Class III	Marked limitation of physical activity. Comfortable at rest but less-than-ordinary activity results in fatigue, palpitation or dyspnoea.
Class IV	Unable to carry out any physical activity without discomfort. Symptoms at rest. If any physical activity is undertaken, discomfort is increased.

and secondary care services, to support patients living with left ventricular systolic dysfunction (British Heart Foundation, 2008). The objectives of the Heart Failure Nurse Service include: education to patients and informal carers; support and advice to patients, informal carers and healthcare professionals; reduction of unnecessary admissions and readmissions to hospital; improving quality of life for patients; and encouraging patients to self-manage their condition. Referrals to the service can be made by secondary care services, GP services and community nurse services and the referral criteria include patients with symptomatic and complex needs.

Support can also be provided to heart failure patients more informally by family, friends and neighbours. An informal carer can be defined as being an unpaid person providing physical, practical and/or emotional care and support to a relative or friend (Candy et al., 2011). The informal carer does not have to be a family member or living with the patient; it is the level of physical and psychological support being provided that is important. Evidence indicates that there are a higher proportion of female carers and, whilst there are younger carers providing support to heart failure patients, predominantly the informal carer population consists of older carers (Barnes et al., 2006a; Dracup et al., 2004). Due to this profile, carers often have their own health problems and evidence suggests that many neglect their own healthcare needs as a result of a focus on meeting the needs of the patient (Usher and Cammarata, 2009).

Patient–professional communication in heart failure

In the United Kingdom, older people living with chronic conditions such as heart failure are mainly cared for in the community by their primary care team, including GPs, who are central in providing communication about the condition. Research has traditionally shown negativity around communication with doctors (Hanratty et al., 2002; Fried, Bradley and O'Leary, 2003) and, whilst GPs are generally considered positively as competent and sensitive, it is acknowledged that they have a lack of time to spend with their patients. The consequences of poor communication with heart failure patients can result in increased anxiety amongst both patients and their families due to inadequate information provision about their condition. In the advanced stages of heart failure, this poor communication can result in inappropriate hospitalisations, unwanted interventions, and patients having little choice in their desired place of death (Barnes et al., 2012). Appropriate, targeted and sensitive communication between older people with heart failure and healthcare professionals, however, can lead to improved case management as well as the ability to plan end-of-life care.

Communicating the diagnosis and prognosis in heart failure

Research in the United Kingdom has explored the attitudes of older people and primary care professionals towards communication of diagnosis, prognosis and symptoms in heart failure (Barnes et al., 2006b). The research team carried out 44 in-depth interviews with older people and 10 focus groups with primary healthcare professionals. The research found that one of the main factors contributing to the problem of communication was that most GPs found diagnosing heart failure and giving a prognosis particularly challenging, making it difficult for them to relay information back to patients (Barnes et al., 2006b). The difficulty in diagnosing heart failure is exacerbated because presenting symptoms, such as shortness of breath and fatigue, can be caused by a variety of different diseases. This confusion over diagnosis can result in patients being repeatedly sent to different specialists for investigation or treatment for a variety of conditions. In the United Kingdom, echocardiograms are increasingly becoming available in community settings, but the service is somewhat fragmented, with many patients being referred to secondary care. This can make access particularly difficult for older people who may by relying on others for transport.

Once diagnosis has been established, the terminology of heart failure can become a barrier to effective communication. For example, whilst for healthcare professionals the term 'heart failure' itself covers a wide-spectrum of the disease, for patients the term has a ring of finality (Taylor and Ogden, 2005). Healthcare professionals acknowledge that the term 'heart failure' is not satisfactory and needs careful explanation, as pointed out by a GP in the Barnes et al. (2006b) study:

> [I]t's sometimes a diagnosis that we almost carry around on our systems and in our heads about people. We don't necessarily share it. When you do share it, you've got to be very careful. It's a shocking and an anxiety-laden piece of news. Failure feels acute rather than chronic.
>
> *(Male GP)*

GPs have suggested alternative labels for the condition including 'tired heart syndrome', 'heart dysfunction' and 'cardiac impairment' (Barnes et al., 2006b; Lehman, Doust and Glasziou, 2005) and, whilst these can all be interpreted as euphemisms, they are used as an alternative way to describe the condition. Patients have expressed a preference to have discussions with healthcare professionals using lay terms, but research has shown that, paradoxically, GPs have reverted to more complex terminology such as 'ventricular dysfunction' to explain the condition. This can leave patients confused and, in some cases, closed off and losing interest in the diagnosis altogether (Barnes et al., 2006b):

> [I]f they talk in layman's language . . . ordinary language, I can understand it. When they get to the fancy words, that loses me completely . . . It sounds very nice, but it don't mean a damn thing does it, not to me, so, er, I don't like 'em to talk to me like that because it's beyond me.
>
> *(Female patient, age 77)*

Heart failure patients and their informal carers have expressed the need to be told their diagnosis as soon as possible (Ostman, Jakobaaon and Falk, 2015). They have suggested that awareness of their diagnosis opens up opportunities for self-management of the condition, increasing empowerment and enabling all parties to be involved in discussions and decisions around healthcare and planning. It is understood that, whilst discussing diagnosis can be difficult, especially in terms of the timing, it can be made less negative for the patient by discussing ways they can manage the condition themselves.

Another key challenge in effective communication in heart failure is the unpredictable trajectory of the disease, which leaves professionals unwilling to enter into prognostic discussions. Prognosis is important in informing diagnosis and treatment decisions (Christaksi, 1999) but GPs often find it difficult to communicate a poor prognosis and the possibility of death can be glossed over or avoided altogether (Zapka et al., 2006). Improved medication and longer life spans means GPs are understandably reluctant to discuss the life-limiting nature of the disease at an early stage:

> It's very difficult 'cause you don't want to alarm patients unduly when, you know . . . they may be NYHA II, and actually, it could be another 10 years before they

progress and something else would kill them first, so you don't want to give undue alarm, but at the same time . . . in order to entice them to take their medications, you probably do need to explain the gravity of the situation. It's a very fine balance.

(Female GP) [source: Barnes et al., 2006b]

Research indicates that patients and their families often receive limited information about the likely course of their disease and are provided with few opportunities to make decisions about the care they receive, particularly in the advanced stages (Aldred, Gott and Gariballa, 2005; Gott et al., 2008). This can result in patients receiving care they may not have chosen and can incur unnecessary costs to healthcare services (for example due to high rates of hospitalisations prior to death).

Providing information and improving communication in heart failure

Research has reported that patients often have a poor understanding of heart failure and try to make sense of their illness in terms of their increasing age and decreasing physical and mental capacities (Cortis and Williams, 2007). This lack of understanding can be compounded by poor communication with their GPs. In the Barnes et al. (2006b) study, patients reported some knowledge of their symptoms and recognized that they were caused by their heart condition, but overall there was a lack of understanding of heart failure:

Female patient (age 84): *Dr [name] does try and explain to me exactly what it is, you know, why I have good days and why I have bad days.*

Researcher: *Mmm . . . Can you tell me a little bit about what he said?*

Female patient: *Erm . . . I don't think I understand it! [Laughs] Erm . . . it's something that opens and closes. Er . . . oh dear, isn't it awful! I try to concentrate when he's telling me you know . . . [Laughs] . . . he does explain, but I can't remember what he said, to be honest with you.*

Several patients in the study said that, despite attempts by healthcare professionals to explain the condition, they preferred not to know since it would cause them to worry. One of the consequences of the lack of communication with their GPs was that patients reported a variety of gaps in their knowledge of their illness and described panic attacks and fear of being alone. They also demonstrated anxiety about the practicalities of what to do in a crisis. This poor communication can be compounded by confusion and short-term memory loss, which are known to be associated with heart failure, with some patients experiencing difficulty remembering or understanding explanations.

Research within the field of health psychology indicates that people vary enormously in their desire for and need of information (Fallowfield, 2005). Indeed, there is evidence that giving health information to those who do not want it can cause undue anxiety and distress. It is therefore important to balance the information needs of patients. Fallowfield (2005) suggests that, when discussing treatment choices with heart failure patients, it is necessary to determine their own preference about the amount and type of information required. Recent UK guidelines on communicating with heart failure patients suggest that the content and timing of information provision should be tailored to the needs of the individual patient (NICE, 2010). In particular, healthcare professionals should assess how much the patient knows about the disease, how much they are prepared to know and the impact of this knowledge on their well-being. The guidelines also suggest: giving patients the information they ask for or need about their condition, its treatment and prognosis in a way they can understand; making the advice specific, detailed and concrete; using words which the patients will understand; and, with consent, sharing information with patients' informal carers.

Evidence from a systematic review of patient–professional communication interventions suggests that communication with heart failure patients and informal carers should ideally be delivered within the primary care setting by trained professionals (Barnes et al., 2012). The ideal scenario put forward was an initial discussion with a GP, followed up incrementally by another healthcare professional with whom the patient had a close and trusted relationship; for example, a district nurse, community matron or heart failure nurse specialist. Diagnosis should be discussed as soon as possible, an optimum time to open up discussions being on receipt of results from a diagnostic test, such as an echocardiogram.

European research into communication in heart failure has tended to focus on advanced care planning (de Vleminck et al., 2014; Gerlich et al., 2012). It is acknowledged that successful advanced care planning is less likely to occur in heart failure than cancer. De Vleminck et al.'s (2014) focus group study in Belgium highlighted the barriers to advanced care planning in heart failure to be: lack of familiarity with the terminal phase; lack of key moments to initiate advance care planning; the patient's lack of awareness of their diagnosis and prognosis; and the fact that patients did not often initiate such discussions themselves. They recommend the development of practical guidelines and educational interventions to improve communication in heart failure. Gerlich's (2012) work focussing on a German healthcare setting also found a need for improved communication in heart failure.

Strategies for improving communication in heart failure

Evidence suggests that discussions of advanced care planning in heart failure should be face to face and accompanied with an offer of support if needed (for example, details of social services and/or financial assistance) (Barnes et al., 2012). However, an individualized assessment is important as some patients may want to know more than others. The GP should begin discussions by assessing how much the patient knows already and take it from there. Ideally, the discussion should take place at the patient's home, potentially involving the district nurse or heart failure nurse specialist as well, as they are providing regular care. People have a right to know what they are being treated for and some studies have shown that patients want more information than their doctors believe they do (Jenkins, Fallowfield and Saul, 2001; Horne and Payne, 2004).

A key component of a successful communication intervention is the need to enhance patient education to ensure an understanding of the condition and its implications. Patient education is an important and necessary prerequisite to discussions of advanced care planning in heart failure, yet this is often assumed rather than formally addressed in communication models developed to date:

> It's a culture change, I think, that we need to get across, and it needs to happen with health professionals first, I guess, before we can actually start educating the patients about it . . . that it isn't all doom and gloom because we do have treatments that can improve the prognosis. So the thing for me, I guess, is patient education would be enormously helpful, but also that we ensure that all healthcare professionals are singing from the same hymn book.
>
> *(Female GP) [source: Barnes et al., 2006b)*

An empowering approach to communication with heart failure patients put forward by Swedish researchers involves active participation, planning and influence over their own decisions, which gives patients a feeling of greater confidence and self-esteem (Ostman, Jacobsson and Falk, 2015). Person-centredness during the patient–professional encounter helps the patients feel recognized, acknowledged and unique. Here, experience of being an equal is paramount; where personal history and individual situation are taken into account. Current practice is largely represented by a 'drip-drip' of information with some healthcare professionals reporting end-of-life conversations starting after a series of unsuccessful treatments.

Importance of informal care for people with heart failure

Many heart failure patients receive informal support in addition to that provided by health professionals. Informal support encompasses unpaid assistance to patients living in the community. This assistance may be provided by family, friends or neighbours who are acting as informal carers. Common tasks informal carers undertake include personal care, such as washing and dressing the patient, and tasks concerning social care needs including financial management and household chores, such as shopping and cleaning. Informal carers are integral to supporting patients being cared for at home and the social support provided is linked to lower rates of unplanned admissions to acute care (Kang, Li and Nolan, 2011). It is important that patients and their informal carers have a point of contact who can organize timely support according to the changing demands of social care. This may include access to high-quality respite care services, consistent and high-quality social care services, access to equipment and assistance to apply for financial support (Lyons et al., 2015).

Challenges for informal caregivers of heart failure patients

Whilst informal carers of heart failure patients report similar issues to those caring for patients with other chronic conditions, heart failure presents the additional challenge of coping with frequent changes in patient symptoms. This is alongside the responsibility of managing and administering medication, emergency admissions to hospital and difficulties associated with prognostication. These challenges can create demands on informal caregivers' physical and psychosocial well-being (Dracup et al., 2004).

Informal carers have reported that the physical requirements of the role impacts on themselves and that they often neglect their own healthcare needs to focus on meeting the needs of the patient. In a study by Pressler et al. (2009) older carers reported frequently forgetting to take medications leading to poor control of their own conditions. The physical aspects of caring can also affect psychosocial well-being, with carers feeling high levels of responsibility associated with the role. Alongside this there can be a sense of being out of control of what is happening to the patient; both of which can contribute to levels of anxiety and depression (Saunders, 2008; Molloy et al., 2008). The sense of helplessness when patients are symptomatic, particularly when they are struggling to breathe, causes great distress. Informal carers may also experience reduced social activities or a change in working patterns. By having reduced contact with friends, family or work colleagues, the burden of caring can be increased; they can become isolated and have no one to share their concerns with (Usher and Cammarata, 2009). Carers can express concerns about leaving the patient alone to pursue their own social interests and this may be related to lack of access to, or poor quality, respite care services. Burdened, depressed caregivers are more likely to develop health problems of their own (Princes Royal Trust for Carers, 2011).

Informal carers can experience restrictions, day to day, as a result of the physical limitations the patients experience when living with symptomatic heart failure. There can be an inability to forward plan as they may be unsure if the patient would be able to physically cope with the proposed activity. This uncertainty can lead to worry and emotional strain including feelings of irritation and disappointment in both patients and carers. A study conducted in Sweden found that some informal carers described missing the daily life experiences they used to share with their partner before they became unwell (Pihl, Fridlund and Martensson, 2014). They described lacking mutual experiences and shared interests as they are no longer able to participate in activities together. Lack of intimacy both physically and mentally with the patient can enhance feelings of loneliness.

When informal carers feel that their own needs are not being met, this can reinforce a lack of communality between the carer and the patient. If there is lack of recognition by family and healthcare professionals to their needs, as the priority is to manage the physical symptoms of the patients, informal carers may perceive that there is limited acknowledgement of the carer as a positive resource in supporting the patient (Stolz, Willman and Uden, 2006).

Strategies to improve caring in heart failure

Networks of support

Evidence suggests that informal carers who feel well supported and have a sense that a network could help them when they needed it cope better with the demands of caring (Stolz, Willman and Uden, 2006; Agren et al., 2012). This network can be a family member or healthcare professional and can offer great reassurance and engender a feeling of shared responsibility of caring. The manner in which healthcare professionals who are involved in the care of heart failure patients respond when carers ask for help or if, when visiting the patient, they ask how the carer is coping are both viewed as a positive means of making the carer feel a priority (Stolz Stolz, Willman and Uden, 2006). Being seen and being heard allows carers to feel that their needs are recognized as important and this can be enhanced when healthcare professionals acknowledge the struggles that informal carers face and offer proactive support. Participants of research in the United Kingdom which evaluated carer support from a heart failure nurse specialist service identified the nurse as a key source of strength and support (Whittingham and Pearce, 2011):

> She just sat and explained it all to us. Asked us if there was anything to query, she just listened. She's been brilliantly helpful. . . . She did care enough about us, I mean she's really good. She's brilliant, never mind good. It's a joy to see her again and it takes a lot of worry off my mind leaving her you see.
>
> *(Male carer, age 67)*

The support of family and friends is also important to help carers maintain a positive outlook. Carers who have limited social support have been shown to find the role more demanding and have increased carer burden (Hwang et al., 2011). It is therefore important that healthcare professionals involved in the patient's care assess the availability of wider social support.

New knowledge and skills

Informal carers who report a good understanding of the condition have been shown to display lower levels of anxiety and better emotional well-being (Bakas et al., 2006). Evidence indicates that partners of heart failure patients desire more information from healthcare providers, particularly in relation to the treatment of symptoms (Imes et al., 2011). Providing basic information can show positive benefits to the informal carer in a short period of time (Harding and Higginson, 2003). Swedish research has shown that spouses of heart failure patients who had information provided by a healthcare professional felt more prepared to help the patient. In particular, advice around medication assisted in their understanding of the condition and its management and, in doing so, this made them feel more effective in their role as carers (Martensson, Dracup and Fridlund, 2001).

A particular challenge that heart failure presents for informal carers is coping with frequent unpredictable symptoms and the subsequent responsibility of managing and administering medication (Dracup et al., 2004). Informal carers are often responsible for altering the dose of diuretic medication according to symptoms and this requires assessment of the patient on a daily basis, alongside the management of supplies to ensure adequate stock if medication is increased. This is supported by research carried out by Barnes et al. (2006a), who carried out interviews with 16 heart failure patients and their informal carers:

> I do all his tablets for him . . . he hasn't a clue what he's taking, really. I try to involve him in putting 'em in boxes . . . Some of these places they get 'em and they're all packed up . . . what they have each day, morning, afternoon and night . . . I enquired about them but we couldn't have 'em . . . Dealing with all them tablets for him . . . to me I thought it were wrong . . . It gave me a headache sorting all these tablets out for him. I says what happens if something happens to him and I've given him these tablets, you know what I mean . . . So I'm like t'nurse and doctor and all combined, you see.
>
> *(Female carer, aged 71)*

Effective communication for informal carers

Alongside access to information required to develop new knowledge and skills, informal carers report a need to have open and honest dialogue to promote understanding of the disease progression (Walden et al., 2001; Aldred, Gott and Gariballa, 2005). Whilst carers acknowledge that heart failure is a serious medical condition, there is limited understanding of it being a chronic, incurable disease (Walden et al., 2001; Clark et al., 2008). The reassurance and rapport provided by heart failure nurse specialist services can facilitate appropriate ongoing support from the point of referral of the patient to the end of life. In doing so, the carer burden can be reduced, therefore impacting positively on both the physical and mental well-being of the carer.

Creating carer authority and confidence can be achieved by them deputizing for their relative and claiming their rights to be actively involved in their healthcare (Gusdal et al., 2016). This includes being the decision-maker as to when to access emergency services, filing complaints about healthcare services and participating in multi professional meetings. Research in Sweden conducted by Gusdal et al. (2016) found that this involvement was also positively received by the healthcare professionals.

Whittingham and Pearce's (2011) evaluation found that informal carers are more confident when they have a point of contact, in particular a heart failure nurse specialist nurse, to discuss patient care:

> She sat and talked. She talked, that sounds daft doesn't it? But it's not because he (the patient) doesn't understand that there's lots of things I can't tell him now. We get talking, to me, not just about him, but about me. I'm not being selfish, I don't mean that in a selfish way, but talk does help and she wanted to know how I felt and I could tell her, which you can't do with a lot of people can you.
>
> *(Female carer, aged 75)*

Additional factors that increase confidence amongst informal carers are support from home care services, adjustments to the home to assist mobility and alarm call systems.

Adapting to the caring role

Informal carers often discuss how they are fearful of the future but, at the same time, are accepting that it would become increasingly necessary for them to take responsibility for activities to support the daily living of the patient (Pihl, Fridlund and Martensson, 2014). In viewing the situation as something that could not be changed, an informal carer interviewed for the Whittingham and Pearce (2011) study reflected on the future:

> I'm thinking that somewhere along the line, I'm going to have to start thinking about giving up work. So then I will have to see what help I can get with that.
>
> *(Male carer, aged 65)*

Adapting in this manner serves to limit the patient's exposure to the carer's own sadness over their loved one's life and compromising physical symptoms (Pihl, Fridlund and Martensson, 2014).

The need to take more responsibility in daily life can be viewed positively, with some informal carers embracing the new challenges they face, taking one day at a time. Carers may prioritize being with their loved one but find new ways of conducting their own activities, or adjust the activities they previously did with their partners in order for them to participate despite physical limitations.

Congruence in patient and informal carer relationship

Research in Sweden found that informal carers developed ways to restore their strength and move forward with their lives (Gusdal et al., 2016). The carers often reported that they were pleased that they had their loved one with them at home and this was associated with increased closeness and solidarity. Particularly important was the need for carers to feel valued and not taken for granted by the patients, and this was associated with enabling carers to remain motivated. Relationships that are reciprocal, in that on occasions the patient becomes the caregiver, help both the informal carer and patient to understand the other's perspective and increase the will to care. To sustain a positive outlook, carers learn to take one day at a time and not to take life for granted; they try not to think too far ahead. This is supported by a patient and his informal carer in the Barnes et al. (2006a) study:

Male patient (aged 56): We do talk, we've always talked. I've never sort of sat in a corner and felt really ill and not said anything. If I've had any sort of pain I've not winged about it, well I don't think so anyway, but I've told [wife] because if anything did go wrong at least she could tell somebody what I'd felt like.

Female carer (aged 65): I think it was last week we had a bit of a down and we talked about it and you felt a lot better didn't you?

An evidence review indicates that, where patients and informal carers have strong emotional relationships and effective communication, patients experience improved health status and carers report feeling less burdened and distressed in relation to the demands of the role (Hooker et al., 2015). Therefore, it is important to acknowledge the importance of nurturing quality relationships, accompanied by effective and structured health and social support, to enable both patients and carers to engage positively with the challenges and complexities of living with heart failure.

Conclusion

It is important that heart failure patients and their informal carers have access to a range of support services, both formal and informal, in order to sustain care in the community and to reduce carer burden. Research outlined in this chapter indicates that patients and informal carers who have positive relationships and access to the support of extended family and friends tend to cope better. Additionally, patients and carers who have a good understanding of their condition display lower levels of anxiety and better emotional well-being. This can be achieved with appropriate, targeted and sensitive communication between older people with heart failure and their healthcare professionals. Support from heart failure nurse specialists has been shown to improve the patient and carer experience, particularly in relation to education and understanding of the condition and its management.

This chapter highlights the importance of positive and meaningful communication between patients, carers and healthcare professionals. Primary healthcare professionals play an important role in caring for patients and their informal carers and this role will continue to expand as care is increasingly delivered to heart failure patients in the community. Ultimately the evidence in this chapter has illustrated the need for primary healthcare professionals to establish relationships with patients and carers that are reliable, dependable and with clearly identified pathways to access resources. By doing so it is hoped that a partnership can be created with recognition of the importance of engagement with patients and their informal carers to promote positive aging with heart failure.

References

Agren, S., Evangelista, L., Hjelm, C., and Stromberg, A. (2012). Dyads affected by chronic heart failure: A randomised study evaluating the effects of education and psychosocial to patients with heart failure and their partners. *Journal of Cardiac Failure*, 18(5), 350–366.

Aldred, H., Gott, M., and Gariballa, S. (2005). Advanced heart failure: Impact on older patients and informal carers. *Journal of Advanced Nursing*, 49(2), 116–124.

Bakas, T., Pressler, S. J., Johnson, E. A., Nauser, J., and Shaneyfelt, T. (2006). Family caregiving in heart failure. *Nursing Research*, 55(3), 180–188.

Barnes, S., Gott, M., Chady, B., Seamark, D., and Halpin, D. (2012). Enhancing patient-professional communication about end-of-life issues in life limiting conditions: A critical review of the literature. *Journal of Pain and Symptom Management*, 44(6), 866–879.

Barnes, S., Gott, M., Payne, S., Parker, C., Seamark, D., Gariballa, S., and Small, N. (2006a). Characteristics and views of family carers of older people with heart failure. *International Journal of Palliative Nursing*, 12(8), 380–389.

Barnes, S., Gott, M., Payne, S., Seamark, D., Parker, C., Gariballa, S., and Small, N. (2006b). Communication in heart failure: Perspectives from older people and primary care professionals. *Health and Social Care in the Community*, 14(6), 482–490.

British Heart Foundation. (2008). *Heart failure nurse services in England: Executive summary*. www.bhf.org.uk/publications/about-bhf/g234-heart-failure-nurse-services-in-england – *full-final-report-2008* (accessed November 8, 2015).

Bui, A. L., Horwich, T. B., and Fonarow, G. C. (2011). Epidemiology and risk profile of heart failure. *Nature Reviews Cardiology*, 8, 30–41.

Candy, B., Jones, L., Drake, R., Leurent, B., and King, M. (2011). Interventions for supporting informal caregivers of patients in the terminal phase of a disease. *Cochrane Database of Systematic Reviews*, 6. Art. ID: CD007617. doi:10.1002/14651858.CD007617.pub2

Christaksi, N. A. (1999). *Death foretold: Prophecy and prognosis in medical care*. Chicago IL: University of Chicago Press.

Clark, A. M., Reid, M. E., Morrison, C. E., Capewell, S., Murdoch, D. L., and McMurray, J. J. (2008). The complex nature of informal care in home-based heart failure management. *Journal of Advanced Nursing*, 61(4), 373–383.

Connolly, M., Beattie, J., Walker, D., and Dancy, M. (2010). *End of life care in heart failure: A framework for implementation.* www.nhsiq.nhs.uk/media/2574509/end-of-life-care-in-heart-failure-framework-for-implementation.pdf (accessed November 9, 2015).

Cortis, J. D., and Williams, A. (2007). Palliative and supportive needs of older adults with heart failure. *International Nursing Review*, 54, 263e70.

Cowie, M. (2010). Commentary. *Evidence-Based Medicine*, 15(1), 9–10.

Criteria Committee of the American Heart Association. (1994). *Nomenclature and criteria for diagnosis of diseases of the heart and great vessels.* Boston, MA: Littlebrown Medical Division.

De Vleminck, A., Pardon, K., Beernaert, K., Deschepper, R., Houttekier, D., Van Audenhove, C., Deliens, L., and Vander Stichele, R. (2014). Barriers to advance care planning in cancer, heart failure and dementia patients: A focus groups study on General Practitioners' views and experiences. *PLOS one*, 9(1), 1–9. http://journals.plos.org/plosone/article?id=10.1371/journal.pone.0084905 (accessed November 10, 2015).

Dracup, K., Evangelista, L., Doering, L., Tullman, D., Moser, D. K., and Hamilton, M. (2004). Emotional well-being in spouses of patients with advanced Heart Failure. *Heart and Lung*, 33(6), 354–361.

Fallowfield, L. (2005). Participation of patients in decisions about treatment for cancer. *British Medical Journal*, 323, 1144.

Fried, T. R., Bradley, E. H., and O'Leary, J. (2003). Prognosis communication in serious illness: Perceptions of older patients, caregivers and clinicians. *Journal of the American Geriatric Society*, 51(10), 1398–1403.

Gerlich, M. G., Klindtworth, K., Oster, P., Pfisterer, M., Hager, K., and Schneider, N. (2012). 'Who is going to explain it to me so that I understand?': Health care needs and experiences of older patients with advanced heart failure. *European Journal of Ageing*, 9, 297–303.

Gott, M., Barnes, S., Payne, S., Parker, C., Seamark, D., Gariballa, S., and Small, N. (2007). Patient views of social service provision for older people with advanced Heart Failure. *Health and Social Care in the Community*, 15(4), 333–342.

Gott, M., Small, N., Barnes, S., Payne, S., and Seamark, D. (2008). Older people's views of a good death in heart failure: Implications for palliative care provision. *Social Science and Medicine*, 67, 1113–1121.

Gusdal, A. K., Josefsson, K., Adolfsson, E. T., and Martin, L. (2016). Informal caregivers' experiences and needs when caring for a relative with heart failure: An interview study. *Journal of Cardiovascular Nursing*, 31(4), 1–8.

Hanratty, B., Hibbert, D., Mair, F., May, C., Ward, C., Capewell, S., Litva, A., and Corcoran, G. (2002). Doctors' perceptions of palliative care for heart failure: Focus group study. *British Medical Journal*, 325, 581–585.

Harding, R., and Higginson, I. J. (2003). What is the best way to help caregivers in cancer and palliative care? A systematic literature review of interventions and their effectiveness. *Palliative Medicine*, 17, 63–74.

Hooker, S. A., Grigsby, B. A., Riegl, B., and Bekelman, D. B. (2015). The impact of relationship quality on health related outcomes in heart failure patients and informal family caregivers. *Journal of Cardiovascular Nursing*, 30(45), 52–63.

Horne, G., and Payne, S. (2004). Removing the boundaries: Palliative care for patients with heart failure. *Palliative Medicine*, 18, 291–296.

Hwang, B., Fleischmann, K. E., Howie-Esquivel, J., Stotts, N. A., and Dracup, K. (2011). Caregiving for patients with heart failure: Impact on patients' families. *American Journal of Critical Care*, 20(6), 431–441.

Imes, C. C., Dougherty, C. M., Pyper, G., and Sullivan, M. D. (2011). Descriptive study of partners' experiences of living with severe heart failure. *Heart and Lung: The Journal of Acute and Critical Care*, 20(3), 208–216.

Jenkins, V., Fallowfield, L., and Saul, J. (2001). Information needs of patients with cancer: Results from a large study in UK cancer centres. *British Journal of Cancer*, 84, 48–51.

Kang, X., Li, Z., and Nolan, M. T. (2011). Informal caregivers' experiences of caring for patients with chronic heart failure: Systematic review and metasynthesis of qualitative studies. *Journal of Cardiovascular Nursing*, 25(5), 386–394.

Lehman, R., Doust, J., and Glasziou, P. (2005). Cardiac impairment or heart failure? *British Medical Journal*, 331, 415–416.

Lyons, K. S., Vellone, E., Lee, C. S., Cocchiere, A., Bidwell, J. T., D'Agostino, F., Hiatt, S. O., Alvaro, R., Juarez-Vela, R., and Eiegel, B. (2015). A dyadic approach to managing heart failure with confidence. *Journal of Cardiovascular Nursing*, 30(Suppl. 1), S64–S1.

Martensson, J., Dracup, K., and Fridlund, B. (2001). Decisive situations influencing spouses' support of patients with heart failure: A critical incident technique analysis. *Heart and Lung*, 30(5), 341–350.

Molloy, G. J., Johnston, D. W., Johnston, M., Gao, C., Witham, M. D., Struthers, A. D., and McMurdo, M. E. (2008). Using the demand-control model of job strain to predict caregiver burden and caregiver satisfaction in the informal caregivers of Heart Failure patients. *British Journal of Health Psychology*, 13, 401–417.

Murray, S. A., and Sheikh, A. (2008). Palliative Care beyond cancer: Care for all at the end of life. *British Medical Journal*, 336, 958.

National Institute for Health and Care Excellence (NICE). (2010). *Chronic heart failure in adults: Management*. www.nice.org.uk/guidance/cg108 (accessed November 8, 2015).

O'Leary, N., Murphy, N. F., O'Loughlin, C., Tiernan, E., and Mcdonald, K. (2009). A comparative study of the palliative care needs of heart failure and cancer patients. *European Journal of Heart Failure*, 11(4), 406–412.

Ostman, M., Jakobsson, E., and Falk, K. (2015). Health-care encounters create both discontinuity and continuity in daily life when living with chronic heart failure: A grounded theory study. *International Journal of Qualitative Studies on Health and Well-Being*, 10, 1–12.

Pihl, E., Fridlund, B., and Martensson, J. (2014). Spouses' experiences of impact on daily life regarding physical limitations in the loved one with heart failure: A phenomenographic analysis. *Canadian Journal of Cardiovascular Nursing*, 20(3), 9–17.

Pressler, S. J., Gradus-Pizlo, I., Chubinski, S. D., Smith, G., Wheeler, S., Wu, J., and Sloan, R. (2009). Family caregiver outcomes in Heart Failure. *American Journal of Critical Care*, 18(2), 150–159.

Princes Royal Trust for Carers. (2011). *Always on call, always concerned: A survey of the experiences of older carers*. www.carers.org (accessed November 8, 2015).

Saunders, M. M. (2008). Factors associated with caregiver burden in Heart Failure family caregivers. *Western Journal of Nursing Research*, 30(8), 943–959.

Stolz, P., Willman, A., and Uden, G. (2006). The meaning of support as narrated by family carers who care for a senior relative at home. *Qualitative Health Research*, 16, 594–610.

Taylor, M. and Ogden, J. (2005) Doctors' use of euphemisms and their impact on patient's beliefs about health: an experimental study of heart failure. *Patient Educ Couns*, 57(3), 321–326.

Usher, B. M., and Cammarata, K. (2009). Heart Failure and family caregiver burden: An update. *Progress in Cardiovascular Nursing*, 24(3),113–114.

Walden, J. A., Dracup, K., Westlake, C., Erickson, V., Hamilton, M. A., and Fonarow, G. C. (2001). Educational needs of patients with advanced heart failure and their caregivers. *The Journal of Heart and Lung Transplantation*, 20(7), 766–769.

Whittingham, K., and Pearce., D. E. (2011). Carer support from a community-based heart specialist nurse service. *British Journal of Nursing*, 20(20), 1302–1307.

Woltz, P. C., Chapa, D. W., Friedmann, E., Akintade, B., and Thomas, S. (2012). Effects of interventions on depression in heart failure: A systematic review. *Heart and Lung*, 41(5), 469–483.

Zapka, J. G., Carter, R., Carter, C. L., Hennessy, W., Kurent, J. E., and Desharnais, S. (2006). Care at the end of life: Focus on communication and race. *Journal of Aging Health*, 18, 791–813.

7

EXPLORING EXPERIENCES OF AGING WITH TYPE 2 DIABETES (T2D)

The case for a whole-system approach

Paul Newton, Koula Asimakopoulou, Mustafa Al-Haboubi and Sasha Scambler

This chapter discusses:

- Type 2 Diabetes (T2D) in context
- Managing T2D as a long-term condition
- Type 2 Diabetes and empowerment
- Day-to-day management of T2D
- Social, familial, interpersonal and healthcare professional roles in T2D self-management
- The role of health system factors in T2D self-management
- T2D-related factors and their influence on self-management
- Socio-contextual factors and their influence on self-management

Introduction

Diabetes is a long-term condition that affects multiple areas of daily life, and as such must be managed on a day-to-day basis by the diagnosed individual, often with the help of their family and/or carers. The prevalence of Type 2 Diabetes (T2D) is growing amongst the older population with risk factors for T2D increasing with age; hence, overall rates rise as the population ages (Diabetes UK, 2010). T2D is a growing issue for older people and supporting the self-management needs of older people living with T2D is one way of helping people to experience their later years positively. Day-to-day management of T2D includes self-care tasks such as monitoring blood sugars, regular exercise, following prescribed dietary measures and medication-taking (taking tablets as well as other exogenous insulin therapies). When this set of behaviours occurs the patient is said to be self-managing their condition. However, as this chapter explains, attaining T2D self-management is not as simple as it may appear as a multitude of factors shape older people's ability to self-manage T2D. The chapter begins by looking at recent research on older people's day-to-day perspectives, understanding the experiences of self-managing T2D. The chapter then moves on to explore how social, familial, interpersonal and healthcare professional relationships impact on how older people self-manage T2D. However, we also demonstrate that the healthcare system plays a role in the factors that shape T2D self-management, as do T2D-related factors such as progression of the illness and the presence of co-morbidities. We then briefly look at wider socio-contextual factors – such as income and ethnicity – and their influence on self-management. We conclude by arguing that to truly empower older people to self-manage and age positively with T2D, it is important to address all the factors that shape self-management.

Type 2 Diabetes (T2D) in context

Diabetes Mellitus is a definition given to a group of heterogeneous metabolic disorders characterized by elevated blood glucose concentration (Foundation of European Nurses in Diabetes (FEND) et al., 2011). Diabetes Mellitus is classified in a number of ways, the most prevalent categories being Type 1 Diabetes (T1D) and Type 2 Diabetes (T2D). Generally T1D occurs when there is no production of insulin in the beta-cells of the pancreas, which results in elevated blood glucose levels and the need to frequently administer exogenous insulin (O'Rahilly, 2006). In the majority of cases the onset of T1D occurs in childhood. T2D, on the other hand, is generally associated with onset in later life (aged 50+) – and is a loss of response to the action of insulin, known as 'insulin resistance' as well as beta cell destruction (FEND et al., 2011). In 2010, Diabetes UK estimated that there were 2.6 million people diagnosed with diabetes in the United Kingdom, 90 per cent (n=2,213,136) of whom had T2D.

In all types of Diabetes Mellitus, it is the body's inability to produce or respond to insulin which increases blood glucose concentration; this causes the blood to thicken, which adversely affects the systemic functioning of the body – particularly the circulatory system (FEND et al., 2011). This leads to the symptoms and further pathologies of Type 2 Diabetes. The morbidities of diabetes are predominantly micro- and macro-vascular in nature and can result in severe complications such as cardiovascular disease, blindness and amputation (O'Rahilly, 2006). T2D is, hence, associated with higher morbidity rates across the lifespan (Diabetes UK, 2010). Diabetes was the eighth most common cause of death globally between 2000 and 2012 (World Health Organization (WHO), 2014), and in England, for example, more than one in 10 (11.6 per cent) deaths amongst 20- to 79-year-olds can be attributed to diabetes (Diabetes UK, 2010).

Internationally there is growing concern surrounding the high prevalence of T2D, in particular high mortality rates and shortened life expectancy (O'Rahilly, 2006; Diabetes UK, 2010). In the United Kingdom (UK) life expectancy is shortened on average by 10 years by living with T2D (Diabetes UK, 2010). As a long-term condition, T2D represents a case where early diagnosis is crucial to good health outcomes and where the subsequent ability to respond to the illness through 'lifestyle changes' and medication-taking – as well as access to healthcare information and the support of health service provision – has an ameliorative effect on health outcomes in terms of quality of life, morbidity and mortality (British Medical Association (BMA), 2004; Diabetes UK, 2010; FEND et al., 2011). The adverse impact of T2D also extends to the effects that complications can have on people's lives – around half of all people living with T2D are living with complications of the condition, many of whom often developed these complications before diagnosis (Diabetes UK, 2010). The burden of the disease that T2D represents for health systems is also a concern – for example, the costs to the UK National Health Service (NHS) was estimated to be around £1 million an hour (Diabetes UK, 2010).

One factor contributing to high prevalence of T2D is the aging population. One in 20 people over 65 years of age have T2D, rising to one in five for those 85 years or above. Therefore, internationally, initiatives have focused on screening the older population at the primary care level (FEND et al., 2011). Focusing on the prevalence and treatment informs service provision and the deployment of health resources; hence it is important to note that social factors have been shown to play a role in T2D-related prevalence. For example, in the United Kingdom, ethnicity has been identified as a factor in the prevalence of T2D, particularly in those of an African Caribbean or Asian origin – a three- to six-fold increased prevalence respectively when compared to the white population (Department of Health, 2001). T2D has a more common prevalence in socio-economic groups with lower incomes – the British Medical Association link these two demographic factors to low birth weights and obesity brought about by poor diet (BMA, 2004). Interventions tend to target individuals who are seen to have 'deficits' in healthy behaviours. However, the social patterning of wider illness by socio-economic status is well established in the UK literature; the main factor implicated being unequal access to health-protective resources due to mal-distribution of wealth (Scambler, 2009). In the north-east of England, for example, T2D prevalence is 28 per cent higher for men and 45 per cent higher for women in the most deprived areas, compared to the regional average. Also in terms of health outcomes, people living with T2D have a higher risk of both morbidity and mortality, which is further exacerbated and confounded by ethnicity, social class and increased age (Connolly, 2006; NHS National Diabetes Service, 2013). It is important to note that the vast majority of managing T2D is conducted on a day-to-day basis by people living with diabetes (self-management of T2D). However, more recent data suggest that variations in morbidity and mortality are not associated with lifestyle alone, but rather access to health-promoting resources and disparities in healthcare provision (NHS National Diabetes Service, 2013). This suggests that factors shaping the prevalence of, and outcomes for, T2D are multifactorial and need to be addressed through a whole-system approach if people are to have positive experiences of aging whilst living with T2D.

Managing T2D as a long-term condition

As we have seen the determinants of T2D are multifactorial, yet systematic reviews of the literature show that blood glucose level is the most commonly researched dimension of diabetes management (Van Dam et al., 2003; Nam et al., 2011). In fact this aspect of diabetes research is the primary focus of some of the largest national studies of diabetes such as the Diabetes Control and Complications Trial Research Group and the United Kingdom Prospective Diabetes Study. The main thrust of these studies being that maintaining control of the metabolism – through strict adherence to dietary, insulin and non-insulin therapy, and regular exercise – can ameliorate symptoms of diabetes, as well as delay and decelerate complications. Therefore, within the research literature there is also growing concern with the frequently poor 'adherence' or 'compliance' to clinically recommended diabetes-related regimens, in spite of public health interventions as well as concern about the impact of T2D on the quality of life of the older people affected (Lawton et al., 2003).

Psychological research points to affective, cognitive and behavioural aspects that influence the capacity to self-care. Research in this vein investigates how factors such as personality and behavioural dispositions (Knight, Dornan and Bundy, 2006), belief in the ability to perform a task (or self-efficacy) (Funnell and Anderson, 2004; Anderson et al., 2009) and perception of risk (Asimakopoulou et al., 2008) – to name but a few – all influence patients' capacity to self-manage. As such, 'control' and 'management' of T2D are measured as maintaining a blood glucose level as close to that of the population without diabetes as possible. In contrast, Diabetes UK (2010) note that although such studies show utility in justifying or evaluating clinical courses of action, they do not take into consideration the *personal and social barriers* people experience in attaining and maintaining adherence to the T2D therapeutic regime. A growing body of research is also developing which seeks to enhance studies of prevalence and adherence by looking at psycho-social aspects of T2D (i.e. how people live with T2D on a day-to-day basis). A key drive in these studies is to explore factors that inhibit or enhance the capacity of older people living with T2D to self-manage, and age positively, with a long-term condition, and to investigate factors that constrain and enable access to supportive social environments that improve health (Gomersall, Madill and Summers, 2011).

T2D and empowerment

Over the past 15 years, the adherence approach to patient care has been supplanted by empowerment models which seek to create an equipoise situation whereby professionals' clinical and bio-medical expertise, and patients' 'lay' expertise, complement one another in the management of T2D (Asimakopoulou et al., 2012). Empowerment, as a concept, is based on the assumption that individuals, if given the freedom to choose and the opportunity to reflect, will be able and willing to select appropriate diabetes goals – which can then be facilitated by the healthcare professionals' knowledge of the clinical realm.

This emphasis on patient-led, self-directive approaches which promote shared decisions with healthcare professionals – a direct challenge to the adherence model – can be linked to wider trends in international healthcare which seek to involve people living with T2D in healthcare decision-making (Coulter, 2002). Its adoption in T2D management is also linked to the oft-cited assertion that although professionals are the clinical experts in T2D management, patients are experts in living with diabetes by virtue of managing T2D on a day-to-day basis (Nam et al., 2011; Corser et al., 2010). Hence, within the approach the experiences of older people living with T2D are a key focus of attaining positive self-management of the condition.

Older people's day-to-day perspectives, understanding and experiences of managing T2D

The bulk of the work looking at the 'day-to-day' strategies people adopt to manage T2D are explored from the perspective of the patient (Nam et al., 2011). Kelleher's (1988) seminal work on managing diabetes suggested that maintaining a 'normal' life was a key concern for people managing diabetes. A central construct of the study was exploring the ways people managed their illness to minimize disruption to their lives – that is, ways the condition "impinged" on their day-to-day lives (Kelleher, 1988). The study found three main styles in which people managed diabetes: copers who 'strategically managed' their illness by pre-emptively adjusting diabetes-related activities – such as timings of food to reduce 'impingement'. Normalisers organized their daily routines and activities around their symptoms and care responsibilities, and hence were seen as complying to advice rather than 'taking charge' of the condition. The final sub-group were worriers/agonisers who tended to report being unwell and having poor control over their condition, leading to heightened anxiety.

Maclean's (1991) seminal work explored the factors that people living with diabetes had for 'adhering' or 'not adhering' to self-management dietary advice. The research also found that, with experience, people living with diabetes were able to use their knowledge and awareness of changes in their body to inform management of diabetes, as opposed to more didactic information. Maclean also charted further factors found to influence patients' responses to dietary requirements and their self-care. These being:

- Individual factors: food history, coping skills, character traits, and gender
- Diabetes factors: severity, duration, experience and threat of complications

- Contextual factors: family support, peer support, professional support, social norms, access and availability of self-monitoring equipment, and occupation.

Maclean (1991) developed a continuum of dietary-management styles ranging from: those who followed a strict diet plan; to those who introduced a moderate to high degree of flexibility; to those who never, or rarely, adhered to dietary advice. It was noted that participants' views consistently reflected an inherent tension with regard to following dietary measures. This tension related to conflicts between the benefits for biological health (usually expressed as a bio-medical measure or increasing longer life expectancy) and feelings of well-being (a subjective sense of normalization, self-esteem and belonging through social integration). The underlying principle Maclean formulated was that where the pursuit of biological health did not compromise well-being, adherence was seen by respondents as less problematic. However, when the pursuit of health conflicted with well-being, individuals became more flexible with their care in order to minimize the perceived restrictions on well-being. This suggests that the people develop underlying perceptual schema relating to how to manage their condition, based on balancing how recommended self-management practices conflict with participating in everyday life; that is, that positive experiences of self-management involve people adapting clinically recommended behaviours when they feel it necessary.

This idea of overcoming the 'restrictions' that T2D self-management places on day-to-day living is a key premise of numerous studies (e.g. Collins et al., 2009 and Ockleford et al., 2008). In fact, the process of balancing clinical concerns against well-being concerns has been a consistent finding in T2D-related patient experience research (Campbell et al., 2003). Brewer-Lowry et al. (2010) sought to explore the perceptual differences between those who did and did not meet clinically recommended behaviours. The study found that those who met clinical targets gauge their self-management tasks in concrete terms and specific terms, as opposed to less structured descriptions given by those who did not meet clinical targets. This concept of an ability to purposively and strategically respond to T2D as a mediator of T2D self-management is a theme in the literature on day-to-day management.

More recent work has continued to develop typologies based on the degree of purposive action undertaken by the individual with T2D. Collins et al. (2009) explored perceptions of self-care coping strategies in people living with T2D according to self-care health value (the value the patient placed on their diabetes self-care in relation to their health); self-care responsibility (how self-care tasks were divided between self and others); and how the individual planned for, monitored and responded to the necessities of self-care. Three self-management types were identified:

- 'Proactive managers' who were self-directed, valued improving long-term health through self-care and could independently maintain metabolic control through planning.
- 'Passive followers' followed their prescribed self-care regime and valued it, but did not react pre-emptively or autonomously to make changes to metabolic control; and
- "Nonconformist" patients who do not follow recommended self-care practices (ibid.).

Although looking at what people do 'well' to achieve self-management targets is a useful exercise, it is questionable whether people's perceived success in self-managing T2D should be underpinned by the ability to hit externally defined clinical targets which are experienced as a barrier to participating in day-to-day life. As such, it would appear that older people experience barriers that require them to make sacrifices in aspects of their well-being they perceive as positive in order to successfully 'adhere' to clinically recommended behaviours.

Day-to-day management of T2D

Thus far, we can see studies have focused on codifying and categorizing behaviours based on how people normalize the management of the day-to-day restrictions of T2D, and how purposively or strategically people living with T2D manage these restrictions. Equally, studies have looked at patients' perspectives of T2D self-management to explore barriers and enablers experienced in the day-to-day aspects of the T2D self-management regimen – with some commentators such as Maclean (1991) fusing both elements together. Exploration of barriers and enablers to T2D management are usually conjoined with suggestions of how to support patients to self-manage. Hayes et al. (2006) explored the task of T2D medicine management from the perspective of older people living with T2D, and found three main issues:

- The inconvenience that administration of T2D treatments had on patients' lives,
- Patients' desire to avoid injections and insulin therapy, and
- The physical and emotional side effects of T2D medications.

Conversely, Morris, Povey and Street (2005) in a longitudinal study found that people who made the transition to insulin injections were initially shocked and reticent, but later grew to accept insulin injections – many finding it empowering to be able to control their treatment. The study concludes that healthcare professionals, by not addressing patients' initial fears about insulin, create barriers of resistance to adopting insulin. This suggests that, with support, older people living with T2D can overcome their fears and integrate T2D management into their day-to-day lives in a positive way.

The adoption of exercise and dietary control has also been found to be restrictive for people living with T2D (Fagerli et al., 2007; Casey, De Civita and Dasgupta, 2010; Wycherley et al., 2012) and on the diets of the household (Wellard, Rennie and King, 2008). Casey, De Civita and Dasgupta (2010) found that older people living with T2D preferred structured support with exercising, in this case an educational programme, but tended to drift away from regular exercise when required to maintain the exercise regime under their own volition. They found that those living with co-morbidities were most likely to be 'derailed' from maintaining regular exercise following structured education. Wycherley et al. (2012) found that maintenance of dietary recommendations and regular exercise was not wholly an issue of motivation (as per Minet et al., 2011), but rather educational programmes offered free access to exercise and support on dietary change. Hence, older people living with T2D who engage with structured education and exercise, experience financial and access barriers to the continuation of exercise and dietary practices when structured programmes end. However, Malpass, Andrews and Turner (2009) found that exercise was found to frequently act as a 'gateway-behaviour' to wider self-management behaviour. It would thus seem that older people do experience both barriers and enablers to day-to-day management but may be able to overcome them with consistent and accessible support.

Social, familial, interpersonal and healthcare professional roles in T2D self-management

A tranche of studies expand the notion of 'people living with diabetes' beyond purposive, self-directed action to demonstrate how management of T2D is influenced by social networks and health service-related factors (Gomersall, Madill and Summers, 2011). Rajaram (1997) explored how families struggle to normalize diabetes within their lives and maintain social acceptability – a process of adaption. Similarly, the work of Hunt, Valenzuela and Pugh (1998) explored the relationship between personal understandings and self-care activity for people with diabetes and found that people were either self-active, other-active (others took care of treatment) or non-active. The study concluded that those who saw their illness as hereditary, or as the result of 'events', were least likely to be self-active. Other studies have shown that spousal support is a key element of successful T2D management (Trief et al., 2003; Beverly, Penrod and Wray, 2007). Trief et al. (2003) found that spousal support was a greater predictor of engagement with dietary control and exercise. However, Beverly, Penrod and Wray (2007, 2008) found both congruence and differences in the perspectives of older people living as couples who managed the condition. Equally, it is easy to see that family and spousal support is an enabler of successful self-management – but it is important to note that older people often live alone, are bereaved and live away from immediate family.

Parry et al. (2005) explored 'cause and control' beliefs related to T2D and found that these shape the way that people living with T2D divide tasks and responsibilities between themselves and others. They suggest that people living with T2D are required to grasp that both the cause and treatment outcomes of T2D are partly, but not wholly, within their control; and that the resulting understanding sometimes leads to inappropriate delegation of care and treatment responsibilities by the person living with T2D. Oftedal, Karlsen and Bru (2010) looked at patients' experiences of support by healthcare professionals and concluded that motivating healthcare professionals can enable patients to self-manage. People living with T2D reported that support should be underpinned by: i) an empathetic approach; ii) practical advice and information; iii) involvement in decision-making; iv) accurate and individualized information; and v) ongoing group-based support. Lawton et al. (2008) have found that personal understanding of T2D is informed by health service delivery. The study (ibid.) showed that patients' health beliefs were intertwined with the healthcare services they receive; for example, patients may feel that their illness is not as serious as it is managed by their general practitioner (GP) rather than a diabetologist. The study also found where T2D was asymptomatic, medical tests (and self-monitoring devices) often actualized the illness for patients through showing physical effects and potential consequences. Indeed, there are numerous studies showing improvements in patient self-management relating to which healthcare professional leads their care. Studies have shown that regular and sustained access to multi-disciplinary teams (Cuddihy, Philis-Tsimikas and Nazeri, 2011), practice nurses (Bartol, 2012; Edwall et al., 2008; Kruger, 2008), diabetes specialist nurses (Edwall, Danielson and Öhrn, 2010; Moser et al., 2008), community health workers (Otero-Sabogal et al., 2010) and telehealth interventions (Wu, Forbes and While, 2010; Jennings et al., 2009) are all associated with positive changes in self-management activity and outcomes. Other studies have also explored how experiences of T2D management can be influenced by use of complementary medicine (Chang, Wallis and Tiralongo, 2012, 2011; Wang, Chuang and Bateman, 2011) and improved through self-help and peer-support mechanisms (Lindenmeyer et al., 2010; Baksi, 2010; Rygg et al., 2010; Simmons et al., 2010).

Day-to-day management of T2D is also shaped by experiences of clinical approaches, health services and organisational/systemic issues informing: i) perceptions of T2D and its management; ii) how responsibilities for care and treatment are divided up; and iii) that these social relations inform self-management styles (Nam et al., 2011). This suggests that the management of T2D at the patient/provider interface involves delegating, or assigning, roles and responsibilities which create different styles, methods and strategies of self-management (Nam et al., 2011). Gomersall, Madill and Summers (2011, p. 14) note that in the T2D literature, self-management as a construct is frequently viewed as a means "to regulate the self", as "[t]here is also a moral dimension in that, after education and empowerment, should diabetes continue to be poorly managed, it is the individual patient who is construed as having failed". The assumption of self-management as relating solely to an individual's capacity for purposive action or as a matter of educating patients to overcome the personal barriers they experience can be seen as reductionist. As has been shown, how empowered the person is to self-manage is also shaped by factors outside the individual, including how facets of healthcare systems inform people's perspectives, understanding and experiences of managing T2D in a day-to-day context (Newton and Asimakopoulou, 2008; Gomersall, Madill and Summers, 2011).

Studies in the doctor–patient relationship, particularly those focused on patient-centring, argue that better health and well-being can – or ought to – be attained in professional–patient encounters where information – both personal and technical – as well as treatment and option-deliberation are shared between participants (Morgan, 2003; Coulter, 2002). Hiscock, Legard and Snape (2001, p. 25) note five main expectations patients had of their encounters:

- Friendly, warm and 'equal' approach to the patient
- Willingness to understand the impact of diabetes
- 'Partnership approach' to treating the condition
- Willingness to make time to answer questions
- Proactive approach to making referrals to other healthcare professionals.

Studies have also highlighted the role of communication between healthcare providers and those living with diabetes. Communication barriers have been found to be exacerbated by cultural and ethnic difference (Kokanovic and Manderson, 2007; Jones et al., 2008; Chlebowy, Hood and LaJoie, 2010; Peek et al., 2010) and by gender (Matthews, Peden and Rowles, 2009; Morris, Povey and Street, 2005). In terms of empowerment a more central concern has developed around the doctor–patient relationship – that of the assumption of an equipoise relationship: that is, the notion that all options available are made available to both parties in the 'empowering' medical encounter (Newton and Asimakopoulou, 2008). Paterson (1999) interviewed patients considered to be expert in managing diabetes. The authors defined 'expert' as: "having the ability to make trustworthy decisions about self-management and maintain good overall glycaemic control" (Paterson et al., 1999, p. 576). A key finding was that people living with diabetes reported that equipoise relationships could be undermined in two key ways: i) experiential knowledge was felt to be routinely discounted by professionals; ii) professionals often failed to provide the resources necessary for people to make informed decisions. This situation could also be further exacerbated by ageism.

The role of health system factors in T2D self-management

Alazria et al. (2007) looked at the role that wider health system factors (such as service organisation and delivery) have on patient management of T2D. The study used focus groups to explore how people living with T2D valued continuity of care in their relationships with healthcare professionals. Patients reported valuing three types of continuity:

- Relational continuity – care from the same health professional
- Cross-boundary (team) continuity – effective transition and good communication between services
- Informational continuity – where information about the patient followed the patient during cross-boundary transfers.

Patients rarely reported experiencing these types of continuity. Alazria et al.'s (2007) study suggests a greater role for systemic factors, such as service organisation, in shaping patients' experiences and expectations of services, and informing their capacity to self-management. Wellard, Rennie and King (2008) showed that systemic factors such as long waiting times and lack of appointments influenced patients' self-management decisions.

T2D-related factors and their influence on self-management

One largely overlooked area of research into patient experiences of T2D is how illness itself creates physical changes in the body which impact on experiences of people living with T2D. One important aspect of Murphy and Kinmouth's (1995) seminal study is the notion of 'embodiment' where it is argued that a key catalyst to self-care behaviour is the ability of respondents to observe and respond to their own bodies. The authors noted that people living with T2D judge the utility of medical advice by interpreting the efficacy of the advice through impact on the physical manifestations of T2D. This suggests physical changes in the body can impact on perceptions and experiences by people living with T2D. People living with T2D also manage multiple conditions and illnesses (Nam et al., 2011). Numerous studies of patient experiences (Bayliss et al., 2003; Jerant et al., 2005; Visram et al., 2008) have found that co-morbidities are a major barrier to self-care activities in T2D. People living with T2D can be managing multiple conditions which pre-existed their diabetes diagnosis. They can also be managing conditions resulting from living with T2D, which can be micro-vascular (e.g. diabetic neuropathy or retinopathy) or macro-vascular (e.g. cardiovascular disease, cerebro-vascular disease and coronary artery disease). Equally, co-morbidities can be any non-diabetes-related acute illnesses or morbidities diagnosed following T2D diagnosis. Depression, for example, is also linked to all of these aforementioned categories, and has been shown to alter perception of T2D self-management and is associated with increased morbidity, mortality and functional limitation – these physical outcomes (co-morbidities) are seen to have a bi-directional relationship with depression (Nam et al., 2011; Chao et al., 2005; Jennings et al., 2009).

However, managing co-morbidity is, for example, seen to impact positively on symptom interpretation. Beverly et al. (2011b) found that older women living with T2D who developed myocardial infarction spotted the symptoms earlier as not their 'typical' T2D symptoms. Similarly, Kreyenbuhl et al. (2011) found that people managing mental illness were better able to control blood glucose than those without mental illness; this skill was an advantage conferred from managing multiple conditions. However, Kerr et al. (2007) found that patients with greater numbers of co-morbidities, such as older people, placed lower priority on managing T2D and had low diabetes self-management ability. Kerr et al. (2007) also found that only macro-vascular and non-diabetes-related co-morbidities were associated with de-prioritizing self-management of T2D. In contrast, living with higher numbers of micro-vascular, macro-vascular and non-diabetes-related conditions were associated with poor self-management. Severity of macro-vascular conditions was negatively correlated with prioritizing T2D self-management; that is, the more severe the condition, the less the person self-managed. This suggests that managing T2D itself may not be the priority in patients' perceptions where a range of co-morbidities exist – such as in older people. Although the realm of physical manifestations may impact in numerous ways on the perceptions of people living with T2D, it must be taken in the context of other illnesses. Although physical manifestations are an important influence on perception, they are also interpreted through people's subjective experiences, as well as systemic and socio-contextual conditions (Song and Lipman, 2008).

Socio-contextual factors and their influence on self-management

Far removed from exploring perceptions and understanding of the physical manifestations of T2D, studies have sought to identify socio-contextual factors that shape self-care practices and 'adherence' to T2D therapies (Brown et al., 2004). Maclean's study (discussed above), for example, found people's responses were influenced by individual factors such as character traits and gender, diabetes factors such as duration and severity of the condition, and contextual factors such as degree of family support available. Newton, Scambler and Asimakopoulou (2015) looked at self-management styles by degree of purposive action by the individual invested, the type of support they drew on, stage of the condition and co-morbidities, as well as relationships with healthcare professionals. Newton, Scambler and Asimakopoulou (2015) found six self-management styles relating to the experiences of older people living with T2D. Older people self-managed T2D: i) through routinisation; ii) as a burden; iii) as maintenance; iv) through delegation; v) through co-management; and vi) through autonomy. The self-management styles identified also shaped the criteria people used to judge the success of their self-management practices. The findings showed that styles of T2D self-management were mediated and moderated by socio-contextual issues and that there was some association between income group and style of self-management. This suggests that socio-contextual resources (e.g. familial and health service support and income) may precede, enable and hinder how people self-manage, and hold greater influence over people's ability to self-manage than their day-to-day, individual purposive efforts to overcome the immediate barriers and restrictions they experience.

Other studies have looked at ethnic and cultural differences (e.g. Kokanovic and Manderson, 2007 and Peek et al., 2010) highlighting how culture influences a person's perception of their illness. These range from exploring how ethnic and cultural difference shape the patient–professional relationship (Peek et al., 2010; Jowsey, Gillespie and Aspin, 2011), compliance with recommended clinical behaviours and the unique lay understandings of T2D in different cultures (Lippa and Klein, 2008; Skelly et al., 2008). Elstad et al. (2008) used focus groups to explore experiences of living with T2D in American Samoan communities. The study found that four factors perceived to cause T2D-related stress could be divided into:

- Individual stressors – physical symptoms
- Familial stressors – lack of support at home
- Environmental stressors – changes in food sources and dietary practices as access to food has changed from a subsistence way of life to one of living and working in a cash economy
- Cultural stressors – cultural stress was associated with adapting to a rapid cultural and economic change in their community.

Studies exploring experiences of T2D self-management and wider structural and social-contextual factors frequently see culture as a confounding variable in health outcomes which are to a greater extent influenced by socio-economic factors. This is because cultural and ethnic minorities tend to be over-represented in poorer socio-economic groups, which is a causal factor in poorer health (Brown et al., 2004; Fagerli, Lien and Wandel, 2007).

Conclusion

In conclusion, we can see that the growth in the prevalence of T2D, which is a growing and particular issue for the older population, has led to concerns about how individuals adhere and comply with clinically recommended behaviours. One key response has been the empowerment approach, which seeks to empower patients to self-manage their condition. The empowerment approach fits well with a body of work focusing on the strategies people adopt to purposively manage their condition. However, it has also been shown that people living with T2D have common barriers and enablers they experience in their efforts to self-manage. These barriers and enablers relate to levels and types of social support, the quality of healthcare support as well as access to, and quality of, health services and continuity of care. However, it is evident that experiences of self-management are further shaped by the stage of the condition and the presence of any co-morbidities. As with all illness and disease, outcomes as well as experiences are shaped by socio-contextual factors which precede and inform people's ability to self-manage the condition, and by the resources they can devote to self-management. Given the evidence discussed above, it is clear that a 'whole-system approach' is required that supports older people by enhancing their socio-contextual resources, which builds on their existing social support and takes into consideration the effects of T2D and its co-morbidities on their ability to self-manage. This, in itself, is perhaps a more universal way to ensure that living with T2D in older age becomes a positive aging experience. Better understanding of older people's experiences of self-management at all levels – not just focusing on the individual's ability to meet clinically recommended behaviours – will enable more effective support of older people in managing their condition, avoid or reduce the likelihood of complications and maximize their chances of aging positively.

References

Alazria, M. H., Heywood, P., Neal, R. D., and Leese, B. (2007). UK GPs' and practice nurses' views of continuity of care for patients with type 2 diabetes. *Family Practice*, 24(2), 128–137.

Anderson, R. M., Donnelly, M. B., and Dedrick, R. F. (1990). Measuring the attitudes of patients towards diabetes and its treatment. *Patient Education Counseling*, 16, 231–245.

Anderson, R. M., Funnell, M. M., Aikens, J. E., Krein, S. L., Fitzgerald, J. T., Nwankwo, R., and Tang, T. S. (2009). Evaluating the efficacy of an empowerment-based self-management consultant intervention: Results of a two-year randomized controlled trial. *Education Therapeutique Du Patient*, 1(1), 3–11.

Asimakopoulou, K. G., Fox, C., Marsh, S., Spimpolo, J., and Skinner, T. C. (2008). The effects of different time frames of risk communication on type 2 diabetes patients' understanding and memory for risk of Coronary Heart Disease and stroke. *Diabetic Medicine*, 25, 811–817.

Asimakopoulou, K. G., Newton, P., Sinclair, A. J., and Scambler, S. (2012). Health care professionals' understanding and day-to-day practice of patient empowerment in diabetes; time to pause for thought? *Diabetes Research and Clinical Practice*, 95(2), 224–229.

Baksi, A. K. (2010). Experiences in peer-to-peer training in diabetes mellitus: Challenges and implications. *Family Practice*, 27(Suppl. 1), i40–i45.

Bartol, T. (2012). Improving the treatment experience for patients with type 2 diabetes: Role of the nurse practitioner. *Journal of the American Academy of Nurse Practitioners*, 24(Suppl. 1), 270–276.

Bayliss, E. A., Steiner, J. F., Fernald, D. H., Crane, L. A., and Main, D. S. (2003). Descriptions of barriers to self-care by persons with comorbid chronic diseases. *Annals of Family Medicine*, 1, 15–21.

Beverly, E. A., Miller, C. K., and Wray, L. A. (2008). Spousal support and food-related behaviour change in middle-aged and older adults living with type 2 diabetes. *Health Education and Behaviour*, 35, 707–720.

Beverly, E. A., Penrod, J., and Wray, L. A. (2007). Living with type 2 diabetes: Marital perspectives of middle-aged and older couples. *Journal of Psychosocial Nursing and Mental Health Services*, 45, 24–32.

Beverly, E. A., Wray L. A., Chiu C. J., and Weinger, K. (2011). Perceived challenges and priorities in co-morbidity management of older patients with Type 2 diabetes. *Diabetes Medicine*, 28(7), 781–784.

Brewer-Lowry, A. N., Arcury, T. A., Bell, R. A., and Quandt, S. A. (2010). Differentiating approaches to diabetes self-management of multi-ethnic rural older adults at the extremes of glycemic control. *Gerontologist*, 50, 657–667.

British Medical Association. (2004). *Diabetes mellitus: An update for healthcare professionals*. London: BMA Publishing.

Brown, A. F., Ettner, S. L., Piette, J., Weinberger, M., Gregg, E., Shapiro, M. F., Karter, A. J., and Beckles, G. L. (2004). Socioeconomic position and health among persons with diabetes mellitus: A conceptual framework and review of the literature. *Epidemiologic Reviews*, 26, 63–77.

Campbell, R., Pound, P., Pope, C., Britten, N., Pill, R., Morgan, M., and Donovan, J. (2003). Evaluating meta-ethnography: A synthesis of qualitative research on lay experiences of diabetes and diabetes care. *Social Science and Medicine*, 56, 671–684.

Casey, D., De Civita, M., and Dasgupta, K. (2010). Understanding physical activity facilitators and barriers during and following a supervised exercise programme in type 2 diabetes: A qualitative study. *Diabetic Medicine*, 27, 79–84.

Chang, H.-Y. A., Wallis, M., and Tiralongo, E. (2011). Use of complementary and alternative medicine among people with type 2 diabetes in Taiwan: A cross-sectional survey. *Evidence-Based Complementary and Alternative Medicine*. Art. ID. 983792.

Chang, H.-Y. A., Wallis, M., and Tiralongo, E. (2012). Predictors of complementary and alternative medicine use by people with type 2 diabetes. *Journal of Advanced Nursing*, 68(6), 1256–1266.

Chao, J., Nau, D. P., Aikens, J. E., and Taylor, S. D. (2005). The mediating role of health beliefs in the relationship between depressive symptoms and medication adherence in persons with diabetes. *Research in Social and Administrative Pharmacy*, 1, 508–525.

Chlebowy, D. O., Hood, S., and LaJoie, A. S. (2010). Facilitators and barriers to self-management of type 2 diabetes among urban African American adults: Focus group findings. *Diabetes Educator*, 36, 897–905.

Collins, M. M., Bradley, C. P., O'Sullivan, T., and Perry, I. J. (2009). Self-care coping strategies in people with diabetes: A qualitative exploratory study. *BMC Endocrine Disorders*, 9, 6.

Connolly, V. (2006). Diabetes, deprivation and outcomes in the wealthy world. *Diabetes Voice*, 51(1), 37–40.

Corser, W., Lein, C., Holmes-Rovner, M., and Gossain, V. (2010). Contemporary adult diabetes mellitus management perceptions. *Patient*, 3(2), 101–111.

Coulter, A. (2002). *The autonomous patient: Ending paternalism in medical care*. London: The Stationary Office.

Cuddihy, R. M., Philis-Tsimikas, A., and Nazeri, A. (2011). Type 2 diabetes care and insulin intensification: Is a more multidisciplinary approach needed? Results from the modify survey. *Diabetes Educator*, 37(1), 111–123.

Department of Health. (2001). National service framework for diabetes. London: Department of Health.

Diabetes UK. (2010). *Diabetes in the UK 2010: Key statistics on diabetes*. www.diabetes.org.uk/Documents/Reports/Diabetes_in_the_UK_2010.pdf (accessed July 16, 2013).

Edwall, L.-L., Danielson, E., and Öhrn, I. (2010). The meaning of a consultation with the diabetes nurse specialist. *Scandinavian Journal of Caring Sciences*, 24(2), 341–348.

Edwall, L.-L., Hellström, A. L., Öhrn, I., and Danielson, E. (2008). The lived experience of the diabetes nurse specialist regular check-ups, as narrated by patients with type 2 diabetes. *Journal of Clinical Nursing*, 17(6), 772–781.

Elstad, E., Tusiofo, C., Rosen, R. K., and McGarvey, S. T. (2008). Living with Ma'i Suka: Individual, familial, cultural, and environmental stress among patients with type 2 diabetes mellitus and their caregivers in American Samoa. *Preventing Chronic Disease*, 5, A79.

Europe, I.D.F., & FEND, P. EURADIA. (2011). *Diabetes, the policy puzzle: Is Europe making progress*. www.fend.org/projects/policy-puzzle (accessed July 16, 2013).

Fagerli, R. A., Lien, M. E., and Wandel, M. (2007). Health worker style and trustworthiness as perceived by Pakistani-born persons with type 2 diabetes in Oslo, Norway. *Health*, 11(1), 109–129.

Funnell, M. M., and Anderson, R. M. (2004). Empowerment and self-management of diabetes. *Clinical Diabetes*, 22(3), 123–127.

Gomersall, T., Madill, A., and Summers, L. K. M. (2011). A meta-synthesis of the self-management of type 2 diabetes. *Qualitative Health Research*, 21(6), 853–871.

Hayes, R. P., Bowman, L., Monahan, P. O., Marrero, D. G., and McHorney, C. A. (2006). Understanding diabetes medications from the perspective of patients with type 2 diabetes: Prerequisite to medication concordance. *Diabetes Educator*, 32(3), 404–414.

Hiscock, J., Legard, R., and Snape, D. (2001). *Listening to diabetes service users: Qualitative findings for the diabetes national service framework*. London: Department of Health.

Hunt, L. M., Valenzuela, M. A., and Pugh, J. A. (1998). Porque me toco a mi? Mexican American diabetes patients' causal stories and their relationship to treatment behaviours. *Social Science & Medicine*, 46(8), 959–969.

Jennings, A., Powell, J., Armstrong, N., Sturt, J., and Dale, J. (2009). A virtual clinic for diabetes self-management: Pilot study. *Journal of Medical Internet Research*, 11(1), 10.

Jerant, A. F., Friederichs-Fitzwater, M. M. von, and Moore, M. (2005). Patients' perceived barriers to active self-management of chronic conditions. *Patient Education and Counseling*, 57, 300–307.

Jones, R. A., Utz, S. W., Williams, I. C., Hinton, I., Alexander, G., and Moore, C. (2008). Family interactions among African Americans diagnosed with type 2 diabetes. *The Diabetes Educator*, 34(2), 318–326.

Jowsey, T., Gillespie, J., and Aspin, C. (2011). Effective communication is crucial to self-management: The experiences of immigrants to Australia living with diabetes. *Chronic Illness*, 7(1), 6–19, March.

Kelleher, D. (1988). Coming to terms with diabetes: Coping strategies and non-compliance. In R. Anderson and M. Bury (Eds.), *Living with chronic illness* (pp. 137–155). London: Unwin Hyman.

Kerr, E. A., Heisler, M., Krein, S. L., Kabeto, M., Langa, K. M., Weir, D., and Piette, J. D. (2007). Beyond comorbidity counts: How do comorbidity type and severity influence diabetes patients' treatment priorities and self-management? *Journal of General Internal Medicine*, 22, 1635–1640.

Knight, K. M., Dornan, T., and Bundy, C. (2006). The diabetes educator: Trying hard, but must concentrate more on behaviour. *Diabetic Medicine*, 23(5), 485–501.

Kokanovic, R., and Manderson, L. (2007). Exploring doctor-patient communication in immigrant Australians with type 2 diabetes: A qualitative study. *Journal of General Internal Medicine*, 22, 459–463.

Kreyenbuhl, J., Leith, J., Medoff, D. R., Fang, L., Dickerson, F. B., Brown, C. H., Goldberg, R. W., Potts, W., and Dixon, L. B. (2011). A comparison of adherence to hypoglycemic medications between type 2 diabetes patients with and without serious mental illness. *Psychiatry Research*, 188(1), 109–114.

Kruger, D. F. (2008). Integrating innovative tools into the management of type 2 diabetes to improve patient self-management. *Journal of the American Academy of Nurse Practitioners*, 20(Suppl. 1), 17–21.

Lawton, J., Peel, E., Parry, O., Araoz, G., and Douglas, M. (2003). Lay perceptions of type 2 diabetes in Scotland: Bringing health services back in. *Social Science & Medicine*, 60, 1423–1435.

Lawton, J., Peel, E., Parry, O., and Douglas, M. (2008). Shifting accountability: A longitudinal qualitative study of diabetes causation accounts. *Social Science & Medicine*, 67(1), 47–56.

Lindenmeyer, A., Whitlock, S., Sturt, J., and Griffiths, F. (2010). Patient engagement with a diabetes self-management intervention. *Chronic Illness*, 6(4), 306–316.

Lippa, K. D., and Klein, H. A. (2008). Portraits of patient cognition: How patients understand diabetes self-care. *Canadian Journal of Nursing Research*, 40(3), 80–95.

Maclean, H. M. (1991). Patterns of diet related self-care in diabetes. *Social Science and Medicine*, 32(6), 689–696.

Malpass, A., Andrews, R., and Turner, K. M. (2009). Patients with type 2 diabetes experiences of making multiple lifestyle changes: A qualitative study. *Patient Education and Counseling*, 74(2), 258–263.

Matthews, S. M., Peden, A. R., and Rowles, G. D. (2009). Patient-provider communication: Understanding diabetes management among adult females. *Patient Education and Counseling*, 76 (1), 31–37.

Minet, L. K. R., Lønvig, E.-M., Henriksen, J. E., and Wagner, L. (2011). The experience of living with diabetes following a self-management program based on motivational interviewing. *Qualitative Health Research*, 21(8), 1115–1126.

Morgan, M. (2003). The doctor-patient relationship. In G. Scambler (Ed.), *Sociology as applied to Medicine* (pp. 49–65). London: Elsevier Science Ltd.

Morris, J. E., Povey, R. C., and Street, C. G. (2005). Experience of people with type 2 diabetes who have changed from oral medication to self-administered insulin injections – a qualitative study. *Practical Diabetes International*, 22(7), 239–243.

Moser, A., Van Der Bruggen, H., Widdershoven, G., and Spreeuwenberg, C. (2008). Self-management of type 2 diabetes mellitus: A qualitative investigation from the perspective of participants in a nurse-led, shared-care programme in the Netherlands. *BMC Public Health*, 8. Art. No. 91.

Murphy, E., and Kinmouth, A. L. (1995). No symptoms, no problem? Patients understandings of non-insulin dependent diabetes. *Family Practice*, 12(2), 184–192.

Nam, S., Chelsa, C., Stotts, N. A., Kroon, L., and Janson, S. L. (2011). Barriers to diabetes management: Patient and provider factors. *Diabetes Research and Clinical Practice*, 93, 1–9.

Newton, P., and Asimakopoulou, K. G. (2008). A response to Professor Anderson's commentary on Empowerment article by Asimakopoulou, K. *European Diabetes Nursing*, 5(1), 36.

Newton, P., Scambler, S., and Asimakopoulou, K. (2015). A qualitative exploration of motivation to self-manage and styles of self-management amongst people living with type 2 diabetes. *Journal of Diabetes Research*. Art. ID. 638205, 9. doi:10.1155/2015/638205

NHS Diabetes. (2013). *Best practice for commissioning diabetes services – An integrated care framework*. www.diabetes.org.uk/Documents/Position%20statements/best-practice-commissioning-diabetes-services-integrated-framework-0313.pdf (accessed January 9, 2013).

Ockleford, E., Shaw, R. L., Willars, J., and Dixon-Woods, M. (2008). Education and self-management for people newly diagnosed with type 2 diabetes: A qualitative study of patients' views. *Chronic Illness*, 4(1), 28–37.

Oftedal, B., Karlsen, B., and Bru, E. (2010). Perceived support from healthcare practitioners among adults with type 2 diabetes. *Journal of Advanced Nursing*, 66, 1500–1509.

O'Rahilly, R. (2006). Evidence-based definition and classification: A commentary. In R. Williams, W. Herman, A. Kinmouth, and N. J. Wareham (Eds.), *The evidence base for diabetes care* (pp. 37–42). Chichester: John Wiley & Sons Ltd.

Otero-Sabogal, R., Arretz, D., Siebold, S., Hallen, E., Lee, R., Ketchel, A., Li, J., and Newman, J. (2010). Physician-community health worker partnering to support diabetes self-management in primary care. *Quality in Primary Care*, 18(6), 363–372.

Parry, O., Peel, E., Douglas, M., and Lawton, J. (2005). Issues of cause and control in patient accounts of type 2 diabetes. *Health Education Research*, 21(1), 97–107.

Paterson, B., Thorne, S., Crawford, J., and Tarko, M. (1999). Living with diabetes as a transformational experience. *Qualitative Health Research*, 9, 786–802.

Peek, M. E., Odoms-Young, A., Quinn, M. T., Gorawara-Bhat, R., Wilson, S. C., and Chin, M. H. (2010). Race and shared decision-making: Perspectives of African-Americans with diabetes. *Social Science & Medicine*, 71(1), 1–9.

Rajaram, S. S. (1997). Experience of hypoglycemia among insulin dependent diabetics and its impact on the family. *Sociology of Health and Illness*, 19, 281–296.

Rygg, L. Ø., Rise, M. B., Lomundal, B., Solberg, H. S., and Steinsbekk, A. (2010). Reasons for participation in group-based type 2 diabetes self-management education: A qualitative study 328. *Scandinavian Journal of Public Health*, 38(8), 788–793.

Scambler, G. (2009). Capitalists, workers and health: Illness as a 'side-effect' of profit-making. *Social Theory and Health*, 7(2), 117–128.

Simmons, D., Voyle, J., Rush, E., and Dear, M. (2010). The New Zealand experience in peer support interventions among people with diabetes. *Family Practice*, 27(Suppl. 1), i53–i61.

Skelly, A. H., Leeman, J., Carlson, J., Soward, A. C. M., and Burns, D. (2008). Conceptual model of symptom-focused diabetes care for African Americans. *Journal of Nursing Scholarship*, 40(3), 261–267.

Song, M., and Lipman, T. H. (2008). Concept analysis: Self-monitoring in type 2 diabetes mellitus. *International Journal of Nursing Studies*, 45(11), 1700–1710.

Trief, P. M., Sandberg, J., Greenberg, R. P., Graff, K., Castronova, N., Yoon, M., and Weinstock, R. S. (2003). Describing support: A qualitative study of couples living with diabetes. *Family System & Health*, 21, 57–67.

Van Dam, H. A., Van Der Horst, F., Van Den Borne, B., Ryckman, R., and Crebolder, H. (2003). Provider-patient interaction in diabetes care: Effects on patient self-care and outcomes – A systematic review. *Patient Education and Counseling*, 51(1), 17–28.

Visram, S., Bremmer, A. S., Harrington, B. E., and Hawthorne, G. (2008). Factors affecting uptake of an education and physical activity programme for newly diagnosed type 2 diabetes. *European Diabetes Nursing*, 5(1), 17–22.

Wang, Y., Chuang, L., and Bateman, W. B. (2011). Focus group study assessing self-management skills of Chinese Americans with type 2 diabetes mellitus. *Journal of Immigrant and Minority Health*, 14(5), 869–874.

Wellard, S. J., Rennie, S., and King, R. (2008). Perceptions of people with type 2 diabetes about self-management and the efficacy of community based services. *Contemporary Nurse*, 29(2), 218–226.

World Health Organization. (2014). *The top 10 causes of death*. www.who.int/mediacentre/factsheets/fs310/en/ (accessed December 15, 2015).

Wu, L., Forbes, A., and While, A. (2010). Patients' experience of a telephone booster intervention to support weight management in type 2 diabetes and its acceptability. *Journal of Telemedicine and Telecare*, 16(4), 221–223.

Wycherley, T. P., Mohr, P., Noakes, M., Clifton, P. M., and Brinkworth, G. D. (2012). Self-reported facilitators of, and impediments to maintenance of healthy lifestyle behaviours following a supervised research-based lifestyle intervention programme in patients with type 2 diabetes. *Diabetic Medicine*, 29, 632–639.

8
DEMENTIA

Joanne Brooke

This chapter discusses:

- Dementia syndromes, prevalence, incidence, symptoms and treatment
- National and international strategies and policies
- Living well with dementia and positive approaches to dementia care, including theoretical approaches of person-centred and relationship-centred care
- Non-pharmacological interventions to support living well with dementia
- Nutrition and dementia
- End-of-life care and dementia

Definition of dementia

The World Health Organization in the ICD-10 Classification of Mental and Behavioural Disorders: Clinical Descriptions and Diagnosis Guidelines (2007) define dementia as:

> Dementia is a syndrome due to disease of the brain, usually of a chronic or progressive nature, in which there is disturbance of multiple higher cortical functions, including memory, thinking, orientation, comprehension, calculation, learning capacity, language, and judgement. Consciousness is not clouded. The impairments of cognitive function are commonly accompanied, and occasionally preceded, by deterioration in emotional control, social behaviour, or motivation.

In the United Kingdom dementia was defined in 2009 in *Living well with dementia: a national dementia strategy*:

> The term 'dementia' is used to describe a syndrome which may be caused by a number of illnesses in which there is progressive decline in multiple areas of function, including decline in memory, reasoning, communication skills and the ability to carry out daily activities. Alongside this decline, individuals may develop behavioural and psychological symptoms such as depression, psychosis, aggression and wandering, which cause

problems in themselves, which complicate care, and which can occur at any stage of the illness.

(*Department of Health, 2009, p. 15*)

Both definitions include aspects of memory loss, but dementia is also the disruption of problem-solving activities which impacts on a person's ability to perform tasks that are required for daily living. The loss of higher cortical functioning changes how the person can interact with the world, impacting on their behaviour. The changes in a person's behaviour may be referred to as non-cognitive symptoms of dementia; when these behaviours include agitation or aggression they may be classified as 'behaviour and psychological symptoms of dementia' (BPSD) (Hughes, 2011).

Prevalence and incidence

Worldwide dementia is estimated to affect 25 million people (Ferri et al., 2005). In the United Kingdom 850,000 people are estimated to be living with dementia, which is a prevalence of one in 14 people aged 65 years and over (Prince et al., 2014a). Early onset dementia, which is diagnosed before the age of 65 years, is estimated to account for 2 to 10 per cent of all cases. Early onset dementia is slightly more common in men than women; however of the total of people living with dementia, there are significantly more women than men. The prevalence of dementia doubles with every five-year increment in age and is one of the main causes of disability and dependence in older people (Prince et al., 2014b).

Types of dementia

Dementia is an umbrella term for a syndrome, which is a collection of symptoms that may be caused by a number of diseases. There are more than 200 diseases and conditions that can impact on the brain and cause the symptoms of dementia. The most prevalent form of dementia is Alzheimer's disease, followed by vascular dementia and then mixed dementia (see Figure 8.1).

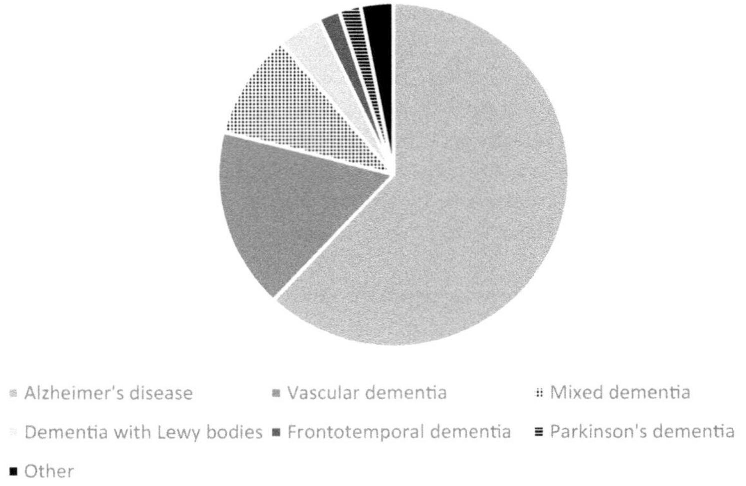

Figure 8.1 Subtypes of dementia.

Adapted from: Alzheimer's Society Dementia UK: Update (2014).

Alzheimer's disease

Dr Alois Alzheimer, a German physician, was the first to link changes in brain tissue to the mental illness of one of his patients in 1906. Auguste Deter, a 51-year-old lady presented with memory loss, unpredictable behaviour and language problems. Dr Alzheimer found abnormalities of the neurons in her brain during her post mortem, which included amyloid plaques attached to the cell bodies and tangles of the axons (Stelzmann, Schnitzlen and Murtagy, 1995). These abnormalities are now commonly referred to as plaques and tangles. Plaques tend to be found in higher concentrations in the amygdala, hippocampus and some regions of the cortex (Wenk, 2003). Plaques and tangles inhibit communication between neurons, ultimately causing their death. Other neuropathological changes include a reduction in activity of the neurotransmitter acetylcholine and neuroinflammation (Wenk, 2003).

The first symptom of Alzheimer's disease typically noticed is a problem with episodic memory (Gold and Budson, 2008). The disease is progressive with a slow decline, which is unique to each individual and difficult to predict. Any sudden decline in cognitive impairment would indicate an acute illness rather than part of the Alzheimer's disease process. However as impairments in memory become greater, this impacts on the person's thinking, reasoning, perception and communication.

Vascular dementia

Vascular dementia is the result of the death of neurons in the brain due to an inadequate blood supply caused by large vessel disease and large infarctions (such as a stroke), small blood vessel disease (such as weakening and narrowing of the blood vessel walls by arteriosclerosis) or small infarctions and lacunar infarcts (Hughes, 2011). The risk factors for the development of atherosclerotic changes causing vascular dementia have been identified as hypertension, cigarette smoking, myocardial infarction, diabetes mellitus and hyperlipidaemia (Gorelick, 2004).

The initial symptoms of vascular dementia include a decline in executive functioning or problem-solving, such as being unable to plan and complete a course of action (Hughes, 2011). The progression of vascular dementia occurs in a step-wise fashion; therefore cognition may be stable for a period of time before an event such as multiple small infarcts occur that will cause an acute decline.

Mixed type dementia

Mixed dementia has been defined as the combination of the pathological processes of both Alzheimer's disease and vascular dementia and is more prevalent in older people (Langa, Foster and Larson, 2004). The progression of mixed dementia is a significant cognitive decline more so than either Alzheimer's disease or vascular dementia alone. The incidence and prevalence of mixed dementia may be underestimated due to the challenges in obtaining an accurate diagnosis; however this is imperative for appropriate treatment (Zekry, Hauw and Gold, 2002).

Dementia with Lewy bodies

In 1912 Dr Friedrich Lewy, a neurologist, was the first to link roundish protein bodies within cell bodies to the cause of Parkinson's disease (Rodrigues e Silva et al., 2010). However, it wasn't until new staining techniques were developed that cortical Lewy bodies were also discovered that led to the identification of dementia with Lewy bodies (DLB).

A prominent symptom of DLB is significant fluctuation in confusion and alertness that can change from hour to hour and day to day, although there is less memory loss in the early stages. Visual hallucinations, difficulty in interpreting visual information, Rapid Eye Movement (REM) sleep disorder, the acting out of dreams may also occur, impacting significantly on the person's behaviour.

Frontotemporal dementia

Frontotemporal dementia is the impact of pathological changes in the front and temporal lobes of the brain, sometimes referred to as Pick's disease or frontal lobe dementia. Frontotemporal dementia is more common in people under the age of 65 (Mercy et al., 2008). There are three clinical presentations of frontotemporal dementia:

- Frontotemporal behaviour variant – particularly noticeable are changes in the person's personality and behaviour, such as reward-seeking behaviours including overeating and alcohol use (Perry et al., 2014).
- Progressive non-fluent aphasia – the main impact is on a person's speech, which becomes slow and hesitant, with errors in grammar and understanding complex sentences.
- Semantic dementia – the development of problems understanding the meaning of words, and finding the right word, which progresses to difficultly recognising familiar people or objects (Alzheimer's Society, 2013a).

Treatment of dementia

Drug treatment to slow the progression of dementia

There is currently no cure for dementia, but different drugs are available to slow the progression and alleviate some of the symptoms. A clear diagnosis of the type of dementia is required prior to the commencement of drug treatment due to the mechanism of the drugs that impact on the changes in the brain caused by each disease. The commencement of drug treatment in the United Kingdom occurs in specialist memory services (National Institute for Health and Care Excellence, 2006).

Alzheimer's disease

Drugs include acetylcholinesterase inhibitors: Aricept (donepezil), Exelon (rivastigmine), Reminyl (galantamine) (Wilcock et al., 2000) or Ebixa (memantine), which works in a different way to the acetylcholinesterase inhibitors (Wenk et al., 2000).

Vascular dementia

Treatment of the underlying conditions is required, with the commencement or regulation of secondary prevention. The drugs used in Alzheimer's disease are not recommended for vascular dementia, unless there is a diagnosis of mixed dementia.

Dementia with Lewy Bodies

Treatment with one of the three acetylcholinesterase inhibitors may occur if the person is experiencing distressing hallucinations or delusions (McKeith et al., 2000).

Frontotemporal dementia

Treated with antidepressant medication, which has been found to reduce some difficult behaviours; acetylcholinesterase inhibitors should not be prescribed, as they have been found to be harmful in some cases (Mendez et al., 2007).

Drug treatments for behaviour and psychological symptoms of dementia (BPSD)

BPSD describes behaviour including agitation, aggression, wandering, shouting, repeated questioning and sleep disturbance. A person with dementia exhibiting BPSD will require a full assessment by their GP and a specialist psychiatrist. Clear guidelines in the United Kingdom have been produced to ensure a robust assessment and trial of non-pharmacological interventions prior to drug prescription (National Institute for Health and Care Excellence, 2015). However, should the need arise, antipsychotic drugs may be prescribed. The adverse side effects of these drugs are well documented (Banerjee, 2009; Muench and Hamer, 2010). This is not to suggest that antipsychotic drugs should not be used, but they must be prescribed and reviewed appropriately (National Institute of Clinical Excellence, 2015). A UK national audit from GP data suggests that the number of people with dementia receiving a prescription of antipsychotic drugs has reduced by 51.8 per cent from 2008–2011 (Health and Social Care Information Centre, 2012). Due to the reduction in antipsychotic drugs and a focus on well-being for people with dementia, there has been a large growth in non-pharmacological interventions that are now viewed as important to support the person with dementia to live well, some of which will be discussed later in the chapter.

National and international strategies, policies and third-sector activity

Dementia has been estimated to cost Europe $239 billion, Asia Pacific $124 billion and North America $213 billion (World Alzheimer's Report, 2010). The economic impact of dementia in the United Kingdom is estimated by the Alzheimer's Society (2014) to be £26.3 million. In the United Kingdom, the National Dementia Strategy (2009) focused on three areas to develop significant improvement: dementia awareness, earlier diagnosis and intervention, and higher quality of care. The strategy has been followed by the Prime Minister's Challenge on Dementia (2012 and 2020), which is a framework for driving improvements in health and social care, creating dementia-friendly communities that understand how to help and conducting robust comprehensive research (Department of Health, 2012).

In the United States, the National Plan to Address Alzheimer's disease (2012) focuses on preventing and effectively treating Alzheimer's disease by 2025, optimising care quality and efficiency, expanding support for people with Alzheimer's disease and their families, enhancing public awareness and engagement, and tracking progress and driving improvement. The National Plan Updates (2013, 2014, 2015) document the progress. President Obama signed the National Alzheimer's Project Act in 2011, which was ground-breaking legislation that established a framework for a national strategic plan to address the prevalence of Alzheimer's disease and to coordinate a multifaceted approach including research, care and support.

In the United Kingdom, policy has also focused on education of the workforce, the 'Making a Difference in Dementia: Nursing Vision and Strategy' (Department of Health, 2013). A model of dementia nursing was introduced with three levels of training: dementia awareness, dementia skilled and dementia specialist. Training for all the health and social care workforce in England has been mapped across three levels/tiers encompassing 14 competencies in the 'Dementia Core Skills Education and Training Framework' (Department of Health, 2015). However, training the workforce is only one element of the UK and US strategies.

The Prime Minister's Challenge on Dementia (Department of Health, 2012) supported the work by the Alzheimer's Society with the aim of creating one million 'Dementia Friends' across England and Wales, which was achieved in 2015. A central objective of being a Dementia Friend is the creation of local communities where people living with dementia are understood and included, thereby removing stigma, lack of understanding, loneliness and social exclusion.

Another initiative is the development of dementia-friendly communities (DFC), which is supported by the Prime Minister Challenge on dementia and the Alzheimer's Society (2013a). DFCs support people with dementia and their families in their local communities so they feel involved with their community as well as supported to live well independently for longer. DFCs are not just supported by the Alzheimer's Society; many other organisations have become involved such as Age UK, public services, churches, superstores, banks, schools, NHS Trusts and many more.

Dementia Action Alliances (DAA) were formed in the United Kingdom to engage and bring together different organisations to work collaboratively to develop DFCs. DAAs are voluntary organisations hosted by the Alzheimer's Society. The aim of DAAs is to develop a society-wide change concerning dementia, both at a national level with regard to policies and attitudes and at a local level by coordinating and supporting local DAAs. A local DAA that been recognised as a successful example of this approach, and has been adopted by other regions, is the Crawley DAA. Crawley DAA included their local NHS Clinical Commissioning Group, Borough Council, County Council, NHS Foundation Trust, Alzheimer's Society, Carers Support Service, Age UK, Local Strategic Partnership, Pensioners Active and Older People's Forum, Town Centre Partnership and Economic Action Group, St Catherine's Hospice, Sussex Police, local schools and colleges. All of the partners in the alliance supported and collaborated to develop Crawley into a dementia-friendly community.

The development of DFCs is not restricted to England and Wales, with examples from the United States and 'A tool kit for building dementia friendly communities' (Wisconsin Department of Health Services et al., 2015), a collaboration of work from Wisconsin Department of Health Services, Alzheimer's Association, AARP Wisconsin and Dementia-Capable Wisconsin in 2015. Leaders at the G8 Dementia Summit (2013) acknowledged the importance of dissemination of successful approaches within dementia care and this included community-based programmes fostering inclusion for people with dementia and their families/carers to improve their quality of life.

Positive approaches to care: person-centred and relationship-centred models

Person-centred care

Person-centred care for people living with dementia is now considered as gold standard (Slater, 2006) and is essential in supporting people with dementia to live well. Person-centred care, or person-centeredness, was first applied to dementia care by Kitwood, who adopted the terminology from Carl Roger's humanistic approach to psychology (Edvardsson, Fetherstonhaugh and Nay, 2010). Person-centred care focuses on caring for the person as an individual, responding to their actual needs and not assuming their needs will follow a certain set criteria (Kitwood and Bredin, 1992). Person-centred care from the perspectives of people with dementia, their family and residential aged care staff included knowing the person, providing meaningful activities, being in a personalised environment, and experiencing flexibility and continuity of care (Edvardsson, Fetherstonhaugh and Nay, 2010).

An essential aspect of person-centred care, according to Kitwood (1997), is 'personhood'. Kitwood (1997) defined personhood as: "*A status or standing bestowed upon one human being, by others, in the context of social relationship and social being. It implies recognition, respect and truth*" (emphasis in original). Personhood is essentially a social process, whereby an individual's personhood develops in or by the presence of others (Kitwood and Bredin, 1992). The aim of dementia care according to Kitwood (1997) is to "*maintain personhood in the face of failing mental powers*" (emphasis in original). Therefore, treating a person with dementia only for their biological disease will ultimately cause harm (Epp, 2003). Kitwood (1997) outlines positive and negative impacts on personhood. The concept of *malignant social psychology* (Kitwood, 1990) describes how health and social care professionals, as well as friends and family, interact with the person with dementia in a depersonalised manner. This type of interaction is not malignant through malice or intent to harm, but due to trying to do their best for the person with dementia and in doing so inadvertently trying to protect them by making decisions or performing tasks for them. However, Kitwood (1997) also described positive person work that can assist to maintain and enhance the personhood, dignity and well-being of the person with dementia. One form of positive person work is celebration, which can be achieved by carers recognising, supporting and endorsing successful achievements of the person with dementia. Validation can be achieved through families and carers recognising and supporting the reality of the person with dementia, by focusing on the person's feelings and emotions rather than the facts they may be providing (Brooker, 2006).

A number of interventions to support person-centred care within different care settings have been described and evaluated, and they are discussed below.

Biographical approach

One biographical approach, which recognises an individual's uniqueness, is storytelling. In a UK NHS hospital, life stories were found to help practitioners to understand their patient in greater depth and to see their patient as people, as well as supported staff to form closer relationships with families (Clarke, Hanson and Ross, 2003). An element of this work that has become standard practice across NHS provision is the completion of short documents to understand the needs, preferences, likes, dislikes and interests of a person with dementia. The most commonly used format is the 'This is Me' booklet (Alzheimer's Society, 2013c).

Reminiscence

Reminiscence therapy for people with dementia living in various community settings have demonstrated a significant positive impact for the person with dementia (Tadaka and Kanagawa, 2007; Hsieh et al., 2010). However, these studies were criticised for not being robust (Blake, 2013). More recently, a meta-analysis of reminiscence therapies for people with dementia found small improvements in cognitive function and a significant reduction in depressive symptoms (Huang et al., 2015). Anecdotal evidence also suggests reminiscence therapy can engage people with dementia, allowing them to become involved and communicating or singing, perhaps for the first time in many months.

Validation therapy

The aims of validation therapy is the validation of the person with dementia through: restoration of self-worth; engaging with the person to promote communication and social connections with others; reducing stress, agitation and anxiety; and supporting the resolving of unfinished life tasks (Feil, 1993). Validation therapy involves the categorisation of behaviours of people with dementia into one of four stages on the continuum of dementia from mild to severe. Then the methods of communication used by the person with dementia such as verbal and non-verbal are allocated to a stage. The four stages include: malorientation, time confusion, repetitive motion and vegetation (Feil, 1993). However, this approach has been heavily criticised, although Feil argues strongly for the effectiveness of this approach (Neal and Briggs, 2000). A Cochrane systematic review by Neal and Barton White (2003) found some evidence to support validation therapy.

Assessment of person-centred care for people with dementia across different settings can be completed through a number of frameworks such as Dementia Care Mapping (Brooker and Surr, 2006) and the VIPS (V – values people, I – individual's needs, P – perspective of service user, S – supportive psychology) Framework (Brooker, 2006). A final aspect of the provision of person-centred care is the impact on the carers; although there is only a relatively small number of studies that have explored this, a systematic review of seven studies concluded the impact tended to be positive (Barbosa et al., 2015).

Relationship-centred care

The theoretical approach of person-centred care envisaged by Kitwood has become diluted and is frequently ill defined in many policy documents and academic literature, particularly within the field of nursing (Nolan et al., 2004; McCormack, 2004). From this perspective, the concept of relationship-centred care emerged, with the 'Senses Framework' (Nolan et al., 1997; Nolan et al., 2001, 2004). The framework endorses person-centred care, but also encapsulates the wider relationships of giving and receiving care (Adams, 2008a). The Senses Framework emphasises the importance of the person with dementia, their families/carers and formal care providers; these relationships should promote a sense of security, belonging, continuity, purpose, achievement and significance. Everyone involved in these relationships needs to experience these senses for good care to be provided. Relationship-centred care is more than just the relationship of the person with dementia and the care provider (McCormack, 2004). In the United Kingdom the relationship-centred approach is reflected in 'The Triangle of Care' (Hannan et al., 2013), which emphasises three people in the relationship: the person with dementia, the family/carer and the professional carer.

Person-centred and relationship-centred care are important concepts with the field of dementia care. A broader and inclusive approach to dementia care has been suggested through a whole-systems approach that accommodates both approaches, where these concepts become the building blocks in a dementia-care framework (Adams, 2008a, 2008b).

Art and dementia

The focus of non-pharmacological interventions has been to find meaningful and engaging activities. Engagement of both the person with dementia and their families/carers in activities can help them to adapt to changes in memory, communication skills, problem-solving and behaviour by focusing on remaining abilities rather than losses (Genoe and Dupuis, 2014).

Recognised and evaluated non-pharmacological interventions include art viewing and object handling at galleries and museums, singing, storytelling at libraries and Dementia Cafés.

Art

Innovative art interventions for people with dementia and their families/carers have steadily increased in the last decade both in the United Kingdom and the United States (Roe et al., 2014; Zeisel, 2009). Participative arts refer to interventions that are led by professional artists for people with dementia and their families/carers (Zeilig, Killick and Fox, 2014). Group facilitated art viewing found people with dementia and their families/carers reported feeling more socially included, improved cognitive functioning and an overall sense of an improved quality of life (Camic, Tischler and Pearman, 2014). Even participants with more severe dementia remembered it as a pleasurable experience and expressed a wish for the intervention to continue, and families/carers discussed the importance of living for the moment (MacPherson et al., 2009). Art viewing and object handling at a national museum for people with mild to moderate dementia and their families/carers significantly increased their well-being following both the art viewing session and the object handling session (Johnson et al., 2015). Many galleries and museums are now working closely with people with dementia and their families/carers to provide support and to engage them in meaningful activities. A systematic review examining the impact of art and dementia found most studies were small, with methodological limitations. However, all studies reported a positive impact for people with dementia including an improvement in their attention, communication and ability to engage with creative activities, but also the spontaneous stimulation of memories (Young, Camic and Tischler, 2016).

Singing

'Singing for the Brain'™ was originally developed by the Alzheimer's Society, with the aim of bringing people with dementia and their families/carers together in a stimulating friendly social environment for the enjoyment of singing, but also to provide a support group unlike traditional support groups. It is of no surprise that people with dementia and their families/carers reported an improvement in memory as the impact of music on memory has been well documented (Larkin, 2001). However, attendees also reported feeling socially included, improvement in their relationships, enjoyment of attending and more importantly feeling supported to accept and cope with the dementia (Bannan and Montgomery-Smith, 2008; Osman, Tischler and Schneider, 2014). Other music interventions are regularly used, especially in care home environments. Singing as well as listening to music has been reported to have a positive impact on the person with dementia through improvement in depressive symptoms, spontaneous singing, recall of old memories and reduced agitation or restlessness (Sarkamo et al., 2013). Singing and music listening has also been found to have a positive impact on care providers, as they gain skills to communicate with people who are mostly uncommunicative (Sarkamo et al., 2013).

Dance/movement

Studies involving the impact of dance and movement for people with dementia have been limited to residential settings. Similar to the issues with understanding the impact of arts on dementia, methodological limitations again make it difficult to provide robust evidence of the effectiveness of this approach (Guzman-Garcia et al., 2013). However, a dance and movement intervention delivered by care home staff resulted in improvements in creative self-expression, communication and, most importantly, pleasure and enjoyment of the people with dementia participating (Rylatt, 2012). A daily dance therapy with the aim to reduce agitation demonstrated some positive results, although an important element was changing the culture of the care home staff to support such a programme (Duignan and Milverton, 2009).

Libraries

Public libraries across England have launched a scheme 'Reading Well, Books on Prescription' in 2013. The scheme was designed to provide self-help reading for people with common mental health conditions; however this has now been extended to include dementia. The books from the Reading Well on Prescription reading list are freely available in public libraries. In addition, many public libraries have created memory boxes or information on how to develop a memory box that can be borrowed by health and social care professionals or individuals.

Dementia Café

The original concept for an Alzheimer Café, commonly referred to now as a Dementia Café, was the idea of Dr Bère Miesen in the Netherlands in 1997, although it has been adopted in the United Kingdom, Greece, Italy, United States and Australia (Miesen and Jones, 2006). The original model proposed by Miesen included a structured programme of themed topics, which would provide information in the form of talks and discussions. The talks were provided by invited speakers from a range of backgrounds and provided in a supportive atmosphere of the café. Miesen and Jones (2006) have described their model of an Alzheimer Café as somewhere between group therapy and a self-help group. People with dementia and their families/carers are able to meet others is the same situation as themselves and to talk openly and freely about issues concerning them. The final, but important, element of an Alzheimer Café is that everyone is aware of dementia and people can attend without having to worry or feel embarrassed for themselves or their loved ones.

Nutrition and dementia

Older people are at risk of weight loss and undernutrition, which results in a decrease of their wound healing, bone density, immune and cognitive functioning, as well as higher rates of admission to hospital, readmissions and mortality (Chapman, 2006). An older person with a diagnosis of dementia is at a higher risk, with weight loss and undernutrition occurring in over half of all people with dementia (Gillette-Guyonnet et al., 2000). A reason for weight loss and undernutrition in people with dementia may be the result of an imbalance between nutritional intake and physical need; for example, wandering or restlessness may increase energy use (Knopman, 2008). There is also a positive correlation between weight loss and the severity of dementia; therefore the greater the weight loss the more severe the dementia (Albanese et al., 2013). Another reason of weight loss and undernutrition is the development of eating and drinking problems, which impact on over half of the people diagnosed with dementia (LeClerc et al., 2004). In the earlier stages of dementia these can include changes in taste, difficulties in planning, coordination, processing sensory information, development of attention deficits and possibly a lack of recognition of hunger and thirst (Volkert, 2014). During the later stages of dementia, problems with swallowing may occur, leaving the person at risk of aspiration pneumonia (Dodds, Stewart and Logemann, 1990).

Interventions to support nutritional intake for people with dementia have been described by Brooke and Ojo (2015) under four categories: environment, support with feeding difficulties, nutritional supplements, and education and training. Each of these will briefly be discussed below, but recognition of person-centred care remains important and not to assume all interventions are suitable or even necessary for all people with dementia.

Environment

Four elements of the environment essential to support nutrition in people with dementia include the fabric, ambience, psychological impact and sociological impact (Cooper, Boyko and Codinhoto, 2008; Yates-Bolton et al., 2012). Therefore the need for a dining room that 'looks like' a dining room – with the table traditionally set with a table cloth and place settings, the use of coloured crockery, good lighting, music, the smell of freshly cooked food and social dining with an optimum of four people around one table – can impact on the nutritional intake of people with dementia (Perivolaris et al., 2006; Rossiter et al., 2014; Brush, Meehan and Calkins, 2002; Thomas and Smith, 2009; Cleary et al., 2008; Timlin and Rysenbry, 2010).

Support with feeding difficulties

Studies exploring interventions to support people with dementia with feeding difficulties have tended to use different outcome measures, thus limiting comparisons of interventions (Jackson et al., 2011). However, complex interventions are required and would need to include elements of small meals throughout the day, finger foods, meals with enhanced energy-dense foods, texture of the food appropriate to the person's swallowing abilities and mid-morning supplements (Jackson et al., 2011).

Nutritional supplements

Food fortification and supplementation may become necessary to ensure adequate amounts are consumed. While high-calorie and protein supplements may promote weight gain and maintain some functional status (Milne et al., 2009; Hanson et al., 2011), there is no evidence to suggest that either macro- or micronutrient supplementation may be beneficial in slowing down the cognitive decline (Prince et al., 2014a).

Education and training

The provision of education and training programmes for families/carers of people with dementia are routinely provided by nutritionists and speech and language therapists, and are well received by those who attend (Salvà et al., 2011). However, the programmes do not impact on the nutritional intake of the person with dementia or reduce families'/carers' burden (Prince et al., 2014b). The provision of the Alzheimer's Society (2013b) Eating and Drinking Factsheet can support both the person with dementia and their families/carers to understand the importance of good nutrition, and includes practical suggestions to support nutritional intake.

End-of-life care and dementia

End-of-life care is important in all terminal diseases and is supported through planning care in advance, commonly referred to as Advance Care Planning (ACP). ACP includes advance statements, advance directives for refusal of treatment and lasting power of attorney (refer to Chapter 11 for more information). For people with dementia, discussions regarding ACP are required in the early stages of the disease, when the person has capacity to be fully involved in these conversations. These discussions are paramount to include the person's thoughts, wishes and preferences; if this does not occur, evidence suggests this leads to fragmented and non-person-centred end-of-life care (Livingston et al., 2010).

Traditionally, healthcare professionals have not viewed dementia as a terminal illness requiring ACP, and this is reflected in the result of studies exploring completion of ACP by disease. Patients with cancer or organ failure are more likely to complete ACP than people with dementia (Evans et al., 2014). In the United States, Gerand et al. (2011) reported only 39 per cent of people with a diagnosis of mild cognitive impairment completed ACP in the five years following their diagnosis.

In the United Kingdom, the provision of discussions regarding end-of-life care and the development of ACP for people with dementia is not uniformly initiated by one particular service. Therefore, it is paramount that healthcare professionals across primary and community care are aware of the provision of their local memory services and engage in the process of ACP with their patients. Processes and documentations have been created to support ACP for people with dementia and their families/carers as well as healthcare professionals, and are currently being evaluated (Poppe, Burleigh and Banerjee, 2013).

However, further training and awareness of ACP in dementia is still required. A review of barriers to the use of ACP with people with dementia identified three themes: lack of ACP knowledge of people with dementia, their families/carers and healthcare professions, lack of understanding regarding the right time to initiate ACP discussions, and reluctance/avoidance of people with dementia and their families/carers to engage in ACP discussions (Brooke and Kirk, 2014).

Conclusion

Definitions of dementia include aspects of memory loss, but also the disruption of problem-solving activities which impacts on a person's ability to perform tasks that are required for daily living. The loss of higher cortical functioning changes how the person can interact with the world, impacting on their behaviour. Dementia is an umbrella term for a syndrome, which is a collection of symptoms that may be caused by a number of diseases. There is currently no cure for dementia, but different drugs are available to slow the progression and alleviate some of the symptoms. Dementia has a huge economic impact internationally. National and international strategies, policies and third-sector initiative have been launched to increase dementia awareness, earlier diagnosis and intervention, and higher quality of care. Person-centred and relationship-centred care are important concepts with in the field of dementia care. A broader and inclusive approach to dementia care has been suggested through a whole-systems approach that accommodates both approaches, where these concepts become the building blocks in a dementia-care framework. The focus of non-pharmacological interventions has been to find meaningful and engaging activities. Engagement of both the person with dementia and their families/carers in activities can help them to adapt to changes in memory, communication skills, problem-solving and behaviour by focusing on remaining abilities rather than losses. Recognised and evaluated non-pharmacological interventions include art viewing and object handling at galleries and museums, singing, storytelling at libraries and Dementia Cafés. An older person with a diagnosis of dementia is at a higher risk of weight loss, with undernutrition occurring in over half of all people with dementia. Interventions to support nutritional intake for people with dementia have been categorised as environment, support with feeding difficulties, nutritional supplements, and education and training. End-of-life care is important in all terminal diseases. For people with dementia, discussions regarding ACP are required in the early stages of the disease, when the person has capacity to be fully involved in these conversations. These discussions are paramount to include the person's thoughts, wishes and preferences; if this does not occur evidence suggests this leads to fragmented and non-person-centred end-of-life care.

References

Adams, T. (2008a). A whole-systems approach for dementia care. *Nursing Older People*, 20(10), 24–26.

Adams, T. (2008b). *Dementia care nursing: Promoting the well-being of people with dementia and their families*. Basingstoke: Palgrave Macmillan.

Albanese, E., Taylor, C., Siervo, M., Stewart, R., Prince, M. J., and Acosta, D. (2013). Dementia severity and weight loss: A comparison across eight cohorts. The 10/66 study. *Alzheimer's Dement*, 9(6), 649–656.

Alzheimer's Society. (2013a). *Building dementia friendly communities: A priority for everyone*. www.alzheimers.org.uk/site/scripts/download_info.php?fileID=1916

Alzheimer's Society. (2013b). *Factsheet: Eating and drinking*. www.alzheimers.org.uk/site/scripts/download_info.php?fileID=1799

Alzheimer's Society. (2013c). *This is me: This leaflet will help you support me in an unfamiliar place*. www.alzheimers.org.uk/site/scripts/download_info.php?fileID=1604

Alzheimer's Society. (2014). *Dementia UK: Update*. www.alzheimers.org.uk/site/scripts/download_info.php?fileID=2323

Banerjee, S. (2009). *The use of antipsychotic medication: Time for action*. www.rcpsych.ac.uk/pdf/Anti psychotic%20Bannerjee%20Report.pdf

Bannan, N., and Montgomery-Smith, C. (2008). 'Singing for the Brain': Reflections on human capacity for music arising from a pilot study of group singing with Alzheimer's patients. *Journal of Royal Society for the Promotion of Health*, 128(2), 73–78.

Barbosa, A., Sousa, L., Nolan, M., and Figueiredo, D. (2015). Effects of person-centred care approaches to dementia care on staff: A systematic review. *American Journal of Alzheimer's Disease and Other Dementias*, 30(8), 723–722.

Blake, M. (2013). Group reminiscence therapy for adults with dementia: A review. *British Journal of Community Nursing*, 18(5), 228–233.

Brooke, J. M., and Kirk, M. (2014). Advance care planning for people living with dementia. *British Journal of Community Nursing*, 19(10), 422–427.

Brooke, J. M., and Ojo, O. (2015). Oral and enteral nutrition in dementia: An overview. *British Journal of Nursing*, 24(12), 624–628.

Brooker, D. J. (2006). *Person-centred dementia care: Making services better*. London: Jessica Kingsley Publishers.

Brooker, D. J., and Surr, C. (2006). Dementia Care Mapping (DCM): Initial validation of DCM 8 in UK field trials. *International Journal of Geriatric Psychiatry*, 21(11), 1018–1025.

Brush, J. A., Meehan, R. A., and Calkins, M. P. (2002). Using the environment to improve intake for people with dementia. *Alzheimer's Care Quarterly*, 3(4), 330–338.

Camic, P. M., Tischler, V., and Pearman, C. H. (2014). Viewing and making art together: A multi-session art-gallery-based intervention for people with dementia and their carers. *Aging and Mental Health*, 18(2), 161–168.

Chapman, I. M. (2006). Nutritional disorders in the elderly. *Medical Clinics of North America*, 90(5), 887–907.

Clarke, A., Hanson, E. J., and Ross, H. (2003). Seeing the person behind the patient: Enhancing the care of the older person using a biographical approach. *Journal of Clinical Nursing*, 12, 697–706.

Cleary, S., Soest, D. van, Milke, D., and Misiaszek, J. (2008). Using the smell of baking bread to facilitate eating in residents with dementia. *Canadian Nursing Home*, 19(1), 6.

Cooper, R., Boyko, C., and Codinhoto, R. (2008). *State-of-science review SR-DR2: The effect of the physical environment on mental wellbeing*. [Commissioned for Foresight Project on Mental Capital and Wellbeing: Making the most of ourselves in the 21st Century.]. London: Government Office for Science.

Department of Health. (2009). *Living well with dementia: A national dementia strategy*. www.gov.uk/government/uploads/system/uploads/attachment_data/file/168220/dh_094051.pdf

Department of Health. (2012). *Prime Minister's challenge on dementia: Delivering major improvements in dementia care and research by 2015*. www.gov.uk/government/uploads/system/uploads/attachment_data/file/215101/dh_133176.pdf

Department of Health. (2013). *Making a difference in dementia: Nursing vision and strategy*. www.gov.uk/government/uploads/system/uploads/attachment_data/file/147956/Making_a_Difference_in_Dementia_Nursing_Vision_and_Strategy.pdf

Department of Health. (2015). *Dementia core skills education and training framework*. www.skillsforhealth.org.uk/images/projects/dementia/Dementia%20Core%20Skills%20Education%20and%20Training%20Framework.pdf

Dodds, W. J., Stewart, E. T., and Logemann, J. A. (1990). Physiology and radiology of the normal oral and pharyngeal phases of swallowing. *AJR. American Journal of Roentgenology*, 154(5), 953–963.

Duignan, D., and Milverton, R. (2009). Exploring dance as a therapy for symptoms and social interaction in a dementia care unit. *Nursing Times*, 105(30), 19–22.

Edvardsson, D., Fetherstonhaugh, D., and Nay, R. (2010). Promoting a continuation of self and normality: Person-centred care as described by people with dementia, their family members and aged care staff. *Journal of Clinical Nursing*, 19(17–18), 2611–2618.

Epp, T. D. (2003). Person-centred Dementia Care: A vision to be refined. *The Canadian Alzheimer Disease Review*, 5(3), 14–19.

Evans, N., Roeline, H., Pasman, W., et al. on behalf of Euroimpact. (2014). End-of-life care in general practice: A cross-sectional, retrospective survey of 'cancer', 'organ failure' and 'old age/dementia' patients. *Palliative Medicine*, 28(7), 967–975.

Feil, N. (1993). Validation therapy with late-onset dementia populations. In G. Jones and B. M. L. Miesen (Eds.), *Care giving in dementia: Research and Applications* (pp. 199–218). Chatham: Mackays of Chatham.

Ferri, C. P., Prince, M., Brayne, C., et al. (2005). Alzheimer's Disease International: Global prevalence of dementia: A Delphi consensus study. *Lancet*, 366, 2112–2117.

G8 UK. (2013). *Global action against dementia*. G8 Dementia Summit Communique. www.gov.uk/government/publications/g8-dementia-summit-global-action-against-dementia/g8-dementia-summit-global-action-against-dementia-11-december-2013

Garand, L., Dew, A., Lingler, H., and DeKoskey, S. T. (2011). Incidence and predictors of advance care planning among persons with cognitive impairment. *The American Journal of Geriatric Psychiatry*, 19(8), 712–720.

Genoe, M. R., & Dupuis, S. L. (2014). The role of leisure within the dementia context. *Dementia*, 13(1), 33–58.

Gillette-Guyonnet, S., NourhashemI, F., Andrieu, S., et al. (2000). Weight loss in Alzheimer disease. *The American Journal of Clinical Nutrition*, 71(2), 637S–642S.

Gold, C. A., and Budson, A. E. (2008). Memory loss in Alzheimer's disease: Implications for development of therapeutics. *Expert Review Neurotherapeutics*, 8(12), 1879–1891.

Gorelick, P. P. (2004). Risk factors for Vascular Dementia and Alzheimer's disease. *Stroke*, 35(Suppl. 1), 2620–2622.

Guzman-Garcia, A., Hughes, J. C., James, I. A., and Rochester, L. (2013). Dancing as a psychosocial intervention in care homes: A systematic review of the literature. *Geriatric Psychiatry*, 28(9), 914–924.

Hannan, R., Thompson, R., Worthington, A., and Rooney, P. (2013). *The triangle of care. Carers included: A guide to best practice for dementia care*. London: Carers Trust.

Hanson, L. C., Ersek, M., Gilliam, R., and Carey, T. S. (2011). Oral feeding options for patients with dementia: A systematic review. *Journal of the American Geriatric Society*, 59(3), 463–472.

Health and Social Care Information Centre. (2012). *National dementia and antipsychotic prescribing audit 2012*. www.hscic.gov.uk/catalogue/PUB06624/nati-deme-anti-pres-audi-summ-rep.pdf

Hsieh, C-J., Chang, C., Su, S-F., et al. (2010). Reminiscence group therapy on depression and apathy in nursing home residents with mild-to-moderate dementia. *Journal of Experimental and Clinical Medicine*, 2(2), 72–78.

Huang, H. C., Chen, Y. T., Chen, P. Y., Huey-Lan Hu, S., Liu, F., Kuo, Y. L., and Chiu, H. Y. (2015). Reminiscence therapy improves cognitive functions and reduces depressive symptoms in elderly people with dementia: A meta-analysis of randomized controlled trials. *Journal of American Medical Directors Association*, 16(12), 1087–1094.

Hughes, J. C. (2011). *Alzheimer's and other dementias*. Oxford: Oxford University Press.

Jackson, J., Currie, K., Graham, C., and Robb, Y. (2011). The effectiveness of interventions to reduce undernutrition and promote eating in older adults with dementia: A systematic review. *JBI Library of Systematic Reviews*, 9(37), 1509–1549.

Johnson, J., Culverwell, A., Hulbert, S., Robertson, M., and Camic, P. M. (2015). Museum activities in dementia care: Using visual analog scales to measure subjective wellbeing. *Dementia*. Doi: 10.1177/1471301215611763.

Kitwood, T. (1990). The dialectics of dementia: With particular reference to Alzheimer's disease. *Ageing and Society*, 10, 177–196.

Kitwood, T. (1997). *Dementia revisited: The person comes first (rethinking ageing)*. Buckinghamshire: Open University Press.

Kitwood, T., and Bredin, K. (1992). Towards a theory of Dementia Care: Personhood and well-being. *Ageing and Society*, 12, 269–287.

Knopman, D. (2008). Go to the head of the class to avoid vascular dementia and skip diabetes and obesity. *Neurology*, 71(14), 1046–1047.

Langa, K. M., Foster, N. L., and Larson, E. B. (2004). Mixed Dementia: Emerging concepts and therapeutic implications. *JAMA*, 292(23), 2901–2908.

Larkin, M. (2001). Music tunes up memory in dementia patients. *Lancet*, 357, 47.

LeClerc, C. M., Wells, D. L., Sidani, S., Dawson, P., and Fay, J. (2004). A feeding abilities assessment for people with dementia. *Alzheimer's Care Quarterly*, 5(2), 123–133.

Livingston, G., Leavey, G., Manela, M., et al. (2010). Making decisions for people with dementia who lack capacity: Qualitative study of family carers in UK. *BMJ*, 341, c4184.

McCormack, B. (2004). Person-centredness in gerontological nursing: An overview of the literature. *International Journal of Older People Nursing*, 13(3a), 31–38.

McKeith, I., Del Ser, T., Spano, P. F., Emre, M., Wesnes, K., Anand, R., Cicin-Sain, A., Ferrara, R., and Spiegel, R. (2000). Efficacy of rivastigmine in dementia with Lewy bodies: A randomised, double-blind, placebo-controlled international study. *Lancet*, 356(9247), 2031–2036.

MacPherson, S., Bird, M., Anderson, K., Davis, T., and Blair, A. (2009). An art gallery access programme for people with dementia: 'You do it for the moment'. *Aging and Mental Health*, 13(5), 744–752.

Mendez, M. F., Shapira, J. S., McMurtray, A., and Licht, E. (2007). Preliminary Findings: Behavioural worsening on Donepezil in patients with Frontotemporal dementia. *The American Journal of Geriatric Psychiatry*, 15(1), 84–87.

Mercy, L., Hodges, J. R., Dawson, K., Barker, R. A., and Brayne, C. (2008). Incidence of early-onset dementias in Cambridgeshire, United Kingdom. *Neurology*, 71(19), 1496–1499.

Miesen, B., and Jones, G. M. M. (2006). The Alzheimer café concept. In G. Jones and B. M. L. Miesen (Eds.), *Care giving in dementia: Research and applications volume 4* (pp. 454–469). London: Brunner-Routledge.

Milne, A. C., Potter, J., Vivanti, A., and Avenell, A. (2009). Protein and energy supplementation in elderly people at risk from malnutrition. *Cochrane Database of Systematic Reviews 2009*, Issue 2. Art. No.: CD003288. DOI: 10.1002/14651858.CD003288.pub3.

Muench, J., and Hamer, A. M. (2010). Adverse effects of antipsychotic medications. *American Family Physician*, 81(5), 617–622.

National Institute for Health and Care Excellence. (2006). *Dementia: Supporting people with dementia and their carers in health and social care*. www.nice.org.uk/guidance/cg42/chapter/guidance#interventions-for-cognitive-symptoms-and-maintenance-of-function-for-people-with-dementia

National Institute for Health and Care Excellence. (2015). *Low-dose antipsychotics in people with dementia*. www.nice.org.uk/advice/ktt7/resources/lowdose-antipsychotics-in-people-with-dementia-1632175200709.

Neal, M., and Barton White, P. (2003). Validation therapy for dementia. *Cochrane Database Systematic Review*, (3), CD001394.

Neal, M., and Briggs, M. (2000). Validation therapy for dementia. *Cochrane Database Systematic Review*, (2), CD001394.

Nolan, M. R., Booth, A., and Nolan, J. (1997). *New directives in rehabilitation: Exploring the nursing contribution*. Research Report Series No 6. London: English National Board for Nursing, Midwifery and Health Visiting.

Nolan, M. R., Davies, S., Brown, J., Keady, J., and Nolan, J. (2004). Beyond 'person-centred' care: A new vision for gerontological nursing. *International Journal of Older People Nursing*, 13(3a), 45–53.

Nolan, M. R., Davies, S., and Grant, G. (2001). *Working with older people and their families: Key issues in policy and practice*. Buckinghamshire: Open University Press.

Osman, S. E., Tischler, V., and Schneider, J. (2014). 'Singing for the Brain': A qualitative study exploring the health and well-being benefits of singing for people with dementia and their carers. *Dementia*, 15(6), 1326–1339.

Perivolaris, A., LeClerc, C. M., Wilkinson, K., and Buchanan, S. (2006). An enhanced dining program for persons with dementia. *Alzheimer's Care Quarterly*, 7(4), 258–267.

Perry, D. C., Sturm, V. E., Seeley, W. W., Miller, B. L., Kramer, J. H., and Rosen, H. J. (2014). Anatomical correlates of reward-seeking behaviours in behavioural variant frontotemporal dementia. *Brain: A Journal of Neurology*, 137, 1621–1626.

Poppe, M., Burleigh, S., and Banerjee, S. (2013). Qualitative evaluation of Advance Care Planning in Early Dementia (ACP-ED). *PLOS ONE*, 8(4), e60412.

Prince, M., Knapp, M., Guerchet, M., McCrone, P., Prina, M., Comas-Herrera, A., Wittenberg, R., Adelaja, B., Hu, B., King, D., Rehill, A., and Salimkumar, D. (2014a). *Dementia UK* (2nd ed.). London: Alzheimer's Society.

Prince, M., Albanese, E., Guerchet, M., and Prina, M. (2014b). *World Alzheimer report 2014: Dementia and risk and reduction. An analysis of protective and modifiable factors*. www.alz.co.uk/research/WorldAlzheimer Report2014.pdf

Rodrigues e Silva, A. M., Geldsetzer, F., Holdorff, B., Kielhorn, F. W., Balzer-Geldsetzer, M., Oertel, W. H., Hurtig, H., and Dodel, R. (2010). Who was the man who discovered the "Lewy bodies"? *Movement Disorders: Official Journal of the Movement Disorders Society*, 25(12), 1765–1773.

Roe, B., McCormick, S., Lucas, T., Gallagher, W., Winn, A., and Elkin, S. (2014). Coffee, cake & culture: Evaluation of an art for health programme for older people in the community. *Dementia*. 15(4), 539–559.

Rossiter, F. F. A., Shinton, C. A., Duff-Walker, K., Behova, S., and Carroll, C. B. (2014). Does coloured crockery influence food consumption in elderly patients in an acute setting? *Age Ageing*, 43(Suppl. 2), ii1–ii2.

Rylatt, P. (2012). The benefits of creative therapy for people with dementia. *Nursing Standard*, 26(33), 42–47.

Salvà, A., Andrieu, S., Fernandez, E., et al. (2011). Health and nutrition promotion program for patients with dementia (NutriAlz): Cluster randomised trial. *Journal of Nutrition Health and Aging*, 15(10), 822–830.

Sarkamo, T., Laitinen, S., Nummien, A., Kurki, M., and Rantanen, P. (2013). Role of music leisure activities in dementia care: Applicability and benefits perceived by caregivers. *Journal of Communications Research*, 5(3), 331–352.

Slater, L. (2006). Person-centredness: a concept analysis. *Contemporary Nurse*, 23(1), 135–144.

Stelzmann, R. A., Schnitzlen, H. N., and Murtagy, F. R. (1995). An English translation of Alzheimer's 1907 paper, "Uber eine eigenartige Erkankung der Hirnrinde". *Clinical Anatomy*, 8, 429–431.

Tadaka, E., and Kanagawa, K. (2007). Effects of reminiscence group in elderly people with Alzheimer's disease and vascular dementia in a community setting. *Geriatrics and Gerontology International*, 7(2), 167–173.

Thomas, D. W., and Smith, M. (2009). The effect of music on caloric consumption among nursing home residents with dementia of the Alzheimer's type. *Activities, Adaptation & Aging*, 33(1), 1–16.

Timlin, G., and Rysenbry, N. (2010). *Design for dementia: Improving dining and bedroom environments in care homes*. London: Helen Hamlyn Centre, Royal College of Art.

Volkert, D. (2014). ESPEN guidelines on nutrition in dementia. Presentation at the *36th ESPEN Congress*, September 6–9, Geneva, Switzerland.

Wenk, G. L. (2003). Neuropathologic changes in Alzheimer's disease. *Journal of Clinical Psychiatry*, 64(Suppl. 9), 7–10.

Wenk, G. L., Quack, G., Moebius, H. J., and Danysz, W. (2000). No interaction of Memantine with acetylcholinesterase inhibitors approved for clinical use. *Life Sciences*, 66(12), 1079–1083.

Wilcock, G. K., Lilienfeld, S., Gaens, E. on behalf of the Galantamine International-1 Study Group. (2000). Efficacy and safety of galantamine in patients with mild to moderate Alzheimer's disease: Multi-centre randomised controlled trial. *BMJ*, 321, 1–7.

Wisconsin Department of Health Services, Alzheimer's Association, AARP Wisconsin and Dementia-Capable Wisconsin. (2015). *A tool kit for building dementia friendly communities*. www.alz.org/sewi/documents/Dementia_Friendly_Communities_toolkit.pdf

The World Health Organization. (2007). *ICD-10 classification of mental and behavioural disorders: Clinical descriptions and diagnosis guidelines*. http://apps.who.int/classifications/apps/icd/icd10online2007/index.htm?gf00.htm+

Yates-Bolton, N., Yates, K., Williamson, T., Newton, R., and Codinhoto, R. (2012). *Improving hospital environments for people with dementia: Listening event report*. Salford: The University of Salford.

Young, R., Camic, R., and Tischler, V. (2016). The impact of community-based arts and health interventions on cognition in people with dementia: A systematic literature review. *Aging and Mental Health*, 20(4), 337–351.

Zeilig, H., Killick, J., and Fox, C. (2014). The participative arts for people living with a dementia: A critical review. *International Journal of Ageing and Later Life*, 9(1), 7–34.

Zeisel, J. (2009). *I'm still here: A breakthrough approach to understanding someone living with Alzheimer's*. New York: Penguin Group (USA).

Zekry, D., Hauw, J. J., and Gold, G. (2002). Mixed dementia: Epidemiology, diagnosis and treatment. *Journal of the American Geriatrics Society*, 50(8), 1431–1438.

9
FALLS

Leslie Gelling

This chapter discusses:

- The causes of falls amongst older adults
- The consequences of falls
- The importance of thorough falls risk assessment
- Multifactorial approaches to care delivery to minimise falls and their consequences
- The use of assistive technology to help minimise falls and the consequences of falls

Learning outcomes

After reading this chapter you will:

- Understand the importance of minimising falls and the consequences of falls in promoting positive aging
- Be aware of the importance of thorough falls risk assessment for all older people
- Be aware of some of the strategies that might be implemented to minimise falls and the consequences of falls for older people

Introduction

Falls are a relatively common and often serious event for older adults and can have an immense impact on quality of life and positive aging in that population. Despite this, evidence to support the most effective strategies to minimise falls is limited and often inconclusive or contradictory (Cumming et al., 2008; National Institute for Health and Care Excellence, 2013). Aging is a natural process but with increased age comes greater frailty, a higher risk of developing functional impairments and other complex co-morbidities. It is therefore inevitable that falls become a greater risk with advancing years and that the consequences of falls can be more serious (Phelan et al., 2015). It would be a mistake, however, to assume that falls and their consequences are not preventable or that action cannot be taken to minimise the risk of falling, regardless of age.

Falls happen in all environments, including in the individual's home, in hospitals and in other care settings. As many as one third of people over the age of 65 fall each year and this number increases to 50 per cent in those over the age of 80 (Sayer et al., 2006). In the United

Kingdom, 300,000 older people attend Accident and Emergency Departments each year after falling at home and of these 1,500 die as a direct result of their fall (Lightbody et al., 2002). One report from the United States indicates that the incidence of in-hospital falls could be as high as 3.56 for each 1,000 patient days with 26.1 per cent of these resulting in an injury (Bouldin et al., 2013). In the United Kingdom the incidence of in-hospital falls has been reported as being in excess of 280,000 annually (National Patient Safety Agency, 2010). The incidence of falls in hospital settings is often increased because of newly acquired risk factors and unfamiliar surroundings (Carmeron et al., 2010). For example, in stroke rehabilitation wards it has been reported that between 25 per cent and 46 per cent of patients will fall on at least one occasion during their period of hospitalisation (Dromerick and Reding, 1994; Forster and Young, 1995). Having had one fall is also an important indicator of the risk of having subsequent falls with 50 per cent of those experiencing a fall having another in the following year (Lilley, Arie and Chilvers, 1995). In light of the high incidence of falls and the impact they can have on the individual, their family and those providing or funding healthcare, it is not surprising that falls prevention has become a priority area for care provision in many parts of the world (Grealish and Chaboyer, 2015).

Whilst there can be no doubt that falls are a serious problem, the reported figures of the incidence of falls are probably underestimations of the true incidence. It has been well documented that the reporting of falls in the hospital settings fails to capture all that occur and that many people who fall at home do not report or seek help (Haines et al., 2009). As a consequence, the true incidence of falls in older people is probably much higher than reported in the literature and may have a more significant impact on positive aging for more people than has been reported.

The cause of falls

In many instances, the reason someone has fallen might be unclear but in most instances falls are the result of a complex combination of intrinsic and extrinsic factors. To further complicate matters, the combination of factors resulting in someone falling are unique to that individual at that point in time, so someone falling on two occasions might exhibit a different combination of factors at the time of each fall. Intrinsic risk factors that might lead to someone falling can include (Phelan et al., 2015):

- Age-related changes (e.g. worsening vision)
- Cognitive decline (e.g. dementia)
- Gait and balance
- Chronic conditions (e.g. arthritis)
- Acute conditions (e.g. stroke, fracture)
- Incontinence.

Extrinsic risk factors that might lead to someone falling can include (Phelan et al., 2015):

- Medications
- Footwear
- Assistive devices
- Home environment (e.g. poor flooring)
- Alcohol and drugs
- Support from caregivers.

This highlights the complexity of assessing and managing falls prevention strategies. It is, however, important to try to discover why someone has fallen so that appropriate strategies can be put in place to minimise the risk of a subsequent fall.

The impact of falls on positive aging

The consequences of experiencing a fall can be serious for the individual involved and has been described as the third leading cause of chronic disability and mortality in older people (Tchalla et al., 2012). Falls can quickly lead to an irreversible decline in functional status, even in those who were independent prior to their fall (Chu, Chiu and Chi, 2008; Thornlow, Anderson and Oddone, 2009). For those who fall whilst in hospital there can be a considerable delay in being discharged or they might never be able to return to their own home (Grealish and Chaboyer, 2015). For those experiencing a fall, the consequences might include, but are not limited to:

- Fractures
- Head injuries
- Minor injures
- Reduced mobility
- Reduced ability to engage in usual social activities
- Reduced independence.

Approximately 50 per cent of falls result in an injury and 10 per cent of those will experience a serious and potentially life-changing injury (King and Tinetti, 1995; Phelan et al., 2015; Tinetti et al., 1995).

Up to 5 per cent of falls amongst older people lead to fracture and approximately 5 per cent of those lead to complex and difficult-to-treat injuries (Tchalla et al., 2012). One of the commonest fractures resulting from a fall is a fracture to the hip, which is 10.5 times more likely to occur in a nursing home than if the individual was living in their own home. Furthermore, the outcomes for those sustaining a hip fracture at home are also better than if they had been in a nursing home at the time of their fall (Butler et al., 1996). The most likely reason for this is that those living independently at home were probably fitter and more mobile before their injury and so were better prepared to recover from their injury.

When someone has fallen once, they can develop a fear of falling, which has been reported as developing in as many as 20 per cent to 39 per cent of people who fall (Patel et al., 2014; Scheffer et al., 2008). Fear of falling can also become a problem in people who have no history of falling, which impacts on their confidence to perform various activities (Liu, 2015). Fear of falling can impact on someone's confidence to mobilise and could lead to further falls or other health problems.

The accumulative effect of the consequences of a fall can have a significant impact on someone's quality of life as a result (Phelan et al., 2015):

- A decreased ability to self-care and live independently
- A decreased ability to participate in physical activities
- A decreased ability to engage in social activities.

The impact on someone's ability to experience positive aging can be significant and it is not uncommon for someone who experiences a fall to enter an irreversible period of decline, even if they were healthy, mobile and living independently prior to their fall.

As the world's population ages, the increasing number of older people who are living longer with complex co-morbidities is creating unprecedented financial challenges even in the most developed countries (Williams, 2005). The treatment and ongoing care of older people who experience a fall can have significant cost implications for care providers. It is difficult to obtain accurate estimates of cost, but in the United States it is estimated that nearly $30 billion is spent each year in direct medical costs as a result of falls in older adults (Stevens et al., 2006) or 6 per cent of all medical expenditure in the United States (Rajendram et al., 2008). It is clear from even the lowest estimates that falls in the older population add a considerable amount to increasingly limited health budgets.

Assessment of fall risk

Assessing an individual's risk of falling will invariably be a complex process and will require the assessor to consider a wide range of factors (National Institute for Health and Care Excellence, 2013; Rajendram et al., 2008).

Falls are frequently a consequence of an accumulation of overlapping factors so assessment can be a time-consuming and challenging process (Webster et al., 2008). Despite this, undertaking a thorough assessment is important because many of the risk factors can be managed to minimise the risk of falling. One of the most useful predictors of a possible future fall is a history of having fallen in the past (Rajendram et al., 2008), but it is also important to recognise that someone not exhibiting any of the recognised risk factors might still be at risk of falling and suffering serious consequences, so all older people should be considered as being at risk of falling.

Research has demonstrated that undertaking a thorough assessment of fall risk factors can have a positive impact on reducing the number of people falling, the number of repeat fallers and the seriousness of injuries sustained when falling (Gillespie et al., 2012; Ray et al., 1997; Rubenstein et al., 1990). It is, therefore, unsurprising that early assessment of all older people is repeatedly advocated as key to falls prevention strategies. The American Geriatrics Society and the British Geriatrics Society published clinical practice guidelines on falls risk assessment and management in which they recommend the annual screening of all adults over the age of 65 (Panel on Prevention of Falls in Older Persons, 2011). In the United States there is also detailed guidance from the Centre for Disease Control (CDC) on each of the proposed stages in the assessment process, which has been incorporated into a tool kit for practitioners (Stevens, 2013; Stevens and Phelan, 2013). Importantly, the tool kit highlights that even individuals assessed as being at low risk could benefit from some falls prevention intervention, including education, exercise and the prescription of vitamin D supplements.

Validated tools are available to support the assessment of risk of falling, including:

- The Peter James Centre Falls Risk Assessment Tool (Haines et al., 2004; Haines et al., 2006)
- The Risk Assessment for Falls Scale II
- The John Hopkins Fall Risk Assessment Tool (Klinkenberg and Potter, 2016).

These tools give some structure and repeatability to falls assessment but they will each include a number of key elements of the assessment process, including (Gillespie et al., 2012; Panel on Prevention of Falls in Older Persons, 2011; Phelan et al., 2015):

- Falls history (including information from witnesses when possible)
- Physical examination (including assessment for postural hypertension)
- Gait and balance

- Medications
- Environment.

Thorough assessment of falls risk is an ongoing process because older people's health status will invariably change as they age. If assessments are not repeated there is a danger that interventions could become redundant and alternatives not considered.

Interventions to minimise fall risk and maximise positive aging

Interventions to minimise the risk of experiencing a fall and, therefore, maximise positive aging should be based on a thorough assessment so that a multifactorial but individualised falls prevention strategy can be implemented (Carmeron et al., 2010; Grealish and Chaboyer, 2015; National Institute for Health and Care Excellence, 2013). Multifactorial approaches are most commonly reported as having an impact on the number of falls (Tchalla et al., 2012), but this does make it difficult to identify the impact of individual interventions within the multifactorial approach.

Exercise

The increased incidence of falls is associated with increased frailty, with the oldest people frequently described as being the most frail and, therefore, at most risk of falling. Worsening gait will result from decreased step height and decreased proprioception whilst balance will decline as a result of increased postural sway and slowed righting reflexes (Phelan et al., 2015). There will also be generalised decreased muscle strength. These factors might be described as inevitable parts of the natural aging process, but there is evidence to suggest that promoting exercise can improve muscle strength, gait, and balance, and, as a result, reduce the risk of falling. The aim for healthcare professionals should be to maintain the highest possible level of mobility whilst minimising the possible risks (Phelan et al., 2015). At the same time as having an impact on falls, exercise can have other health benefits for older people.

Evidence to support the use of exercise as part of a falls reduction programme is mixed. In a large systematic review they identified six studies that used a single exercise modality and a further four studies that introduced a combination of exercise types (Carmeron et al., 2010). The findings of these individual studies were described as 'inconsistent' and did not always demonstrate a benefit to the use of exercise to minimise fall risk. For example:

- Pooled data from four studies testing a combination of exercise types demonstrated a significant increase in the rate of falls (Faber et al., 2006; Mulrow et al., 1994; Rosendahl et al., 2008; Schoenfelder, 2000).
- Pooled data from three studies testing a supervised exercise programme demonstrated a significant reduction in the risk of falling (Barreca et al., 2004; Donald et al., 2000; Jarvis, Kerr and Mockett, 2007).

These systematic reviewers concluded that individual assessment and careful selection of the type of exercise were essential because there is a possibility that the wrong type of exercise could result in an increased risk of falling (Carmeron et al., 2010). Whilst current evidence provides inconsistent advice about how much exercise or which types of exercise are most beneficial in minimising fall risk, it would appear that any form of exercise is preferable to no exercise at all (Sousa et al., 2016).

Medicines

Several types of medicine can increase the risk of falling, including:

- Psychoactive medicines (e.g. antidepressants)
- Antihypertensives
- Nonsteroidal anti-inflammatories
- Diuretics.

In some instances it might be possible to decrease doses or even stop medicines that are no longer needed or when an alternative therapeutic approach might be available. For example, many older people are prescribed sedative drugs to treat insomnia but this might also increase someone's risk of falling (Pratt et al., 2014; Tannenbaum et al., 2015). Where possible, alternative approaches to managing insomnia should be tried before prescribing sedative drugs. Having pharmacists involved in reviewing medicines prescribed for older people and offering recommendations has been demonstrated to result in a significant reduction in the rate of falls (Zermansky et al., 2006) and in the risk of falling (Crotty et al., 2004). The risk of falling is often a neglected side-effect of prescribing medicines, so there does need to be a balance between such prescriptions and possible consequences, and this should be considered as part of an older person's falls risk assessment.

Vitamin D supplementation

Vitamin D can increase muscle strength through specific vitamin D receptors in human muscle tissue whilst vitamin D deficiency can result in muscle weakness and pain (Sahota, 2009). Vitamin D supplements have been shown to increase muscle strength, reduce pain and reduce the number of falls in older adults (Bischoff et al., 2003; Broe et al., 2007; Burleigh, McColl and Potter, 2007; Flicker et al., 2005). In the most comprehensive systematic review of vitamin D supplementation in those at risk of falling, including eight randomised controlled trials, it was demonstrated that supplemental vitamin D at a dose of 700–1,000 IU daily could reduce the risk of falling amongst older individuals of 19 per cent (Bischoff-Ferrari et al., 2009). Doses below 700 IU daily did not demonstrate the same benefit.

Environmental factors

There are a number of environmental factors that can increase the risk of someone falling, including:

- Furnishings and adaptations made to the home (e.g. poorly positioned hand rails)
- Aids used for mobilising (e.g. walking sticks and frames)
- Aids to communication
- Flooring
- Footwear
- Lighting.

Slippery floors can create a hazard that might be exacerbated by the individual having inappropriate or ill-fitting footwear or poor lighting. These factors might come together at night when someone wakes and urgently needs to go to the toilet. In one study a 'light path' was used to help offer participants a clear path to the toilet but this study is complicated by the fact that all participants were also using tele-assistance to seek help if they needed it (Tchalla et al., 2012).

The study demonstrated a significant reduction in the number of falls and in the number of participants hospitalised following their fall, but it is not clear which of the two technologies had the most impact on these findings or if they need to be combined to have a positive effect. There needs to be more research to explore this further.

Assessment of environmental factors is usually undertaken by a trained occupational therapist who will seek to identify obstacles to safe movement inside and outside the home. Adaptations can be made to make the environment safer.

Cognitive impairment

Cognitive impairment, including dementia, is one of the major causes of falls and strategies to manage cognitive impairment are multifactorial, creating an additional complexity when seeking to minimise falls in these individuals (Grealish and Chaboyer, 2015). Dementia can increase the incidence of falls as a result of impaired gait and poor balance and can also reduce someone's hazard recognition (Phelan et al., 2015). There has been little research around falls prevention in those with cognitive impairment, possibly because of the challenges of research ethics, but there is some evidence to suggest that mobility and balance problems can be improved in this group through exercise programmes (Phelan et al., 2015).

Education

There is a danger that older people might underestimate the personal risk of falling (Yardley et al., 2006). Care providers, healthcare professionals and family members have a key role to play in helping older people to understand the factors that might cause them to fall and what they might do to minimise their risk of falling (Phelan et al., 2015). Information should be given orally and in writing and might include information about (National Institute for Health and Care Excellence, 2013):

- What measures they can take to prevent further falls
- How to stay motivated if referred for falls prevention strategies that include exercise or strength and balancing components
- The preventable nature of some falls
- The physical and psychological benefits of modifying falls risk
- Where they can seek further advice and assistance
- How to cope if they have a fall, including how to summon help and how to avoid a long lie.

Use of assistive technology

Within a multifactorial approach to minimising falls and the consequences of falls, assistive technology has an important role to play. This assistive technology might include:

- Bed pressure sensors
- Chair pressure sensors
- Accelerometers.

The bed and chair sensors are designed to alert healthcare professionals or carers when someone is getting out of bed or standing from their chair so they can intervene to minimise the risk of that individual falling and to support the individual in mobilising as much as they are able. The accelerometer is worn by someone at risk of falling and sends an alert when someone has fallen, thus ensuring that a carer or healthcare professional can get to them as soon as possible and is able to minimise any consequences. Many of the long-term consequences of falls are a result of older people not being found as soon as possible after the fall.

Despite growing interest in the use of technology in this way, the evidence to support it is limited and often inconclusive. Three trials conducted in hospital settings were able to demonstrate that bed and chair pressure pads were able to reduce the number of falls in a hospital population, but not to a statistically significant level (Sahota et al., 2014; Shorr et al., 2012; Tideiksaar, Feiner and Maby, 1993). It is important to note that this technology cannot stop someone from falling and so can only be used as part of a multifactorial approach to falls prevention. Assistive technology will also have limited use for the many people who are being encouraged to mobilise as part of their falls prevention strategy but might be useful in helping to improve someone's confidence to mobilise because they will know they can get help if they need it (Hill et al., 2014; Pietrzak, Cotea and Pullman, 2014). Being able to continue living at home is clearly preferable, so the use of assistive technology can be the difference between someone being able to live at home or needing to remain in hospital or move to a nursing home (Mann et al., 1999; Miskelly, 2001).

One of the main problems with the use of assistive technology has been the attitude of healthcare professionals to its use. Whilst there is a general acceptance of the use of technology in this way (Tideiksaar, Feiner and Maby, 1993), there is also evidence that sometimes healthcare professionals and carers turn alarms off or leave alarms unattended (Sahota et al., 2014). One reason for this might be the high number of false alarms resulting in 'alarm fatigue' (Graham and Cvach, 2010; Shorr et al., 2012). This highlights the need for staff to have confidence in the equipment and to be appropriately trained in the use of the technology. It is also important that older people are carefully assessed to ensure that they have the most appropriate types of assistive technology available to them. For example, bed or chair sensors may not be the best use of technology for individuals who are mobilising with minimal or no assistance. This will require repeated assessment because as someone's confidence and ability to mobilise improves, their need for assistive technology could also change.

Minimising consequences following a fall

Even with the most thorough assessment of fall risk and with the implementation of strategies to minimise falls, it is inevitable that older people will sometimes fall. If the consequences of a fall can be minimised, then the impact on the individual's ability to live independently and positively can also be minimised. One of the most serious injuries resulting from a fall is a hip fracture and one strategy that might be effective in reducing the risk of a fracture is hip protectors. Whilst there is some evidence to demonstrate that hip protectors can be effective in reducing the seriousness of falls in care settings, the same benefit is not reported in community settings (Parker, Gillespie and Gillespei, 2006). This is believed to result from a reluctance to wear this protection at home because they can add considerable bulk under clothing (Rajendram et al., 2008). So like many of the strategies that might be introduced to minimise falls, or the consequences of falls, the individual needs to be comfortable with the intervention, be willing to use it and be knowledgeable in its use.

The most useful way to minimise the consequences of a fall is to reduce the length of time it takes someone to get help after they have fallen. This reduction in response time is best achieved through the use of alarms, which can either be user activated or automatic. Selecting the most appropriate alarm will be guided by the thorough falls risk assessment and may need to be reconsidered as the individual's circumstances change. Most importantly, the alarm system needs to be acceptable to the individual, to carers and, when appropriate, to healthcare professionals.

Conclusion

The assessment of fall risk and the implementation of multifactorial but individualised fall prevention strategies can promote positive aging in a significantly large proportion of our population. The complexity of the causes of falls, the importance of thorough falls risk assessment and some of the multifactorial approaches to minimising falls have been explored in this chapter. Experiencing a fall and the often serious consequences of a fall can have a major impact on someone's life and healthcare professionals have an essential role to play in ensuring that falls are minimised, as much as possible, and that those who have experienced a fall are supported in achieving their pre-fall quality of life. This chapter has highlighted a number of interventions that can be used to help minimise the risk of falling and to promote positive aging, but in isolation they are unlikely to be effective. A thorough assessment and a multifactorial but individualised approach to falls prevention is the most effective way to support people in living positively into their old age.

References

Barreca, S., Sigouin, C. S., Lambert, C., and Ansley, B. (2004). Effects of extra training on the ability of stroke survivors to perform an independent sit-to-stand: A randomized controlled trial. *Journal of Geriatric Physical Therapy*, 27(2), 59–64.

Bischoff-Ferrari, H. A., Dawson-Hughes, B., Staehelin, H. B., Orav, J. E., Stuck, A. E., Theiler, R., Wong, J. B., Egli, A., Kiel, D. P., and Henschkowski, J. (2009). Fall prevention with supplemental and active forms of vitamin D: A meta-analysis of randomised controlled trials. *British Medical Journal*, 339, b3692.

Bischoff-Ferrari, H. A., Stahelin, H. B., Dick, W., Akos, R., Knecht, M., Salis, C., Nebiker, M., Theiler, R., Pfeifer, M., Begerow, B., Lew, R. A., and Conzelmann, M. (2003). Effects of vitamin D and calcium supplementation on falls: A randomized controlled trial. *Journal of Bone and Mineral Research*, 18(2), 343–351.

Bouldin, E. L., Andresen, E. M., Dunton, N. E., Simon, M., Waters, T. M., Liu, M., Daniels, M. J., Mion, L. C., and Shorr, R. I. (2013). Falls among adult patients hospitalized in the United States: Prevalence and trends. *Journal of Patient Safety*, 9(1), 13–17.

Broe, K. E., Chen, T. C., Weinberg, J., Bischoff-Ferrari, H. A., Holick, M. F., and Kiel, D. P. (2007). A higher dose of vitamin d reduces the risk of falls in nursing home residents: A randomized, multiple-dose study. *Journal of the American Geriatrics Society*, 55(2), 234–239.

Burleigh, E., McColl, J., and Potter, J. (2007). Does vitamin D stop inpatients falling? A randomised controlled trial. *Age and Ageing*, 36(5), 507–513.

Butler, M., Norton, R., Lee-Joe, T., Cheng, A., and Campbell, A. J. (1996). The risks of hip fracture in older people from private homes and institutions. *Age and Ageing*, 25(5), 381–385.

Carmeron, I. D., Murray, G. R., Gillespie, L. D., Robertson, M. C., Hill, K. D., Cumming, R. G., and Kerse, N. (2010). Interventions for preventing falls in older people in nursing care facilities and hospitals. *Cochrane Database of Systematic Reviews*, 20(1), 54–65.

Chu, L. W., Chiu, A. Y., and Chi, I. (2008). Falls and subsequent health service utilization in community-dwelling Chinese older adults. *Archives of Gerontology and Geriatrics*, 46(2), 125–135.

Crotty, M., Rowett, D., Spurling, L., Giles, L. C., and Phillips, P. A. (2004). Does the addition of a pharmacist transition coordinator improve evidence-based medication management and health outcomes in older adults moving from the hospital to a long-term care facility? Results of a randomized, controlled trial. *The American Journal of Geriatric Pharmacotherapy*, 2(4), 257–264.

Cumming, R. G., Sherrington, C., Lord, S. R., Simpson, J. M., Vogler, C., Cameron, I. D., and Naganathan, V. (2008). Cluster randomised trial of a targeted multifactorial intervention to prevent falls among older people in hospital. *British Medical Journal*, 336(7647), 758–760.

Donald, I. P., Pitt, K., Armstrong, E., and Shuttleworth, H. (2000). Preventing falls on an elderly care rehabilitation ward. *Clinical Rehabilitation*, 14(2), 178–185.

Dromerick, A., and Reding, M. (1994). Medical and neurological complications during inpatient stroke rehabilitation. *Stroke*, 25(2), 358–361.

Faber, M. J., Bosscher, R. J., Chin, A. P. M. J., and Wieringen, P. C. van. (2006). Effects of exercise programs on falls and mobility in frail and pre-frail older adults: A multicenter randomized controlled trial. *Archives of Physical Medicine and Rehabilitation*, 87(7), 885–896.

Flicker, L., MacInnis, R. J., Stein, M. S., Scherer, S. C., Mead, K. E., Nowson, C. A., Thomas, J., Lowndes, C., Hopper, J. L., and Wark, J. D. (2005). Should older people in residential care receive vitamin D to prevent falls? Results of a randomized trial. *Journal of the American Geriatrics Society*, 53(11), 1881–1888.

Forster, A., and Young, J. (1995). Incidence and consequences of falls due to stroke: A systematic inquiry. *British Medical Journal*, 311(6997), 83–86.

Gillespie, L. D., Robertson, M. C., Gillespie, W. J., Sherrington, C., Gates, S., Clemson, L. M., and Lamb, S. E. (2012). Interventions for preventing falls in older people living in the community. *Cochrane Database of Systematic Reviews*, 9(11).

Graham, K. C., and Cvach, M. (2010). Monitor alarm fatigue: Standardizing use of physiological monitors and decreasing nuisance alarms. *American Journal of Critical Care*, 19(1), 28–34.

Grealish, L., and Chaboyer, W. (2015). Older, in hospital and confused – The value of nursing care in preventing falls in older people with cognitive impairment. *International Journal of Nursing Studies*, 52(8), 1285–1287.

Haines, T. P., Bennell, K. L., Osborne, R. H., and Hill, K. D. (2004). Effectiveness of targeted falls prevention programme in subacute hospital setting: Randomised controlled trial. *British Medical Journal*, 328(7441), 676.

Haines, T. P., Bennell, K. L., Osborne, R. H., and Hill, K. D. (2006). A new instrument for targeting falls prevention interventions was accurate and clinically applicable in a hospital setting. *Journal of Clinical Epidemiology*, 59(2), 168–175.

Haines, T. P., Massey, B., Varghese, P., Fleming, J., and Gray, L. (2009). Inconsistency in classification and reporting of in-hospital falls. *Journal of the American Geriatric Society*, 57(3), 517–523.

Hill, A. M., Waldron, N., Etherton-Beer, C., McPhail, S. M., Ingram, K., Flicker, L., and Haines, T. P. (2014). A stepped-wedge cluster randomised controlled trial for evaluating rates of falls among inpatients in aged care rehabilitation units receiving tailored multimedia education in addition to usual care: A trial protocol. *British Medical Journal Open*, 4(1), e004195.

Jarvis, N., Kerr, K., and Mockett, S. (2007). Pilot study to explore the feasibility of a randomised controlled trial to determine the dose effect of physiotherapy on patients admitted to hospital following a fall. *Practical Evidence*, 2(2), 4–12.

King, M. B., and Tinetti, M. E. (1995). Falls in community-dwelling older persons. *Journal of the American Geriatrics Society*, 43(10), 1146–1154.

Klinkenberg, W. D., and Potter, P. (2016). Validity of the Johns Hopkins fall risk assessment tool for predicting falls on inpatient medicine services. *Journal of Nursing Care Quality*, 32(2), 108–113.

Lightbody, E., Watkins, C., Leathley, M., Sharma, A., and Lye, M. (2002). Evaluation of a nurse-led falls prevention programme versus usual care: A randomized controlled trial. *Age and Ageing*, 31(3), 203–210.

Lilley, J. M., Arie, T., and Chilvers, C. E. (1995). Accidents involving older people: A review of the literature. *Age and Ageing*, 24(4), 346–365.

Liu, J. Y. (2015). Fear of falling in robust community-dwelling older people: Results of a cross-sectional study. *Journal of Clinical Nursing*, 24(3–4), 393–405.

Mann, C. M., Ottenbacher, K. J., Fraas, L., and Tomita, M. (1999). Effectiveness of assistive technology and environmental interventions in maintaining independence and reducing home care costs for the frail elderly. *Archives of Family Medicine*, 8, 210–217.

Miskelly, F. G. (2001). Assistive technology in elderly care. *Age and Ageing*, 30(6), 455–458.

Mulrow, C. D., Gerety, M. B., Kanten, D., Cornell, J. E., DeNino, L. A., Chiodo, L., Aguilar, C., O'Neil, M. B., Rosenberg, J., and Solis, R. M. (1994). A randomized trial of physical rehabilitation for very frail nursing home residents. *Journal of the American Medical Association*, 271(7), 519–524.

National Institute for Health and Care Excellence. (2013). *Falls in older people: Assessing risk and prevention.* Manchester: NICE.

National Patient Safety Agency. (2010). *Slips, trips and falls data update.* London: NPSA.

Panel on Prevention of Falls in Older Persons. (2011). Summary of the Updated American Geriatrics Society/British Geriatrics Society clinical practice guideline for prevention of falls in older persons. *Journal of the American Geriatrics Society*, 59(1), 148–157.

Parker, M. J., Gillespie, W. J., and Gillespie, L. D. (2006). Effectiveness of hip protectors for preventing hip fractures in elderly people: Systematic review. *British Medical Journal*, 332(7541), 571–574.

Patel, K. V., Phelan, E. A., Leveille, S. G., Lamb, S. E., Missikpode, C., Wallace, R. B., Guralnik, J. M., and Turk, D. C. (2014). High prevalence of falls, fear of falling, and impaired balance in older adults with pain in the United States: Findings from the 2011 National Health and Aging Trends Study. *Journal of the American Geriatrics Society*, 62(10), 1844–1852.

Phelan, E. A., Mahoney, J. E., Voit, J. C., and Stevens, J. A. (2015). Assessment and management of fall risk in primary care settings. *Medical Clinics of North America*, 99(2), 281–293.

Pietrzak, E., Cotea, C., and Pullman, S. (2014). Does smart home technology prevent falls in community-dwelling older adults: A literature review. *Journal of Informatics in Primary Care*, 21(3), 105–112.

Pratt, N. L., Ramsay, E. N., Kalisch, Ellett. L. M., Nguyen, T. A., Barratt, J. D., and Roughead, E. E. (2014). Association between use of multiple psychoactive medicines and hospitalization for falls: Retrospective analysis of a large healthcare claim database. *Drug Safety*, 37(7), 529–535.

Rajendram, O., Corcoran, A., Kinosian, B., and Alwan, M. (2008). Falls, fall prevention and fall detection technology. In M. Alwan and R. Felder (Eds.), *Aging medicine, eldercare technology for clinical practitioners* (pp. 187–202). New Jersey: Humana Press.

Ray, W. A., Taylor, J. A., Meador, K. G., Thapa, P. B., Brown, A. K., Kajihara, H. K., Davis, C., Gideon, P., and Griffin, M. R. (1997). A randomized trial of a consultation service to reduce falls in nursing homes. *Journal of the American Medical Association*, 278(7), 557–562.

Rosendahl, E., Gustafson, Y., Nordin, E., Lundin-Olsson, L., and Nyberg, L. (2008). A randomized controlled trial of fall prevention by a high-intensity functional exercise program for older people living in residential care facilities. *Aging Clinical and Experimental Research*, 20(1), 67–75.

Rubenstein, L. Z., Robbins, A. S., Josephson, K. R., Schulman, B. L., and Osterweil, D. (1990). The value of assessing falls in an elderly population: A randomized clinical trial. *Annals of Internal Medicine*, 113(4), 308–316.

Sahota, O. (2009). Vitamin D and in-patient falls. *Age and Ageing*, 38(3), 339–340.

Sahota, O., Drummond, A., Kendrick, D., Grainge, M. J., Vass, C., Sach, T., Gladman, J., and Avis, M. (2014). REFINE (REducing Falls in In-patieNt Elderly) using bed and bedside chair pressure sensors linked to radio-pagers in acute hospital care: A randomised controlled trial. *Age and Ageing*, 43(2), 247–253.

Sayer, A. A., Syddall, H. E., Martin, H. J., Dennison, E. M., Anderson, F. H., and Cooper, C. (2006). Falls, sarcopenia, and growth in early life: Findings from the Hertfordshire cohort study. *American Journal of Epidemiology*, 164(7), 665–671.

Scheffer, A. C., Schuurmans, M. J., Dijk, N. van, Hooft, T. van der, and Rooij, S. E. de. (2008). Fear of falling: Measurement strategy, prevalence, risk factors and consequences among older persons. *Age and Ageing*, 37(1), 19–24.

Schoenfelder, D. P. (2000). A fall prevention program for elderly individuals: Exercise in long-term care settings. *Journal of Gerontological Nursing*, 26(3), 43–51.

Shorr, R. I., Chandler, A. M., Mion, L. C., Waters, T. M., Liu, M., Daniels, M. J., Kessler, L. A., and Miller, S. T. (2012). Effects of an intervention to increase bed alarm use to prevent falls in hospitalized patients: A cluster randomized trial. *Annals of Internal Medicine*, 157(10), 692–699.

Sousa, N., Mendes, R., Silva, A., and Oliveira, J. (2016). Combined exercise is more effective than aerobic exercise in the improvement of fall risk factors: A randomized controlled trial in community-dwelling older men. *Clinical Rehabilitation,* 31(4), 478–486.

Stevens, J. A. (2013). The STEADI tool kit: A fall prevention resource for health care providers. *IHS Primary Care Provider*, 39(9), 162–166.

Stevens, J. A., Corso, P. S., Finkelstein, E. A., and Miller, T. R. (2006). The costs of fatal and non-fatal falls among older adults. *Injury Prevention*, 12(5), 290–295.

Stevens, J. A., and Phelan, E. A. (2013). Development of STEADI: A fall prevention resource for health care providers. *Health Promotion Practice*, 14(5), 706–714.

Tannenbaum, C., Diaby, V., Singh, D., Perreault, S., Luc, M., and Vasiliadis, H. M. (2015). Sedative-hypnotic medicines and falls in community-dwelling older adults: A cost-effectiveness (decision-tree) analysis from a US Medicare perspective. *Drugs and Aging*, 32(4), 305–314.

Tchalla, A. E., Lachal, F., Cardinaud, N., Saulnier, I., Bhalla, D., Roquejoffre, A., Rialle, V., Preux, P. M., and Dantoine, T. (2012). Efficacy of simple home-based technologies combined with a monitoring assistive center in decreasing falls in a frail elderly population (results of the Esoppe study). *Archives of Gerontology and Geriatrics*, 55(3), 683–689.

Thornlow, D. K., Anderson, R., and Oddone, E. (2009). Cascade iatrogenesis: Factors leading to the development of adverse events in hospitalized older adults. *International Journal of Nursing Studies*, 46(11), 1528–1535.

Tideiksaar, R., Feiner, C. F., and Maby, J. (1993). Falls prevention: The efficacy of a bed alarm system in an acute-care setting. *Mount Sinai Journal of Medicine*, 60(6), 522–527.

Tinetti, M. E., Doucette, J., Claus, E., and Marottoli, R. (1995). Risk factors for serious injury during falls by older persons in the community. *Journal of the American Geriatrics Society*, 43(11), 1214–1221.

Webster, J., Courtney, M., O'Rourke, P., Marsh, N., Gale, C., Abbott, B., McRae, P., and Mason, K. (2008). Should elderly patients be screened for their 'falls risk'? Validity of the STRATIFY falls screening tool and predictors of falls in a large acute hospital. *Age and Ageing*, 37(6), 702–706.

Williams, A. (2005). An aging population: Burden or blessing? *Value in Health*, 8(4), 447–450.

Yardley, L., Bishop, F. L., Beyer, N., Hauer, K., Kempen, G. I., Piot-Ziegler, C., Todd, C. J., Cuttelod, T., Horne, M., Lanta, K., and Holt, A. R. (2006). Older people's views of falls-prevention interventions in six European countries. *Gerontologist*, 46(5), 650–660.

Zermansky, A. G., Alldred, D. P., Petty, D. R., Raynor, D. K., Freemantle, N., Eastaugh, J., and Bowie, P. (2006). Clinical medication review by a pharmacist of elderly people living in care homes--randomised controlled trial. *Age and Ageing*, 35(6), 586–591.

10

PAIN MANAGEMENT AND ASSESSMENT

Trevor Thompson, M. Elena Mendoza and Rachael E. Docking

This chapter discusses:

- The problem of pain in an aging population
- Non-pharmacological treatments for pain
- Assessment of pain

Introduction

Millions of people around the world live with chronic pain. Chronic pain, usually defined as pain lasting anything from three to six months or more, can significantly impair mood, sleep, daily activities, relationships, overall quality of life and ability to work (Abdulla et al., 2013; American Geriatrics Society, 2009), and cause misery to even the most stoic of individuals. When pain fails to be controlled, it can compromise immune function, promote tumour growth and inhibit healing following surgery, resulting in increased mortality, and has led some authors to provocatively refute the maxim that 'pain can't kill' (Lynch & Watson, 2006).

There are numerous types of chronic pain, including back pain, headache, abdominal pain and joint pain, and these can be the immediate result of disease or injury. It can be surprising to learn, however, that chronic pain can persist when any injury has long since healed or even when there is no identifiable injury or disease (but a likely malfunction of the nervous system).

Pain experienced at any age group creates difficulties in carrying out the most basic day-to-day tasks, with the impact on older persons even more pronounced, as everyday life activities can often be a challenge for them even without pain. Aside from the individual burden, pain carries a substantial economic burden. Economic costs are driven in part by the costs of lost productivity, absenteeism and early retirement. In the United Kingdom in 2000, back pain alone was found to have cost the economy £12.3 billion (Maniadakis & Gray, 2000). The international figures are even more startling. In the United States, the estimated total incremental cost of healthcare due to pain has ranged from \$261 to \$300 billion (Gaskin and Richard, 2011). In Germany, societal costs of back pain have been calculated to be €16.5 to €50 billion, while in Portugal, the total indirect cost of chronic back and joint pain in 2008 was estimated at approximately €740 million (Gouveia et al., 2012).

Pain in an aging population

While it has been previously hypothesized that the prevalence of pain decreases with age, there is growing evidence to suggest that pain continues to increase in older age, particularly disabling pain or pain sufficient to interfere with day-to-day living (Dionne, Dunn & Croft, 2006; Docking et al., 2011; Thomas et al., 2007). Pain appears to become most common at around 55–65 years (Gibson & Lussier, 2012), with older adults reporting more pain complaints in general as well as increased incidence of chronic pain conditions. International epidemiological studies reveal vulnerability to pain in later life to be a truly global phenomenon. A recent survey suggests that the total number of adults with chronic pain exceeds those with heart disease, cancer and diabetes combined (Steglitz, Buscemi and Ferguson, 2012), with over half of older adults in the United States reporting bothersome pain in the preceding month (Patel et al., 2014). Studies conducted in Europe, Asia and Australia (Jackson et al., 2014; Henderson et al., 2013; Leadley et al., 2012), and across developed and less-developed countries (Tsang et al., 2008) have reported similar findings.

It is evident that pain presents a significant challenge to the goal of positive aging, and one that is only likely to become more pressing given our rapidly aging population. This challenge can only be met with appropriate and effective techniques for pain management. Pharmacological intervention is usually considered the first line treatment, with analgesic medication ranging from milder drugs such as paracetamol (called acetaminophen in the United States and Japan) to stronger, opiate drugs that act on the central nervous system and are designed to treat moderate or severe pain. The ability of medication to deliver effective pain relief is well established (Lynch & Watson, 2006). However, medication use is not without safety concerns, with adverse reactions generally varying with the type and dosage of the drug administered (Reid, Eccleston & Pillemer, 2015). Importantly, physiological changes with age mean these concerns may be especially relevant to older adults. Older patients are generally at higher risk of adverse drug reactions and demonstrate increased sensitivity to standard dosages (American Geriatrics Society, 2009).

Additional worries include an increased likelihood of other health conditions and prescribed medications inviting drug contraindications, as well as a heightened sensitivity to invasive methods of administration (see Abdulla et al., 2013 for a review). Accordingly, recent guidelines have suggested that non-pharmacological interventions should be considered in older people (Abdulla et al., 2013), either as multi-modal strategies in combination with analgesics (Reid, Ecclestion & Pillemer, 2015) or potentially alone when side effects from medication prove prohibitive. Encouragingly, there is optimism about the role of non-drug-based interventions as treatment for older adults with pain (McGuire et al., 2014).

As a 'non-pharmacological intervention' is simply one that does not involve drugs, the term naturally incorporates a range of diverse strategies, ranging from physical therapies such as physiotherapy, massage and exercise to psychological approaches such as cognitive behavioural therapy. Considerable research has been conducted over the last few years to evaluate the efficacy of some of these non-pharmacological approaches to management of the affective, cognitive, behavioural and socio-cultural dimensions of pain in the elderly. Developments in methods for pain management have been accompanied by attempts to develop improved methods of pain assessment. The better we are able to assess and monitor pain, the more accurately we are able to diagnose it and evaluate interventions designed to treat it. Progress in this area may be especially valuable for the aging population given evidence that older adults are more likely to have difficulties communicating their pain (Chapman, 2010; Clarke et al., 2012), have their pain under assessed (Denny & Guido, 2012; Pautex and Vogt-Ferrier, 2006) and be inadequately treated (Tracy & Morrison, 2013). The last few years have seen progress in ways to make the assessment of pain as accurate, reliable and convenient as possible, including technology-assisted self-management interventions, electronic pain diaries, clinical dashboards and interventions delivered using Internet and mobile applications.

In the remainder of this chapter, we will outline psychosocial and physical interventions, review evidence for their efficacy and evaluate their potential as techniques for pain management in older adults. Drug therapies will not be discussed, as these have been well documented elsewhere (e.g. Lynch & Watson, 2006; Bandolier, 2015). We will then briefly review new methods for pain assessment and evaluate their promise for use in an older population.

Psychosocial interventions

Cognitive behavioural therapy (CBT)

CBT consists of a set of psychological techniques to change dysfunctional thoughts and to modify unhelpful beliefs, attitudes and behaviours. The goal is to increase patient's self-control over pain. Multidisciplinary interventions that include CBT and exercise are recommended by the American Geriatrics Society's guidelines for older adults with chronic pain (American Geriatrics Society, 1998, 2002). However, only a few studies have examined the efficacy of CBT in the elderly.

There are two studies that applied a CBT intervention to nursing home residents. One found a significant decrease in pain after treatment (Cipher, Clifford & Roper, 2007). And the second one compared CBT with an attention/support control treatment, and results showed that 80 per cent of patients in the CBT group reported improvements in pain, compared with 34 per cent in the control group (Cook, 1998). These effects remained at four months follow-up.

Another study examined the effects of a CBT pain management program designed for community-dwelling seniors. Both the intervention group and the wait-list control group reported decreases in pain intensity, but CBT resulted in fewer maladaptive beliefs about pain and greater use of relaxation (Green et al., 2009).

Finally, a more recent study compared the effects of an outpatient interdisciplinary pain rehabilitation program based on a CBT model and incorporated opioid withdrawal in different age groups (Darchuk et al., 2010). Results showed that older patients reported reductions in pain severity, depression, catastrophizing and pain interference, as well as an increase in perceived control and physical and social functioning. Improvements were comparable to the middle age group, whereas younger patients had greater effects in these variables; however, the significant analgesic reductions were found in all groups.

Acceptance and commitment therapy (ACT)

ACT is one of the approaches comprised in the so-called third wave of CBT. It involves working with important life values and is based on the acceptance of pain without attempting to control or change it. Results from a study that compared the response to ACT versus CBT of adults of different groups of age with chronic pain showed that older adults were more likely to respond to ACT than younger adults. This may be because older adults have tried more options to reduce pain, as opposed to younger adults who may have still other options to exhaust. Therefore, older adults may be more willing than younger adults to respond to an acceptance approach in which the efforts are focused on living according to personal important values regardless of pain (Wetherell et al., 2015).

There are preliminary findings from two studies indicating that ACT-based interventions may be promising in the elderly with chronic pain. One study examined the effects of an ACT intervention to increase daily functioning by increasing psychological flexibility without trying to decrease pain (McCracken & Jones, 2012). Results showed gains in measures of pain, psychosocial disability, anxiety, depression, psychological acceptance and mindfulness.

Another study with patients living in nursing homes (Alonso-Fernández et al., 2015) combined ACT with the Selective Optimization with Compensation model (SOC; Baltes & Baltes, 1990). This model considers aging as a process of gains and losses to which older adults may achieve a successful adaptation to life changes when using strategies of selection of goals, compensation for losses and optimization of performance. This approach is consistent with ACT and the combination of both may help maximize the elderly's ability to make adjustments in behaviours and decisions consistent with their values. Results indicated a significant increase in chronic pain acceptance after treatment that the control group did not report. This approach may be a suitable option for older people with chronic musculoskeletal pain, although additional research is necessary to provide more evidence about its efficacy and to examine the different contributions of each technique (Alonso-Fernández et al., 2015).

Finally, a recent systematic review and meta-analysis concluded that while there is simply insufficient evidence to provide an authoritative evaluation of the efficacy of ACT for any disorder, it is 'probably efficacious' for chronic pain (Öst, 2014). Therefore, more research is necessary to clarify the benefits of ACT in older adults.

Hypnosis

Hypnosis has a long history in pain management. It is a self-control technique that can be used alone or as an adjunct to other treatments and, when it is combined, it enhances the benefits of the other interventions (Kirsch, Montgomery & Sapirstein, 1995). In clinical settings, it involves a hypnotic induction followed by suggestions targeting the presenting symptoms and includes training in self-hypnosis so that the patients can use it on their own whenever they need it.

Although further research is necessary to clarify the mechanisms of reductions in pain through hypnosis, findings from recent functional neuroimaging studies have found that hypnotic strategies modulate pain, influencing cortical and subcortical activity in those parts of the brain that are involved in pain perception and modulation (Del Casale et al., 2015).

According to the published trials and reviews, there is consistent evidence that hypnosis is an effective and efficient technique in the treatment of pain, both chronic and acute, across several conditions (Dorfman et al., 2013; Elkins, Jensen & Patterson, 2007; Jensen, 2009; Jensen & Patterson, 2006; Stoelb et al., 2009). Evidence also indicates that patients report high rates of satisfaction with treatments that include hypnosis even when that treatment did not result in large decreases in pain intensity (Jensen et al., 2006).

Results from a recent meta-analysis (Adachi et al., 2014) indicated that hypnosis is moderately more efficacious than standard care, wait-list and other psychological interventions, including CBT, for managing non-headache chronic pain. Additional research is needed to examine the efficacy of hypnosis compared to other psychological interventions for headaches.

These studies have been carried out with adults of different age groups. Even though some of the medical conditions studied are more prevalent in older people, specific research focusing in the elderly and the needs of this population is needed.

A recent pilot study with older adults used hypnosis as an analgesic method during photodynamic therapy for the treatment of pre-carcinomatous lesions (Paquier-Valette et al., 2014).

Results showed that hypnosis reduced pain during the procedure, indicating that it may be a promising method for managing the main adverse effect of photodynamic therapy in the elderly.

Overall, studies support the clinical use of hypnotic techniques for pain management since it is cost effective, has minimal side effects and enhances other therapeutic techniques.

Mindfulness and meditation

Meditation is a practice to train the mind or induce a mode of consciousness in which the person realizes some benefit or acknowledges the mental contents without identifying with them (Lutz et al., 2008). Studies of the effectiveness of mindfulness-based meditation specific for the elderly are scarce and results are not consistent. Some benefits have been reported in patients with chronic back pain (Morone et al., 2008), but these effects have not been replicated when patients present a higher severity of pain (Morone et al., 2009).

Further research is necessary to establish the efficacy of mindfulness meditation in older patients.

Guided imagery and relaxation

Guided imagery has been used for centuries to decrease anxiety and pain. Its goal is to focus the attention to evoke and generate mental images that recreate the sensory perceptions on sights, sounds, music and words to elicit emotions and sensations that are helpful for the patient's problem (Antall & Kresevic, 2004).

Guided imagery is often used along with relaxation and some studies have suggested that they may be effective strategies for pain management for postoperative older patients (Antall and Kresevic, 2004) and for older women with osteoarthritis (Baird & Sands, 2004).

Research using neuroimaging technologies has found that imagery can engage the same neural structures that are involved in perception in the same modality and that these structures can also affect the body as the actual perceptual experience (Kosslyn, Ganis & Thompson, 2001). These findings warrant more research on its mechanisms and on the efficacy on different populations to improve its use and benefits.

Biofeedback

Biofeedback is a technique that trains the patients to gain awareness of their physiological functions so that they learn to control them at will. It is used with relaxation and cognitive techniques, and there are reports of comparable results for both young and older adults in the management of pain (Middaugh et al., 1991; Middaugh & Pawlick, 2002). However, the evidence for the efficacy of biofeedback is limited and controlled studies are necessary to evaluate the contribution of this technique to the results obtained in the multicomponent programs that have been examined to date.

Music

Music has a long history of use in medical settings and some studies have suggested that it is promising as an analgesic strategy in patients with fibromyalgia (Linnemann et al., 2015), patients undergoing surgery and its recovery (Hole et al., 2015), and during painful physical therapy (Bellieni et al., 2013).

Findings from reviews have reported that, in older adults, both receptive and active aspects of music have shown improvements in function and symptoms in stroke rehabilitation, several forms of dementia and pain control (Kneafsey, 1997; Myskja & Lindbaek, 2000). Another review reported benefits of music and singing for the older patients in different symptoms and recommended further research to support these findings and to explore how nursing interventions incorporating music should be efficiently implemented (Skingley & Vella-Burrows, 2010).

Finally, a systematic review that focused on home-based music therapy (Schmid & Ostermann, 2010) analysed the research on the programs developed for the long-term care of geriatric patients after they have been discharged from hospital or those who need palliative care. Authors found that, although settings were heterogeneous, music listening programs showed to be beneficial in the reduction of depression and pain, and in improving quality of life. Hence, home-based music therapy can be considered as an innovative service in healthcare for the elderly (Schmid and Ostermann, 2010).

Mirror therapy

The clinical use of mirror visual feedback is used for managing phantom pain by restoring motor function through plastic changes in the primary motor cortex (Michielsen et al., 2011). In a case series, this therapy was used with older adults after recent lower limb amputation (González et al., 2013) and results showed analgesic effects and benefits as a rehabilitation instrument. Although this study does not provide enough evidence, it suggests that mirror therapy, which has shown good results in other populations, can be promising in geriatric patients.

Physical interventions

Exercise

It has been found that, for older people, inactivity is one of the most commonly used strategies to manage pain (Brown et al., 2011). Even though older adults report that inactivity decreases pain, it results in additional problems. Moreover, there is evidence supporting that activity and exercise adapted to the person's physical conditions can provide a number of health benefits, such as improved fitness, lubrication of the joints, less stiffness with movement, increased endorphins and activity diversion (Brown et al., 2011).

In a review of the effects of exercise alone or with psychosocial interventions in managing chronic pain in older adults, Park and Hughes (2012) reported that after these interventions, participants experienced a significant reduction in pain and an enhanced functional capacity.

In order to foster mobility and activity in the elderly with chronic pain, it is important that health providers reassure the patients that physical activity that is adapted to their needs and conditions and within reasonable limits provides benefits in different domains and does not necessarily cause harm. Professionals imparting pain management education should address patient's beliefs, since research has found that fear of movement and re-injury or fall predicts avoidance of activity and causes psychological distress (Lamé et al., 2005).

Qigong

Qigong is a technique from Chinese traditional medicine that integrates physical postures, breathing techniques and focused intention. There is one study with older adults that found this technique as promising in helping manage pain and mood disturbance, and in improving physical function (Trott et al., 2009). However, a different study with the same population did not find significant effects for neck pain (Yang & Kim, 2005). Future studies are necessary to prove the efficacy of this technique for pain management in the elderly.

Transcutaneous electrical nerve stimulation (TENS) and acupuncture

TENS is a form of electrical stimulation with surface electrodes. It is a safe technique that activates a complex neuronal network to modulate pain perception by activating descending inhibitory systems in the central nervous system to reduce hyperalgesia (Vance et al., 2014). A recent systematic review demonstrated a medium-sized statistically significant effect of TENS for management of pain in people with multiple sclerosis (Sawant et al., 2015).

However, evidence of the effectiveness of TENS in community-dwelling older adults with chronic pain is inconsistent. Two randomized controlled trials (RCTs) found significant relief for knee pain (Ng, Leung & Poon, 2003) and for back pain (Grant et al., 1999) in this population, but a third one (Breit & Van der Wall, 2004) concluded that TENS was not effective for chronic low back pain.

TENS has also been used with acupuncture. Results from a RCT that compared these two treatments alone and combined in older adults with chronic low back pain demonstrated a reduction in pain intensity and an improvement in quality of life in the group that received the combined treatment that was superior to the effects in the groups receiving the treatments alone (Itoh et al., 2009).

Finally, the evidence regarding the efficacy of acupuncture for older adults is inconsistent and many of the studies showing positive benefits have methodological weaknesses (Abdulla et al., 2013). Future research is needed to clarify acupuncture efficacy for pain management.

Pain perception and pain management in the elderly

In order to develop effective treatment interventions for chronic pain in older people, it is important to take into account the pertinent research findings.

Distraction is commonly used as a strategy to reduce the perceived pain. However, according to a study by Zhou and colleagues (2015), for older adults there is an increase in the perception of pain during distraction that may be due to limited working memory capacity resulting from the deterioration/degeneration of frontal cerebral networks. This is consistent with studies indicating that cognitive dual processing is sensitive to the effects of aging, limiting executive resources and reducing the resources for pain modulation as a result of cognitive distraction (Beursken & Bock, 2012; Hahn, Wild-Wall and Falkenstein, 2011). Thus, distraction techniques may not be as effective for pain management in the elderly as they are in younger adults.

Moreover, it has been found that pain intensity varies according to ethnicity. In a study with ethnically diverse community-dwelling older adults, African Americans reported the highest levels of pain intensity, followed by Afro-Caribbeans and Hispanics, and European-Americans reported the lowest pain levels (Park et al., 2015).

There is evidence supporting that specific pain-related beliefs, attitudes and coping responses play an important role in patient adjustment to chronic pain and in mediating the way patients engage with treatments (Degood & Tait, 2001; Jensen, Turner and Romano, 2007). Findings indicate that the beliefs and coping strategies most consistently and strongly associated with patient outcomes are the adaptive belief of having control over pain and the maladaptive responses of guarding, resting and catastrophizing (Jensen, Turner & Romano, 2007).

A recent study analysed the relationship between pain-related beliefs and the psychological and daily functioning of the elderly (Miró, Queral & Nolla, 2014). Findings indicated that those patients who believed that one has control over pain reported better psychological functioning and lower levels of pain interference. However, patients who believed that one is unable to function due to pain, that pain is a sign of harm, that activity has to be avoided and that others should provide help in response to one's pain behaviours reported poorer psychological functioning and more pain interference (Miró, Queral & Nolla et al., 2014).

Catastrophizing is a factor consistently associated with both pain intensity and pain interference (Keefe et al., 2004; Quartana, Campbell & Edwards, 2009; Thompson et al., 2008; Thompson et al., 2011). It is the tendency to focus on pain and evaluate pain and its effects in unrealistic and negative ways, and comprises elements of rumination, magnification and helplessness (DeGood & Tait, 2001; Sullivan, 2012).

Clinical interventions that include strategies for decreasing pain-related catastrophizing, such as cognitive therapy, are beneficial for decreasing pain intensity (Ehde & Jensen, 2004). However, research also indicates that catastrophizing may be an exaggerated pain expression aimed to maximize proximity, social assistance and empathic responses from other people (Sullivan, 2012). Thus, the patient's pain catastrophizing is followed by support and help from other people, and it is reinforced by positive consequences, becoming a maladaptive cycle (Burns et al., 2015). Therefore, pain catastrophizing may be considered as a coping strategy in which people express their pain to obtain assistance and support from others. These findings have clinical relevance because interventions that address pain catastrophizing without providing skills for obtaining others' support in an adaptive way may not have the expected effects in pain management. It is necessary to consider the interpersonal processes and psychosocial contexts involved in pain catastrophizing (Burns et al., 2015).

In sum, non-pharmacological approaches for pain management are cost effective, have minimal side effects and have been demonstrated to help improve the results of multidimensional treatments for pain management. When tailoring interventions for pain management in the elderly it is important to consider the specific characteristics of this population reported in the literature, such as their difficulty to use distraction and their better response to acceptance approaches.

Likewise, health professionals should be aware of the beliefs and attitudes that may hinder the elderly's efficient pain management, such as that pain always means harm, that activity causes injury and should be avoided, and that one does not have control over pain. Interventions including educational components addressing these factors are more efficient and suitable to the elderly's needs. Finally, strategies aimed to reduce catastrophizing and, therefore, to decrease pain intensity should also provide skills to ask for help to others, to avoid the use of catastrophizing as a maladaptive coping strategy.

Pain assessment

Although pain becomes increasingly common with advancing age, there is limited research to inform the assessment and management of pain in those >65 years, particularly those with dementia. Evidence suggests that this group may not receive adequate assessment of their pain and pain that is assessed is often under-treated or poorly managed (Closs et al., 2004). However, this is compounded by the fact that pain is less likely to be communicated in a language we can understand (Collett et al., 2007).

Reasons for poor assessment and treatment of pain in older adults include a belief that pain is a normal part of aging, lack of understanding around polypharmacy, and a lack of routine pain assessment and training for healthcare professionals. Previous evidence has found that nurses themselves identify their lack of knowledge as a fundamental barrier to optimal pain management (Brunier, Carson & Harrison, 1995).

Pain is, by its nature, a self-reported measure, and therefore accurate assessment can be a challenge, particularly in a population with sensory deficits and potential difficulties with cognition. However, there have been pain assessment tools developed and tested in the older population which have proved relatively successful. A few of the most widely used scales are the Numeric Rating Scale (NRS; McCafferey & Beebe, 1989), the Verbal Descriptor Scale (VDS; Melzack, 1975), the Faces Pain Scale-Revised (FPS-R; Bieri et al., 1990), the Wong-Baker Faces Pain Scale (Wong & Baker, 1988), the Visual Analogue Scale (VAS: Von Korff et al., 1992) and the McGill Pain Questionnaire (Melzack, 1975). These are described briefly below.

Numeric rating scale (NRS)

The NRS asks participants to rate their current pain intensity from 0 ("no pain") to 10 ("worst possible pain") and is one of the most widely used instruments for pain screening due to the fact that it is simple to administer, easy to score, and readily administered in written or verbal form. The NRS can be oriented either vertically or horizontally; however a vertical presentation can be easier for someone who has problems around abstract thinking.

Verbal descriptor scale (VDS)

The VDS asks patients to describe their pain using three to five numerically ranked words, including "none", "mild", "moderate", "severe" and "unbearable" or "the most intense pain imaginable". The VDS is short, simple and easy to score and analyse; it also shows good reliability and validity when used with older adults. However, evidence has found it is not the best scale to use for older adults with cognitive impairment compared to a descriptor scale where less vocabulary is required (Feldt, Ryden & Miles, 1998).

Faces pain scale-revised (FPS-R)

The FPS-R was initially developed for use with children but has since been used with older adults with cognitive difficulties. It consists of seven faces representing increasing levels of pain from which patients have to choose the face that best represents their own pain.

Wong-Baker faces pain scale

The Wong-Baker Faces Pain Scale, similar to the FPS-R, presents participants with increasingly distressed faces and asks them to choose the face which matches their current pain state most accurately. The Wong-Baker Faces Pain Scale is selected as one of the easiest scales to use for older adults with and without cognitive impairment.

Visual analogue scale (VAS)

The VAS presents participants with a line, for which the left-hand side is labelled "no pain" and the right-hand side is labelled "most intense pain imaginable". However, this scale has challenges related to educational level, cognitive impairment and motor abilities (Herr, Mobily & Richardson, 1998). While it is easy to use, it is not the most appropriate pain assessment tool for older adults.

McGill Pain Questionnaire (MPQ)

The MPQ is a multidimensional pain assessment tool which provides a thorough evaluation of pain, including location, intensity, temporal qualities and sensitivity to change. The MPQ has good validity for use with older adults; however is not ideal for those with cognitive impairment (Helme et al., 1996).

Pain assessment in people with dementia

Dementia affects approximately 35.6 million people globally, with an estimated 7.3 million adults in Europe affected (WHO Europe, 2012). Assuming no change occurs in mortality risk, the prevalence of dementia is likely to double every 20 years (Ferri et al., 2006). With a high prevalence of both pain and dementia, it is not surprising that many older adults experience these concurrently.

As previously discussed, pain is measured through self-report techniques; however cognitive impairment can reduce an individual's ability to communicate, making it a challenge to rely on self-report pain assessment. As a result, over the last decade there has been an increase in the development and use of observational behavioural scales to assess pain in people with dementia (Zwakhalen et al., 2006). Many pain indicators have been identified to help with pain assessment in the older adult with dementia, including non-verbal cues and behaviours (Baker et al., 1996), facial indices (Baker et al., 1996), vocalisations and changes in usual behaviour (Feldt, Ryden & Miles, 1998).

Observational behavioural assessment scales rely entirely on a carer's knowledge and understanding about the individual, including their usual behaviour. Therefore, it is often essential for formal carers (e.g. nursing home staff) to request input from family or close friends of what would be expected for the individual in usual pain experience.

However, even with a range of assessment scales available, pain is still not routinely assessed in older adults with dementia. A recent audit conducted in one hospital in the United Kingdom identified that only two-thirds of older adults admitted into acute care had their pain formally assessed (Niruban et al., 2010).

Some of this under-assessment of pain may be due to a lack of knowledge and training around pain assessment in older adults with dementia. It is therefore essential that we take this opportunity of an aging population to learn more about the barriers to the use of pain assessment tools and work with healthcare staff actively to improve their knowledge and understanding to ensure people with dementia receive the best care from appropriately trained staff.

Pain assessment – technology approach

In our increasingly technological world, we have an exciting opportunity to use technology to improve the assessment of pain and to deliver education and training. A recent report from the Institute of Medicine recommended the promotion of self-management of pain through the use of technology (IoM, 2011). However, it is also essential that we look at innovative new approaches to pain assessment and pain management where possible.

Palermo and Jamison (2015) published a special series which provided a contemporary overview of innovative technologies in pain treatment. Authors reviewed original articles over areas including technology-assisted self-management interventions, electronic pain diaries, clinical dashboards and interventions delivered using Internet and mobile applications. Authors felt that the topic of technology and pain assessment/self-management is one that is timely and they encouraged future research in this vital area. Benefits include improved pain assessment and management for the individual, but also a significant reduction in the economic cost of chronic pain. The reviewed evidence focused on children, adolescents and adults; however none were specific for older adults and none were specific for improving pain assessment from the healthcare perspective.

IPhone pain assessment app

With an aging population who are likely to remain within their own homes in the community, and an increase in pain and dementia, it could be assumed that older adults will be seen more regularly in emergency situations. It would therefore be expected that the staff would be experienced in dealing with the specific problems associated with this population and consequently be more skilled in the techniques associated with assessment and management of pain for the older adult. This, however, is not the case. Barriers and attitudes to pain amongst health professionals towards the older adult pervade along with fears and misconceptions regarding pre-existing comorbidities and the prescribing of drugs.

Pain management in the paramedic setting is increasingly important in UK Ambulance services, where 80 per cent of patients present with pain-related complaints (Williams & Sutton, 2012). Paramedics report barriers to providing adequate pain relief, such as concerns about patient accuracy in evaluating their own pain and the effect of analgesia interfering with clinical assessments. Furthermore, paramedics identified that patients with dementia or cognitive impairments may have problems communicating their pain and, as such, pain may be ignored, overlooked or mistaken for challenging behaviour (Harvey, 2014). Currently national clinical guidelines for paramedics recommend the VRS and Wong-Baker Faces Pain Scale to assess pain. However, these do not account for patients who have difficulty communicating.

We need to consider more innovative and creative ways of delivering care in the future. Pain assessment in adults with cognitive impairment is hampered by communication difficulties on the part of the adult and limited access to assessment tools by paramedic staff. Therefore, researchers at the University of Greenwich (led by Professor Pat Schofield) collaborated with the Computing and Mathematical Sciences Department to develop the iPhone pain assessment app. This was evaluated across South London Ambulance Service NHS Trust and South East Coast Ambulance Service NHS Foundation Trust to explore the feasibility of using the pain assessment app as a tool for the assessment of pain in adults with dementia within the paramedic setting and to explore their ideas on how the app could be improved (Docking et al., 2017). Following this, recommended changes put forward by the paramedic students were presented to an expert panel of paramedics, who selected those most relevant for future implementation.

The results indicated that the iPhone pain assessment app could prove a useful tool in the pre-hospital setting and potentially other populations with communication difficulties. Evidence suggests that one of the most common reasons for dialling 999 is because an individual is experiencing pain (McLean, Maio & Domeier, 2002). By providing access to a tool, within the paramedic setting, that has been specifically developed to help identify pain in a user-friendly format, we are likely to see improvements in pain management and subsequently improved quality of life for the adult with dementia.

Paramedic students and staff involved were open to admit that current pain assessment, within their clinical practice for the older adult with cognitive impairment, is not substantial and at times is ignored. Participants responded, on the whole, very positively to the concept behind the app and were enthusiastic about its use in practice. The most common concern raised was the use of technology within the clinical setting and how appropriate this is, and the lack of adequate support for paramedic staff to allow them the opportunity to use app-based assessment methods in practice. The majority of participants did not feel that use of an electronic device was currently possible within the clinical setting. However, as the technology age continues, there will be an increase in need for technology in the healthcare setting, which will bring with it greater acceptance and understanding from patients of the benefit such methods can bring.

The development of apps can provide new insight into innovative methods for pain assessment for older adults, which appears to be both feasible and welcomed by those within clinical professions. The benefits of implementing such a tool are wide reaching, improving healthcare professionals' knowledge and confidence in pain assessment and also potentially improving pain management for the older person. In addition, there is huge potential for wider application of this tool; along with national implementation across the paramedic emergency services, there are other possible clinical situations where the app could be utilised, such as emergency departments, acute care wards and nursing homes.

Summary

Pain can provide a significant challenge to positive aging and is a challenge only likely to become more widespread given our rapidly aging population. More and more older adults will have to deal with threats to basic day-to-day functioning, mood, sleep and overall quality of life that can result from living with persistent pain.

This challenge can be most effectively met by the availability of the widest possible pool of pain management techniques to facilitate the selection of those which best meet the older adult's individual needs and which provide optimal effectiveness, cost and convenience with minimal side effects. While analgesic drugs may continue to be first line treatment for many older adults, it is important to continue to develop and evaluate non-pharmacological methods of pain management, either as interventions to be used in conjunction with analgesic drugs or when drug treatment is either not possible or not effective. Encouragingly, preliminary research appears to suggest that psychological and physical interventions offer potential as effective pain management in older adults. However, further additional controlled research is needed to identify the most effective treatments, the magnitude of their analgesic effects and what type of older adult with what type of pain will benefit most from their application. With respect to pain assessment, it is time we took advantage of what the technology age has to offer and develop and utilize assessment tools that can potentially improve the quality of life for older adults living with pain to ensure they can remain living in their own homes for as long as possible. While pain does continue to be an issue for older adults, we must challenge ageist and discriminatory attitudes. Pain in older people needs to be seen as a priority and no longer thought of as a normal part of aging.

References

Abdulla, A., Adams, N., Bone, M., Elliott, A. M., Gaffin, J., Jones, D., Knaggs, R., Martin, D., Sampson, L., & Schofield, P. A. (2013). Guidance on the management of pain in older people. *Age and Ageing*, 42(Suppl. 1), i1–i57. doi:10.1093/ageing/afs200

Adachi, T., Fujino, H., Nakae, A., Mashimo, T., & Sasaki, J. (2014). A meta-analysis of hypnosis for chronic pain problems: A comparison between hypnosis, Standard Care, and other psychological interventions. *International Journal of Clinical and Experimental Hypnosis*, 62(1), 1–28. doi:10.1080/00207144.2013.841471

Alonso-Fernández, M., López-López, A., Losada, A., González, J. L., & Wetherell, J. L. (2015). Acceptance and commitment therapy and selective optimization with compensation for institutionalized older people with chronic pain. *Pain Medicine*, 17(2), 264–277.

American Geriatrics Society Panel of Chronic Pain in Older Persons. (1998). The management of chronic pain in older persons: American Geriatrics Society. *Journal of the American Geriatric Society*, 46, 635–651.

American Geriatrics Society Panel on Persistent Pain in Older Persons. (2002). The management of persistent pain in older persons. *Journal of the Americans Geriatric Society*, 50, S205–S224. doi:10.1046/j.1532–5415.50.6s.1.x

American Geriatrics Society Panel on Pharmacological Management of Persistent Pain in Older Persons. (2009). Pharmacological management of persistent pain in older persons. *Journal of the American Geriatric Society*, 57(8), 1331–1346. doi:10.1111/j.1532–5415.2009.02376.x

Antall, G. F., & Kresevic, D. (2004). The use of guided imagery to manage pain in an elderly orthopedic population. *Orthopaedic Nursing*, 23, 335–340.

Baird, C. L., & Sands, L. (2004). A pilot study of the effectiveness of guided imagery with progressive muscle relaxation to reduce chronic pain and mobility difficulties of osteoarthritis. *Pain Management Nursing*, 5, 97–104.

Baker, A., Bowring, L., Brignell, A., & Kafford, D. (1996). Chronic pain management in cognitively impaired patients: A preliminary research project. *Perspectives (Gerontological Nursing Association (Canada))*, 20(2), 4.

Baltes, P. B., & Baltes, M. M. (1990). Psychological perspectives on successful aging: The model of selective optimization with compensation. In P. B. Baltes and M. M. Baltes (Eds.), *Successful aging: Perspectives from the behavioral sciences* (pp. 1–34). Cambridge: Cambridge University Press.

Bandolier. (2015). *Oxford league table of analgesics in acute pain*. www.medicine.ox.ac.uk/bandolier/booth/painpag/acutrev/analgesics/leagtab.html (accessed August 14, 2015).

Bellieni, C. V., Cioncoloni, D., Mazzanti, S., Bianchi, M. E., Morrone, I., Becattelli, R., Perrone, S., & Buonocore, G. (2013). Music provided through a portable media player (iPod) blunts pain during physical therapy. *Pain Management Nursing*, 14, e151–155. doi:10.1016/j.pmn.2011.09.003

Beursken, R., & Bock, O. (2012). Age-related deficits of dual-task walking: A review. *Neural Plasticity*, 131608, 1–9. doi:10.1155/2012/131608

Bieri, D., Reeve, R. A., Champion, G. D., Addicoat, L., & Ziegler, J. B. (1990). The Faces Pain Scale for the self-assessment of the severity of pain experienced by children: Development, initial validation, and preliminary investigation for ratio scale properties. *Pain*, 41(2), 139–150.

Breit, R., & Van der Wall, H. D. (2004). Transcutaneous electrical nerve stimulation for postoperative pain relief after total knee arthroplasty. *The Journal of Arthroplasty*, 19, 45–48. doi:10.1016/S0883-5403(03)00458-3

Brown, S. T., Kirkpatrick, M. K., Swanson, M. S., & McKenzie, I. L. (2011). Pain experience of the elderly. *Pain Management Nursing*, 12, 190–196. doi:10.1016/j.pmn.2010.05.004

Brunier, G., Carson, G., & Harrison, D. E. (1995). What do nurses know and believe about patients with pain? Results of a hospital survey. *Journal of Pain and Symptom Management*, 10(6), 436–445.

Burns, J. W., Gerhart, J. I., Post, K. M., Smith, D. A., Porter, L. S., Schuster, E., Buvanendran, A., Fras, A. M., & Keefe, F. J. (2015). The communal coping model of pain catastrophizing in daily life: A within-couples daily diary study. *Journal of Pain*, 16(11), 1163–1175.

Chapman, S. (2010). Managing pain in the older person. *Nursing Standard*, 25(11), 35–39. doi:10.7748/ns2010.11.25.11.35.c8103

Cipher, D. J., Clifford, A., & Roper, K. D. (2007). The effectiveness of geropsychological treatment in improving pain, depression, behavioral disturbances, functional disability, and health care utilization in long term care. *Clinical Gerontology*, 30, 23–40. doi:10.1300/J018v30n03_02

Clarke, A., Anthony, G., Gray, D., Jones, D., McNamee, P., Schofield, P., . . . Martin, D. (2012). "I feel so stupid because I can't give a proper answer . . ." How older adults describe chronic pain: A qualitative study. *BMC Geriatrics*, 12, 78. doi:10.1186/1471-2318-12-78

Closs, S. J., Barr, B., Briggs, M., Cash, K., & Seers, K. (2004). A comparison of five pain assessment scales for nursing home residents with varying degrees of cognitive impairment. *Journal of Pain and Symptom Management*, 27(3), 196–205.

Collett, B., O'Mahoney, S., Schofield, P., Closs, S. J., & Potter, J. (2007). The assessment of pain in older people. *Clinical Medicine*, 7(5), 496–500.

Cook, A. J. (1998). Cognitive-behavioral pain management for elderly nursing home residents. *Journal of Gerontology Series B: Psychological Sciences Social Sciences*, 53, 51–59.

Darchuk, K. M., Townsend, C. O., Rome, J. D., Bruce, B. K., & Hooten, W. M. (2010). Longitudinal treatment outcomes for geriatric patients with chronic non-cancer pain at an interdisciplinary pain rehabilitation program. *Pain Medicine*, 11, 1352–1364. doi:10.1111/j.1526–4637.2010.00937.x

DeGood, D. E., & Tait, R. (2001). Assessment of pain beliefs and pain coping. In D. C. Turk and R. Melzack (Eds.), *Handbook of pain assessment* (pp. 320–341). New York: Guilford Press.

Del Casale, A., Ferracuti, A., Rapinesi, C., Serata, D., Caltagirone, S. S., Savoja, V., Piacentino, D., Callovini, G., Manfredi, G., Sani, G., Kotzalidis, G. D., & Girardi, P. (2015). Pain perception and hypnosis: Findings from recent functional neuroimaging studies. *International Journal of Clinical and Experimental Hypnosis*, 63, 144–170. doi:10.1080/00207144.2015.1002371

Denny, D. L., & Guido, G. W. (2012). Undertreatment of pain in older adults: An application of beneficence. *Nursing Ethics*, 19(6), 800–809. doi:10.1177/0969733012447015

Dionne, C. E., Dunn, K. M., & Croft, P. R. (2006). Does back pain prevalence really decrease with increasing age? A systematic review. *Age and Ageing*, 35(3), 229–234.

Docking, R. E., Fleming, J., Brayne, C., Zhao, J., Macfarlane, G. J., & Jones, G. T. (2011). Epidemiology of back pain in older adults: Prevalence and risk factors for back pain onset. *Rheumatology*, 50(9), 1645–1653.

Docking, R. E., Lane, M., & Schofield, P. A. (2017). Usability testing of the iPhone app to improve pain assessment for older adults with cognitive impairment (prehospital setting): A qualitative study. *Pain Medicine*, 0, 1–11. doi: 10.1093/pm/pnx028

Dorfman, D., George, M. C., Schnur, J., Simpson, D. M., Davidson, G., & Montgomery, G. (2013). Hypnosis for treatment of HIV neuropathic pain: A preliminary report. *Pain Medicine*, 14(7), 1048–1056. doi:10.1111/pme.12074

Ehde, D. M., & Jensen, M. P. (2004). Feasibility of a cognitive restructuring intervention for treatment of chronic pain in persons with disabilities. *Rehabilitation Psychology*, 49(3), 254–258. doi:10.1037/0090–5550.49.3.254

Elkins, G., Jensen, M. P., & Patterson, D. R. (2007). Hypnotherapy for the management of chronic pain. *International Journal of Clinical and Experimental Hypnosis*, 55(3), 275–287. doi:10.1080/00207140701338621

Feldt, K. S., Ryden, M. B., & Miles, S. (1998). Treatment of pain in cognitively impaired compared with cognitively intact older patients with hip-fracture. *Journal of the American Geriatrics Society*, 46(9), 1079–1085.

Ferri, C. P., Prince, M., Brayne, C., Brodaty, H., Fratiglioni, L., Ganguli, M., Hall, K., Hasegawa, K., Hendrie, H., Huang, Y., Jorm, A., Mathers, C., Menezes, P., Rimmer, E., & Scazufca, M. (2006). Global prevalence of dementia: A Delphi consensus study. *The Lancet*, 366(9503), 2112–2117.

Gaskin, D. J., & Richard, P. (2012). The economic costs of pain in the United States. *The Journal of Pain*, 13(8), 715–724.

Gibson, S. J., & Lussier, D. (2012). Prevalence and relevance of pain in older persons. *Pain Medicine*, 13(Suppl. 2), S23–S26. doi:10.1111/j.1526–4637.2012.01349.x

González, P., Manzano, M. P., Muñoz, M. T., Martín, C., & Forcano, M. (2013). Síndrome del miembro fantasma: Aproximación terapéutica mediante el tratamiento espejo. Experiencia de un Servicio de Geriatría. [Phantom limb pain syndrome: Therapeutic approach using mirror therapy in a Geriatric Department]. *Revista Espanola De Geriatria Y Gerontologia*, 48, 198–201. doi:10.1016/j.regg.2012.11.001

Gouveia, M., & Augusto, M. (2012). Indirect costs of chronic pain in Portugal. Presentation at *Societal Impact of Pain Conference*, Copenhagen, Denmark. www.sip-platform.eu

Grant, D. J., Bishop-Miller, J., Winchester, D. M., Anderson, M., & Faulkner, S. (1999). A randomized comparative trial of acupuncture versus transcutaneous electrical nerve stimulation for chronic back pain in the elderly. *Pain*, 82, 9–13. doi:10.1016/S0304-3959(99)00027-5

Green, S. M., Hadjistavropoulos, T., Hadjistavropoulos, H., Marten, R., & Sharpe, D. (2009). Controlled investigation of a cognitive behavioural pain management program for older adults. *Behavioural and Cognitive Psychotherapy*, 37, 221–226. doi:10.1017/S1352465809005177

Hahn, M., Wild-Wall, N., & Falkenstein, M. (2011). Age-related differences in performance and stimulus processing in dual task situation. *Brain Research*, 1414, 66–76. doi:10.1016/j.brainres.2011.07.051

Harvey, C. (2014). Is there scope for an observational pain scoring tool in paramedic practice? *Journal of Paramedic Practice*, 6(2), 84–88.

Helme, R. D., Katz, B., Gibson, S. J., Bradbeer, M., Farrell, M., Neufeld, M., & Corran, T. (1996). Multidisciplinary pain clinics for older people. Do they have a role? *Clinics in Geriatric Medicine*, 12(3), 563–582.

Henderson, J. V., Harrison, C. M., Britt, H. C., Bayram, C. F., & Miller, G. C. (2013). Prevalence, causes, severity, impact, and management of chronic pain in Australian general practice patients. *Pain Medicine*, 14(9), 1346–1361. doi:10.1111/pme.12195

Herr, K., Mobily, P., & Richardson, G. (1998). Use of experimental pain to compare psychometric properties and usability of pain scales in the adult and older adult populations. In *Annual Meeting of the American Society for Pain Management in Nursing*.

Hole, J., Hirsch, M., Ball, E., & Meads, C. (2015). Music as an aid for postoperative recovery in adults: A systematic review and meta-analysis. *The Lancet*, 386(10004), 1659–1671.

Institute of Medicine (US). Committee on Advancing Pain Research, Care, and Education. (2011). *Relieving pain in America: A blueprint for transforming prevention, care, education, and research*. Washington, DC: National Academies Press.

Itoh, K., Itoh, S., Katsumi, Y., & Kitakoji, H. (2009). A pilot study on using acupuncture and transcutaneous electrical nerve stimulation to treat chronic no-specific low back pain. *Complementary Therapies in Clinical Practice*, 15, 22–25. doi:10.1016/j.ctcp.2008.09.003

Jackson, T., Chen, H., Iezzi, T., Yee, M., & Chen, F. (2014). Prevalence and correlates of chronic pain in a random population study of adults in Chongqing, China. *Clinical Journal of Pain*, 30(4), 346–352. doi:10.1097/AJP.0b013e31829ea1e3

Jensen, M. P. (2009). Hypnosis for chronic pain management: A new hope. *Pain*, 146, 235–237. doi:10.1016/j.pain.2009.06.027

Jensen, M. P., McArthur, K. D., Barber, J., Hanley, M. A., Engel, J. M., Romano, J. M., Cardenas, D. D., Kraft, G. H., Hoffman, A. J, & Patterson, D. R. (2006). Satisfaction with, and the beneficial side effects of, hypnotic analgesia. *International Journal of Clinical and Experimental Hypnosis*, 54, 432–447. doi:10.1080/00207140600856798

Jensen, M. P., & Patterson, D. R. (2006). Hypnotic treatment of chronic pain. *Journal of Behavioral Medicine*, 29, 95–124.

Jensen, M. P., Turner, J. A., & Romano, J. M. (2007). Changes after multidisciplinary pain treatment in patient pain beliefs and coping are associated with concurrent changes in patient functioning. *Pain*, 131, 38–47. http://dx.doi.org/10.1016/j.pain.2006.12.007

Keefe, F. J., Rumble, M. E., Scipio, C. D., Giordano, L. A., & Perri, L. M. (2004). Psychological aspects of persistent pain: Current state of the science. *Journal of Pain*, 5, 195–211.

Kirsch, I., Montgomery, G., & Sapirstein, G. (1995). Hypnosis as an adjunct to cognitive-behavioral psychotherapy: A meta-analysis. *Journal of Consulting and Clinical Psychology*, 63, 214–220. http://dx.doi.org/10.1037/0022-006X.63.2.214

Kneafsey, R. (1997). The therapeutic use of music in a care of the elderly setting: A literature review. *Journal of Clinical Nursing*, 6, 341–346.

Kosslyn, S. M., Ganis, G., & Thompson, W. L. (2001). Neural foundations of imagery. *Nature Reviews Neuroscience*, 2, 635–642. doi:10.1038/35090055

Lamé, I. E., Peters, M. L., Vlaeyen, J. W., Kleef, M. V., & Patijn, J. (2005). Quality of life in chronic pain is more associated with beliefs about pain, than with pain intensity. *European Journal of Pain*, 9, 15–24.

Leadley, R. M., Armstrong, N., Lee, Y. C., Allen, A., & Kleijnen, J. (2012). Chronic diseases in the European Union: The prevalence and health cost implications of chronic pain. *Journal of Pain & Palliative Care Pharmacotherapy*, 26(4), 310–325. doi:10.3109/15360288.2012.736933

Linnemann, A., Kappert, M. B., Fischer, S., Doerr, J. M., Strahler, J., & Nater, U. M. (2015). The effects of music listening on pain and stress in the daily life of patients with fibromyalgia syndrome. *Frontiers in Human Neuroscience*, 9, 1–10. doi:10.3389/fnhum.2015.00434

Lutz, A., Slagter, H. A., Dunne, J. D., & Davidson, R. J. (2008). Attention regulation and monitoring in meditation. *Trends in Cognitive Science*, 12, 163–169. doi:10.1016/j.tics.2008.01.005

Lynch, M. E., & Watson, C. P. (2006). The pharmacotherapy of chronic pain: A review. *Pain Research & Management*, 11(1), 11–38. www.ncbi.nlm.nih.gov/entrez/query.fcgi?cmd=Retrieve&db=PubMed&dopt=Citation&list_uids=16511612

McCafferey, M., & Beebe, A. (1989). Giving Narcotics for pain: A problem solver handbook. *Nursing*, 19(10), 161–165.

McCracken, L.M, & Jones, R. (2012). Treatment for chronic pain for adults in the seventh and eighth decades of life: A preliminary study of Acceptance and Commitment Therapy (ACT). *Pain Medicine*, 13, 860–867. doi:10.1111/j.1526-4637.2012.01407.x

McGuire, B. E., Nicholas, M. K., Asghari, A., Wood, B. M., & Main, C. J. (2014). The effectiveness of psychological treatments for chronic pain in older adults: Cautious optimism and an agenda for research. *Current Opinion in Psychiatry*, 27(5), 380–384. doi:10.1097/YCO.0000000000000090

McLean, S. A., Maio, R. F., & Domeier, R. M. (2002). The epidemiology of pain in the prehospital setting. *Prehospital Emergency Care*, 6(4), 402–405.

Maniadakis, N., and Gray, A. (2000). The economic burden of back pain in the UK. *Pain*, 84(1), 95–103.

Melzack, R. (1975). The McGill pain questionnaire: Major properties and scoring methods. *Pain*, 1(3), 277–299.

Michielsen, M. E., Smits, M., Ribbers, G. M., Stam, H. J., Van Der Geest, J. N., Bussmann, J. B., & Selles, R. W. (2011). The neuronal correlates of mirror therapy: An fMRI study on mirror induced visual illusions in patients with stroke. *Journal of Neurology, Neurosurgery & Psychiatry*, 82(4), 393–398. doi:10.1136/jnnp.2009.194134

Middaugh, S. J., & Pawlick, K. (2002). Biofeedback and behavioural treatment of persistent pain in the older adult: A review and a study. *Applied Psychophysiology and Biofeedback*, 27, 185–202. doi:10.1023/A:1016208128254

Middaugh, S. J., Woods, S. E., Kee, W. G., Harden, R. N., & Peters, J. R. (1991). Biofeedback assisted relaxation training for chronic pain in the ageing. *Biofeedback and Self-Regulation*, 16, 361–377.

Miró, J., Queral, R., & Nolla, M. C. (2014). Pain-related attitudes and functioning in elderly primary care patients. *The Spanish Journal of Psychology*, 17, e104, 1–6. doi:10.1017/sjp.2014.103

Morone, N. E., Lynch, C. S., Greco, C. M., Tindle, H. A., & Weiner, D. K. (2008). 'I felt like a new person': The effects of mindfulness meditation on older adults with chronic pain: Qualitative narrative analysis of diary entries. *Journal of Pain*, 9, 841–848. doi:10.1016/j.jpain.2008.04.003

Morone, N. E., Rollman, B. L., Moore, C. G., Li, Q., & Weiner, D. K. (2009). A mind-body program for older adults with chronic low back pain: Results of a pilot study. *Pain Medicine*, 10, 1395–1407. doi:10.1111/j.1526-4637.2009.00746.x

Myskja, A., & Lindbaek, M. (2000). Examples of the use of music in clinical medicine. *Tidsskr Nor Laegeforen*, 120, 1186–1190.

Ng, M. M. L., Leung, M. C. P., & Poon, D. M. Y. (2003). The effects of electro-acupuncture and transcutaneous electrical nerve stimulation on patients with painful osteoarthritic knees: A randomized controlled trial with follow-up evaluation. *Journal of Alternative and Complementary Medicine*, 9, 641–649. doi:10.1089/107555303322524490

Niruban, A., Biswas, S., Willicombe, S. C., & Myint, P. K. (2010). An audit on assessment and management of pain at the time of acute hospital admission in older people. *International Journal of Clinical Practice*, 64(10), 1453–1457.

Öst, L. G. (2014). The efficacy of Acceptance and Commitment Therapy: An updated systematic review and meta-analysis. *Behaviour Research and Therapy*, 61, 105–121. doi:10.1016/j.brat.2014.07.018

Palermo, T. M., & Jamison, R. N. (2015). Innovative delivery of pain management interventions: Current trends and future progress. *The Clinical Journal of Pain*, 31(6), 467–469.

Paquier-Valette, C., Wierzbicka-Hainaut, E., Cante, V., Charles, S., & Guillet, G. (2014). Évaluation de l'hypnose à visée antalgique dans la photothérapie dynamique: étude pilote. [Evaluation of hypnosis in pain management during photodynamic therapy: A pilot study]. *Annales De Dermatologie Et De Venereologie*, 141, 181–185. doi:10.1016/j.annder.2013.10.046

Park, J., Engstrom, G., Tappen, R., & Ouslander, J. (2015). Health-related quality of life and pain intensity among ethnically diverse community-dwelling older adults. *Pain Management Nursing*, 16(5), 733–742.

Park, J., & Hughes, A. K. (2012). Nonpharmacological approaches to the management of chronic pain in community-dwelling older adults: A review of empirical evidence. *Journal of the American Geriatrics Society*, 60, 555–568. doi:10.1111/j.1532–5415.2011.03846.x

Patel, K.V., Phelan, E. A., Leveille, S. G., Lamb, S. E., Missikpode, C., Wallace, R. B., . . . Turk, D. C. (2014). High prevalence of falls, fear of falling, and impaired balance in older adults with pain in the United States: Findings from the 2011 National Health and Aging Trends Study. *Journal of the American Geriatrics Society*, 62(10), 1844–1852. doi:10.1111/jgs.13072

Pautex, S., & Vogt-Ferrier, N. (2006). Management of chronic pain in older persons. *Revue Medicale Suisse*, 2(71), 1629–1630, 1632. www.ncbi.nlm.nih.gov/entrez/query.fcgi?cmd=Retrieve&db=PubMed&dopt=Citation&list_uids=16878529

Quartana, P. J., Campbell, C. M., & Edwards, R. R. (2009). Pain catastrophizing: A critical review. *Expert Review of Neurotherapeutics*, 9, 745–758. doi:10.1586/ern.09.34

Reid, M. C., Eccleston, C., & Pillemer, K. (2015). Management of chronic pain in older adults. *BMJ*, 350, h532. doi:10.1136/bmj.h532

Sawant, A., Dadurka, K., Overend, T., & Kremenchutzky, M. (2015). Systematic review of efficacy of TENS for management of central pain in people with multiple sclerosis. *Multiple Sclerosis and Related Disorders*, 4(3). doi:10.1016/j.msard.2015.03.006

Schmid, W., & Ostermann, T. (2010). Home-based music therapy – a systematic overview of settings and conditions for an innovative service in healthcare. *BMC Health Services Research*, 10, 291. doi:10.1186/1472-6963-10-291

Skingley, A., & Vella-Burrows, T. (2010). Therapeutic effects of music and singing for older people. *Nursing Standard*, 24, 35–41.

Steglitz, J., Buscemi, J., & Ferguson, M. J. (2012). The future of pain research, education, and treatment: A summary of the IOM report "Relieving pain in America: A blueprint for transforming prevention, care, education, and research". *Translational Behavioural Medicine*, 2(1), 6–8. doi:10.1007/s13142-012-0110-2

Stoelb, B. L., Molton, I. R., Jensen, M. P., & Patterson, D. R. (2009). The efficacy of hypnotic analgesia in adults: A review of the literature. *Contemporary Hypnosis*, 26(1), 24–39. doi:10.1002/ch.370

Sullivan, M. (2012). The communal coping model of pain catastrophizing: Clinical and research implications. *Canadian Psychology*, 53, 32–41. http://dx.doi.org/10.1037/a0026726

Thomas, E., Mottram, S., Peat, G., Wilkie, R., & Croft, P. (2007). The effect of age on the onset of pain interference in a general population of older adults: Prospective findings from the North Staffordshire Osteoarthritis Project (NorStOP). *Pain*, 129(1), 21–27.

Thompson, T., Keogh, E., & French, C. C. (2011). Sensory focusing versus distraction and pain: Moderating effects of anxiety sensitivity in males and females. *The Journal of Pain*, 12, 849–858. doi:10.1016/j.jpain.2011.01.004.

Thompson, T., Keogh, E., French, C. C., & Davis, R. (2008). Anxiety sensitivity and pain: Generalisability across noxious stimuli. *Pain*, 134, 187–196. doi:10.1016/j.pain.2007.04.018

Tracy, B., & Morrison, R. S. (2013). Pain management in older adults. *Clinical Therapeutics*, 35(11), 1659–1668. doi:10.1016/j.clinthera.2013.09.026

Trott, P.V., Wiedemann, A. M., Lűdtke, R., Reishauer, A., Willich, S. N., and Witt, C. M. (2009). Qigong and exercise therapy for elderly patients with chronic neck pain (QIBANE): A randomized controlled study. *Journal of Pain*, 10, 501–508. doi:10.1016/j.jpain.2008.11.004

Tsang, A., Von Korff, M., Lee, S., Alonso, J., Karam, E., Angermeyer, M. C., . . . Watanabe, M. (2008). Common chronic pain conditions in developed and developing countries: Gender and age differences and comorbidity with depression-anxiety disorders. *Journal of Pain*, 9(10), 883–891. doi:10.1016/j.jpain.2008.05.005

Vance, C. G., Dailey, D. L., Rakel, B. A., & Sluka, K. A. (2014). Using TENS for pain control: The state of the evidence. *Pain Management*, 4, 197–209. doi:10.2217/pmt.14.13

Von Korff, M., Ormel, J., Keefe, F. J., & Dworkin, S. F. (1992). Grading the severity of chronic pain. *Pain*, 50(2), 133–149.

Wetherell, J. L., Petkus, A. J., Alonso-Fernández, M., Bower, E. S., Steiner, A. R., & Afari, N. (2015). Age moderates response to acceptance and commitment therapy vs. cognitive behavioral therapy for chronic pain. *International Journal of Geriatric Psychiatry*, 31(3), 302–308.

Williams, E., & Sutton, S. (2012). *Elderly fallers referrals: Update. London Ambulance Service: Clinical update* (Issue 28). www.londonambulance.nhs.uk/health_professionals/gp_information/idoc.ashx?docid=c5ec9929-66a8-41a1-8e9a-28d08fe25278&version=-1

Wong, D. L., & Baker, C. M. (1988). Pain in children: Comparison of assessment scales. *Pediatric Nursing*, 14(1), 9–17.

World Health Organization. (2012). *Dementia: A public health priority*. www.who.int/mental_health/publications/dementia_report_2012/en/ (accessed November 16, 2015).

Yang, K., & Kim, Y. (2005). Efficacy of qi-therapy (external qigong) for elderly people with chronic pain. *International Journal of Neuroscience*, 115, 949–963.

Zhou, S., Després, O., Pebayle, T., & Dufour, A. (2015). Age-related decline in cognitive pain modulation induced by distraction: Evidence from event-related potentials. *Journal of Pain*. Art. ID. S1526-5900(15)00704-X, 16(9), 862–872.

Zwakhalen, S. M., Hamers, J. P., Abu-Saad, H. H., & Berger, M. P. (2006). Pain in elderly people with severe dementia: A systematic review of behavioural pain assessment tools. *BMC Geriatrics*, 6(1), 3.

PART III

Well-being

11
PHYSICAL ACTIVITY AND HEALTHY EATING

Rachel Crockett, Jennifer Stock and Tatiana Christides

Learning outcomes

- To understand the role of physical activity and healthy eating in positive aging
- To gain an overview of the factors that hinder and support engagement in physical activity and healthy eating in older adults
- To appreciate the need to take account of the specific needs of older adults in the development of behaviour change interventions

Introduction

The twentieth century saw substantial breakthroughs in the treatment of acute illnesses which were previously associated with high mortality rates. However, as people have lived longer, the impact of chronic and preventable diseases such as type 2 diabetes, some forms of cancer, cardiovascular disease and chronic obstructive pulmonary disease has become apparent across the population of both developed and developing countries. The rise in chronic and preventable diseases is particularly acute in older adults as aging tends to be associated with higher rates of these diseases. In the latter part of the twentieth century the contribution of behaviours – such as sedentary lifestyles and eating a diet high in energy, fat, salt and sugar but low in fibre and unprocessed foods – to many preventable diseases has been recognised. Consequently, the impact of behaviour change interventions to support engagement in more healthy behaviours such as physical activity and eating a healthful diet has been recognised.

The discipline of health psychology is concerned with the application of psychology to the understanding of health and illness. It has been at the forefront of understanding the psychological, social and environmental factors that may hinder engagement in behaviours to promote health, as well as the development of behaviour change interventions. However, within health psychology the greatest focus in terms of health behaviour change has been in younger populations. When applied to understanding health in older populations, the focus has tended to be on managing ill health and functional decline associated with aging rather than on aging well (Peel, McClure & Barlett, 2005). While managing ill health in older adults is important, as it is at any age, this chapter will present a case for the importance of promoting and supporting health behaviours, specifically physical activity and healthy eating, in older age as a means to maximise health and promote positive aging.

The chapter covers three areas. A summary survey of evidence suggesting beneficial effects of physical activity and healthy eating on positive aging will be presented. While there is considerable evidence linking health-promoting behaviour across the lifespan on well-being and longevity in old age, this summary will draw on evidence linking the effects of engaging in physical activity and healthy eating in later life on outcomes across this life stage. In the subsequent section, an overview of some of the challenges that engaging in physical activity and healthy eating can present to older adults will be outlined. Finally the chapter will present evidence of the effectiveness of behaviour change interventions to promote physical activity and healthy eating in older adults.

Current evidence in the field

The impact of physical activity and healthy eating on health and well-being in older adults

Establishing the beneficial effects of engaging in physical activity and healthy eating across older adulthood is important in building evidence of effective methods to enable older adults to positively influence their health and well-being. There is epidemiological data to indicate that those who are more physically active live for longer than those who do not engage in such activity. For example, data from a cohort of older adults born between 1921 and 1926 and recruited to the Australian Longitudinal study of Women's Health and the Health of Men study showed that, compared to being physically inactive, having been physically active within the last week was associated with a significant survival advantage. A dose-respondent effect was also apparent such that greater physical activity was associated with a greater survival advantage (Brown et al., 2012).

However longer life expectancy may be of reduced value to older adults if it is associated with poor health, high levels of dependency and low levels of psychological well-being. Indeed, qualitative data indicates that older adults themselves define aging well as keeping active, feeling well, having a positive outlook, maintaining independence and the absence of disease and functional limitations (Kendig et al., 2014). There is evidence to indicate that engaging in physical activity can support positive aging. For example a systematic review of longitudinal studies suggested beneficial effects of physical activity on positive aging, including remaining free of poor health and living both independently and longer (Peel, McClure & Barlett, 2005). However, a further study draws attention to the fact that the effects of physical activity may vary across older adults. Data from the Melbourne Longitudinal Studies on Healthy Ageing Program (MELSHA) followed a participant pool of 1000 adults aged over 65 years at baseline in 1994 up to 2006 (n=420 still living in the community). In multivariate analyses, not meeting the criteria for aging well was associated with older age, having more health conditions (such as cognitive impairment, falls or pain) and various lifestyle factors including poor nutrition and being underweight. Physical activity was only associated with aging well in female participants in whom not aging well was predicted by lower levels of physical activity (Kendig et al., 2014). This finding suggests effects of physical activity on positive aging in older adults may be modified by both gender and increasing age (those included the sample at follow-up would have been at least 75 years old), and that our understanding of the effects of physical activity in this group is incomplete.

Engaging in physical activity is also protective against increasing disability, which is a central challenge to being able to live independently. A major problem in older adults is falling and fall-related injury is a substantial source of disability in this group. Falls are associated with admission to hospital, increased dependence and the need for health and social care, thus making falls a major challenge to independence (Hausdorff, Rios & Edelberg, 2001; Scuffham, Chaplin & Legood, 2003). Although, in general, aging is associated with increased disability, longitudinal data from the United States shows that physical activity moderates this relationship such that greater levels of physical activity are associated with lower levels of disability as people age (Cotter & Lachman, 2010). It is notable that while a typical behavioural response to having had a fall is reducing one's mobility as a measure to prevent future falls, maintaining mobility reduces the risks of having a future fall (Boyd & Stevens, 2009; Reelick et al., 2009).

Although the numbers of studies exploring the effects of eating a healthful diet on positive aging are more limited, support is given to the beneficial effects of both physical activity and healthy eating through studies assessing the impact of obesity on outcomes. Specifically, lower levels of obesity that reflect, at least in some part, consumption of lower energy diets and increased energy expenditure through being physically active have been associated with outcomes suggesting positive aging (Cotter & Lachman, 2010; Peel, McClure & Bartlett, 2005; Zamboni et al., 2005). Furthermore, there is an emerging body of evidence that suggests that being overweight or obese is associated with increased risk of dementia with aging (Luchsinger & Gustafson, 2009); unfortunately, studies evaluating whether weight loss in older adults decreases this risk are lacking and needed.

The benefits of physical activity and healthy eating on positive aging are not limited to physical health outcomes, such as reduced levels of obesity, but also to reduced cognitive decline and incidence of Alzheimer's disease. Jak (2011) reviewed and narratively synthesised the evidence relating the impact of physical activity on cognitive aging. Jak found evidence from both longitudinal and cross-sectional studies of an association between greater physical activity and reductions in the decline of cognitive function, with more substantial effects suggested for vigorous activity. However the finding was not uniform, with some studies finding the effect was no longer significant once depression, vascular disease and likely preclinical dementia were controlled for. One suggestion made for the lack of a consistent effect was that the impact of physical activity on cognitive function may be linked to participation in cognitively stimulating activities (Jak, 2011). Since this review, Barnes et al. (2013) examined the combined effects of physical plus mental activity on cognitive function in inactive older adults with cognitive complaints utilising a randomised controlled design. All participants engaged in home-based mental activity and class-based physical activity for 12 weeks and were randomised into one of four groups utilising a 2×2 factorial design: mental activity intervention (intensive computer) or mental activity pseudo-control (educational DVDs) plus exercise intervention (aerobic) or exercise pseudo-control (stretching and toning). The findings showed that 12 weeks of physical plus mental activity was associated with significant improvements in global cognitive function. However, there was no evidence of difference between the intervention and pseudo-control groups. This may reflect practice effects on cognitive tests, or may suggest that the amount of activity is more important than the type in this population. It may also be that a 12-week intervention is not long enough to see benefits in this population or that the sample size was not large enough to detect small but physiologically relevant effects (Lautenschlager & Cox, 2013).

Moderating factors on the beneficial effects of physical activity have also been found for cognitive outcomes and risk of dementia. For instance, numerous reviews have demonstrated that studies which found the largest effects had included a larger proportion of females (>50 per cent) in their samples. Comparatively, studies which included only men in their sample found small or no effects (Clifford, Bandelow &Hogervorst, 2009; Kramer & Erickson, 2007). Further evidence suggests that age and genetic status may also moderate the effect of physical activity on cognitive outcomes, but findings have not been consistent (Miller, Taler & Davidson, 2012; Clifford et al., 2013).

Jak's (2011) review also found evidence that for those who have been diagnosed with Alzheimer's disease, the progress of the disease may be slower not only where patients were more physically active prior to the onset of the disease, but also where they were more physically active following the diagnosis. Indeed, in those diagnosed with Alzheimer's disease, greater physical activity was associated with improved cognitive function and nutritional status as well as reduced falls and behavioural problems resulting from the progression of the disease. An absence of longitudinal studies in this area is noted (Jak, 2011). Such studies would be invaluable in determining the longer term trajectory of those diagnosed with dementia but keeping physically active.

A more recent review, including a meta-analysis, of the effects of various modifiable factors on cognitive function and dementia provides further evidence to suggest that physical activity has beneficial effects on cognition (Beydoun et al., 2014). Of all the possible risks studied, the meta-analyses indicated that the largest population-attributable risk for Alzheimer's disease was lower versus higher physical activity. Specifically, the analyses suggested that 32 per cent of cases of Alzheimer's disease could be prevented if physical activity levels were high across the population. This was similar to the risks for midlife smoking (31 per cent) and somewhat higher than the next largest modifiable risk factor of low education (24 per cent). The review also found meta-analytic evidence for some nutrition-related risks. Higher blood concentrations of homocysteine, which are related to an inadequate intake or absorption of B vitamins, have been associated with an increased incidence of Alzheimer's disease. The meta-analyses found that low, compared to high, blood concentrations of homocysteine were associated with a 22 per cent reduction in the prevalence of Alzheimer's disease. A similar risk reduction was also observed for those who had a greater compared to less-than-weekly consumption of fish, possibly attributable to increased intake of fish-derived essential fatty acids (Whalley et al., 2008).

The impact of risk factors for Alzheimer's disease cannot be considered in isolation from one another and the non-independence of seven commonly identified modifiable risk factors for Alzheimer's disease (diabetes, midlife hypertension, midlife obesity, physical inactivity, smoking, depression and educational attainment) has been noted (Norton et al., 2014). For example, co-occurrence of type 2 diabetes, hypertension and obesity forms what is termed the metabolic syndrome, which is itself related to physical inactivity. Furthermore, six of the risk factors are related to the seventh, specifically low education. In a meta-analysis assuming independence of these risk factors in contributing to the prevalence of Alzheimer's disease, Norton and his colleagues found that close to a half of the prevalence of Alzheimer's disease worldwide could be accounted for by the seven risk factors. In the developed world (specifically the United States, Europe and the United Kingdom) the greatest single risk factor for Alzheimer's disease was physical inactivity accounting for around a third of the prevalence compared to just under 18 per cent worldwide. Worldwide low education accounted for the largest proportion of the prevalence (40 per cent). However, when the analyses were adjusted to account for non-independence between risk factors, the combined population-attributable risk for the seven risk factors reduced to 28 per cent worldwide with physical activity accounting for close to 20 per cent of the population-attributable risk in the developed countries and 13 per cent worldwide (Norton et al., 2014).

While the adjusted figures are lower than the unadjusted figures, they still suggest scope for physical activity interventions to play a significant role in reducing the prevalence of Alzheimer's disease. In addition, the relationships identified between major modifiable risk factors for Alzheimer's disease also highlights the relationships between these risk factors and other preventable diseases, including cardiovascular disease and type 2 diabetes (as a disease in its own right rather than solely as a risk factor for other conditions). This in turn suggests that interventions to increase rates of physical activity will have linked benefits in reducing a range of preventable diseases that are prevalent in older adults. In addition, the major modifiable risk factors of Alzheimer's disease identified by Norton et al. suggest an impact of diet on the development of Alzheimer's disease in relation to the development of type 2 diabetes, hypertension and obesity. This is supported further by research which links consumption of a Western diet, high in energy and saturated fats, to increased obesity and reduced cognitive function (Kanoski & Davidson, 2011). The association of obesity with increased risk of Alzheimer's disease may highlight a role of high-energy diets in the development of cognitive impairment. Indeed there is some evidence that restriction of calorie intake may have a preventative effect on cognitive decline, although it should be noted that being underweight is also a risk for poorer health in old age. Interestingly while Feart et al. (2009) found that a Mediterranean diet (low in red meat, high in vegetable and low in saturated fats) was associated with higher scores on some (but not all) measures of cognitive function in older adults, it was not associated with incidence of dementia over five years. One interpretation of these findings is that rather than a direct protective effect of eating a more healthful diet on risk for Alzheimer's disease, there is an indirect effect in which high energy consumption is associated with preventable conditions which are then in turn associated with risk for Alzheimer's disease.

In addition to the impact of physical activity and healthy eating on objective health outcomes, there is also evidence on benefits to subjective aspects of well-being. In 2001, Rejeski and colleagues reviewed evidence as to the effects of physical activity on quality of life; they found evidence that physical activity has beneficial effects on constructs such as life satisfaction, physical health and psychological well-being. Elavsky et al. (2005) suggest that life satisfaction may represent the cognitive appraisal of well-being by an individual and a number of studies highlighted the impact of cognitive variables, particularly self-efficacy, on the relationship between physical activity and life satisfaction. Self-efficacy is the belief that one has the ability to engage in a specific behaviour and thus indicates a sense of control over important aspects of one's life (Bandura, 1998). It makes intuitive sense therefore that self-efficacy would be associated with life satisfaction. Important behaviours include those to promote health and, indeed, self-efficacy is a consistent predictor of uptake of health behaviours (Frank, Heiby & Lee, 2007). For those without significant physical disability, walking can be a relatively easy behaviour in which to engage to increase physical activity levels. Being able to maintain or improve levels of physical activity is likely to enhance a sense of independence with beneficial effects on life satisfaction. In terms of healthy eating, Rejeski and Mihalko (2001) find that the evidence for the impact of nutrition on quality of life is more limited than that for physical activity, but evidence is available to indicate that a better quality of diet is associated with greater health-related quality of life and greater well-being in older adults (Milte et al., 2015).

Challenges to physical activity and healthy eating in older adults

Aging brings with it a number of challenges to engaging in physical activity and healthy eating which may not be encountered in the same way as at other life stages. Some of these changes relate to changes in health associated with aging, while others relate to changing psychological and social situations. These challenges are not necessarily insurmountable and this section will discuss how various factors may modify the impact of these challenges on physical activity and healthy eating.

A major change for many during the earlier years of older adulthood is the transition brought about by retirement from work. Retirement brings a variety of possible, and significant, changes in day-to-day life including an increased amount of leisure time, reduced economic resources, loss of social group and, perhaps, loss of the personal and social identity developed within the workplace. Unsurprisingly, given the increased onset of disability and disease as people age, overall the evidence suggests that as people age their physical activity reduces (Berger et al., 2005). The period of transition and change associated with retirement may provide an opportunity for the development of new habits, including increased physical activity with the hope that these may then be sustained across older age.

There is, however, somewhat contradictory evidence as to whether the cessation of work consequent to retirement results in reduced physical activity or whether the increase in leisure time results in increased physical activity. Michael Marmot and his colleagues used epidemiological data from the Whitehall II Study to explore the impact of retirement on physical activity in British civil servants. Prior to retirement physical activity levels were lowest in those working 30 or more hours a week; specifically, participants working less than 30 hours a week had 1.27 to 1.59 times greater physical activity levels than those working more than 30 hours a week. Those who were retired had the highest physical activity levels, reporting rates 2.13–2.28 times greater than those working 30 hours or more a week (Mein et al., 2005). While these findings seem to suggest that retirement is associated with an increase in physical activity, this sample may not have been representative of a general population sample at retirement. Most of those included in the study had desk-based jobs and thus relatively small amounts of physical activity were involved in their working life, meaning that following retirement relatively small changes in lifestyle might result in greater physical activity than during the individual's working life.

Longitudinal data from France similarly identified a mean increase in leisure time physical activity of two hours per week following retirement. However, retirement was also associated with an increase in sedentary activity, specifically watching television (Touvier et al., 2010). Sedentary activity is independently associated with poorer health outcomes (Owen et al., 2010), thus suggesting a complex effect of reduced work and increased leisure time on activity and subsequent health. The picture concerning the effect of retirement on activity levels is further complicated by different effects in different social groups. Taking education as an indicator of socioeconomic status, evidence suggests that, while physical activity increases following retirement in those from higher socioeconomic groups, in those from lower socioeconomic groups, activity tends to decline (Chung et al., 2009). This may reflect, at least in part, that those with less education tend to employed in more physically active types jobs such as caring and manual labour while more highly educated workers may have more sedentary, desk-bound jobs. Thus, pre-retirement activity is a likely moderator of the impact of retirement on physical activity levels. Reduced physical activity in those from lower socioeconomic groups may also be associated with economic resources post retirement as pensions in less-skilled, and therefore less well-paid jobs, are likely to be lower than those for people employed in more-skilled jobs. While physical activity as an element of a job role will be free of charge, charges for many leisure time physical activities may make them unaffordable for those with fewer economic resources post retirement (Shaw & Spokane, 2008).

For many, especially those who have commuted during their working life, retirement will mean spending an increasing proportion of their time within their local area. Reduced economic resources and the onset of decreasing mobility may also serve to keep people within their local area. The neighbourhoods in which people live can have a significant effect on day-to-day life, health and well-being and the increased time spent in these following retirement may increase this effect. It is widely recognised that these local environments have an impact on health, including through the effects of the environment on physical activity and eating behaviour (James, Jackson-Leach and Rigby, 2010). For older adults, as for many population groups, walking is an important way to be physically active. It does not require special skills, equipment or economic resources, and can be integrated into activities of daily life such as going shopping or visiting friends. The physical environment can support walking, particularly in older adults through the provision of footpaths that: i) link residential areas with local shops; ii) are even and safe from trip hazards; iii) are well-lit; and iv) keep pedestrians away from those using other forms of transport. While older adults may feel less safe on foot in some built-up areas, there is some evidence that older adults living in rural areas are discouraged from walking by the lack of properly made up footpaths (Wilcox et al., 2000).

The impact of the local environment on walking has been illustrated by Proctor-Gray and her colleagues using data from MOBILIZE Boston. MOBILIZE Boston is an epidemiological study of older adults living in Boston in the United States exploring factors associated with mobility and independent living in this group. This data set was used to explore the determinants of community-level variation in walking behaviour in older adults (Procter-Gray et al., 2015). Walking behaviour was classified as either recreational walking or utilitarian walking. More respondents engaged in recreational walking at least once a week (42 per cent) compared to utilitarian walking at least once a week (28 per cent), with 18 per cent engaging in both types of walking at least once a week. At the individual level the determinants of utilitarian and recreational walking, such as balance, were fairly similar but the two types of walking were associated with different neighbourhood characteristics. Greater distances to local amenities such as public transport, shops, hospital, park and libraries were associated with reduced utilitarian walking but had no association with recreational walking. Greater utilitarian, but not recreational, walking was also associated with more socially deprived neighbourhoods. Furthermore, the communities with the greatest walking prevalence were those with the most utilitarian walkers. These results underline the importance of the neighbourhood environment in determining walking and suggest that enabling older people to integrate walking into their day-to-day lives may be a more effective way of increasing physical activity in this group than encouraging time and effort set aside specifically to engage in physical activity. Health psychologists underline the importance of habit formation in the maintenance of more healthy behaviours over time (Gardner, de Bruijn & Lally, 2011). Habits rooted in day-to-day activities are likely to be more robust than habits created in isolation, given that the repetition associated with daily activities has been associated with habit formation (Lally et al., 2010). While some neighbourhood characteristics can support more healthy behaviour, other characteristics can hinder more healthy behaviour. For example, in the general population, higher obesity has been found to be associated with a greater number of fast food outlets within a local area, suggesting that the ready availability of less healthful food may have adverse effects on diets (Ball et al., 2010). Similar effects have been found for older adults (Pruchno et al., 2014).

Finally, the neighbourhoods in which people live are an important source of social support. Indeed isolation within local communities is frequently highlighted as a major problem for older adults (Stewart et al., 2014). Isolation may have a whole range of effects on the well-being of older adults, including reductions in health behaviour though the association of social support and health behaviour (Harvey & Alexander, 2012). Research supports this suggestion with evidence that both physical activity and good nutrition increase with support from friends (Harvey and Alexander, 2012; McIntosh, Shifflett & Picou, 1989). While support from others is important in enabling physical activity and healthy eating in those who are living independently, it is also important, in different ways, as older adults experience increasing dependency and a greater need for support from others in maintaining well-being. Ensuring good nutrition can be a particular challenge both for older adults themselves and, as they become more dependent, for those who support and care for them. For those living independently in the community, isolation can be associated with inadequate nutrition, as older adults who are eat alone tend to eat a poorer diet (Vesnaver & Keller, 2011). A further problem may be changes in nutritional needs that become more acute as people age – the same time at which many older adults are experiencing increased dependence on others for support with day-to-day activities such as eating. This is illustrated by the case of vitamin D; physiological changes associated with aging increase the need for oral vitamin D intake. However, there is evidence that neither older adults, nor those who provide support for them, are aware of this increased need (Alemu & Varnam, 2012).

Optimal vitamin D status is essential for calcium homeostasis and musculoskeletal health and strength, which are particularly important issues for older adults in enabling healthful aging (Dawson-Hughes, 2008). The body can synthesise vitamin D from sunlight-derived Ultraviolet B (UVB) light waves acting on the skin; however with normal aging, sunlight-induced vitamin D synthesis decreases and the body becomes less sensitive to the effects of vitamin D, effectively increasing requirements (Bell, 1995; Christakos et al., 2011). Dietary vitamin D provides additional intake, but because there are only low levels of vitamin D in most commonly eaten foods, diet may not adequately compensate for the increased needs associated with aging (SACN, 2007; Finch, Doyle & Lowe, 1998). Furthermore, sunlight exposure and dietary intake of vitamin D is typically lower in dependent older adults compared with healthy older people (Finch, Doyle & Lowe, 1998). Older adults in care homes are at especially high risk for vitamin D deficiency, as in addition to the above-mentioned challenges in maintaining normal vitamin D status, they are more likely to be on multiple medications, increasing the risk of drug-induced decreased vitamin D levels (Salazar, Poon & Nair, 2007).

In summary, older dependent adults and those living in care homes have multiple factors that increase their risk for clinically significant vitamin D deficiency leading to recommendations that they receive vitamin D supplementation (SACN, 2007; Committee on Medical Aspects of the Food Nutrition Policy, 1998; Wise, 2014). However, despite these recommendations, in the United Kingdom around a third of older adults living in care homes remain vitamin D deficient. An investigation of possible reasons for this deficiency found that amongst residents of one care home, risks of vitamin D deficiency were high as none of the residents met the required dietary intake of vitamin D, all had minimal sunlight exposure and no resident was on vitamin D supplements (Milligan et al., 2012). Qualitative interviews with care home staff suggested that staff were unaware both of the relationship between bone health and vitamin D and of the increased risk of falls and fracture associated with vitamin D deficiency. This lack of knowledge in those providing support to dependent older adults means that they cannot provide the support needed to ensure adequate levels of vitamin D in dependent older adults. Interventions to increase knowledge of the nutritional and activity needs of older adults, in both older adults themselves, but also in those who care for them, would be an appropriate first step to decrease vitamin D deficiency in this high-risk population.

Interventions to promote physical activity and healthy eating in older adults

Increasing recognition of the role that behaviour has in the development of preventable diseases has given rise to emergence of an extensive evidence base concerning the development and implementation of effective interventions to promote health-related behaviours. This research has been grounded in efforts to understand the predictors of more and less healthy behaviours as a basis for the development of interventions.

Predictors of behaviour may be grouped together as i) those relating to the individual themselves, especially those relating to the individual's cognitions; ii) those relating to the individual's social relationships; and iii) those relating to the wider environment. A wide range of theories of health behaviour have been developed to systematise how these predictors relate to one another and to the target behaviour. A good example of a psychological theory widely applied to understand health behaviour and behaviour change interventions is Social Cognitive Theory (SCT; Bandura, 1997; Graves, 2003). It is a theory that includes predictors that frequently occur, often with different terminology, in other theories applied to health behaviour. This makes it a useful framework to understand current knowledge in regards to health behaviour change. In terms of conceptualising the individual within SCT, key cognitions include *self-efficacy* (as described earlier in this chapter), *goals* (which act as incentives and guides to behaviour) and *outcome expectancies* of engaging in the behaviour (Bandura, 1997). Three dimensions of outcome expectancies have been specified: firstly, the area of the consequences of the behaviour, whether physical, social or self-evaluative; secondly, whether consequences are evaluated as positive or negative (or both); and, thirdly, whether consequences are short or long term (Bandura, 1997). The impact of both the individual's social situation and environment is encapsulated in the third predictor of behaviour identified by SCT, termed socio-structural factors, which comprises the facilitators and barriers to behaviour change that the individual encounters in the social and wider environment in which they live (Bandura, 1998). Typically self-efficacy is understood as central to SCT, having both direct effects on behaviour and indirect effects through its influences on the setting of goals and outcome expectancies (Bandura, 1997). In the remainder of this chapter the way in which theories of health behaviour can be used to develop interventions to be used in older adults will be explored, focusing on SCT. Before doing so, it should be noted that support for the notion that older adults can and do engage in activities to promote their health is supported by meta-synthesis of meta-analytic data, indicating that increasing effectiveness of interventions to promote uptake of health behaviours in older adults is associated with increasing age (Johnson, Scott-Sheldon & Carey, 2010).

The B-NICE (Behavioural Nutrition Intervention for Community Elders) trial serves as an example of the application of theory to the development of interventions to promote healthy eating in older adults (Locher et al., 2011). The intervention was designed to maintain or prevent weight loss following serious illness in older adults living at home and thus focussed on energy (calorie) intake. The intervention was tailored to the individual's needs and levels of self-efficacy and goals for energy intake were set based on these and the individual's preferences. The intervention development also recognised the impact of socio-structural factors on the behaviour of the individual and thus took account of interpersonal, institutional, community and policy-level influences on behaviour. The trial of the intervention randomised 40 adults to a control or intervention group with outcome data on 34 individuals. The study found the intervention was feasible but statistical analyses did not find any significant differences between groups in energy consumption. This may be due to lack of power as, at a descriptive level, 50 per cent (8/16) of the control group had increased their intake over the study period compared to 72 per cent (13/18) in the intervention group. In addition, this was a sample from a vulnerable group with a mean age of 81 years and two-thirds of the sample were not consuming enough energy at the start of the intervention to maintain their weight. These factors made it a challenging, albeit important, group in which to seek to improve nutrition (Locher et al., 2013).

An important issue for behaviour change interventions is maintenance of the behaviour change in the long term beyond the completion of an intervention. There is evidence that theory-based interventions may support more lasting change than standard interventions. A randomised control trial compared the impact of a peer-led intervention using constructs from

SCT with a standard physical activity intervention (Buman et al., 2011). The use of peers to implement an intervention is particularly appropriate in the context of SCT, given that Bandura argues that one of the main ways of increasing self-efficacy is through vicarious learning, which is seeing another successfully implement the behaviour (Bandura, 1998). Although in the short term both the standard and intervention group had similar rates of moderate to vigorous physical activity, at 18 months follow-up (eight months after the end of the intervention), the intervention group had significantly higher rates of such activity than the standard intervention group. A mixed methods study of the experience of those participating in the intervention group suggested that goal-setting and social support for behaviour change were important aspects of the intervention to participants. The salience of these predictors to participants suggests support for the importance of both socio-structural and cognitive predictors in supporting behaviour change (Floegal et al., 2015).

This research summary provides some useful pointers as to the how behaviour change may be supported in older adults. However, as noted at the beginning of this chapter, the evidence base regarding behaviour change in older adults remains a very small part of the overall evidence currently available in regards to effective behaviour change. More evidence is needed to ascertain the extent to which evidence drawn from general populations can be applied to older adults at different stage of the aging process. This issue is highlighted by a recent meta-analysis which aimed to explore which behaviour change techniques were effective in promoting self-efficacy and physical activity following a physical activity behaviour change intervention in older adults. The behaviour change techniques used in each intervention were coded based on the CALO-RE taxonomy. The CALO-RE taxonomy was developed from systematic reviews of behaviour change interventions across general populations (Michie et al., 2011). While the meta-analysis found that overall the interventions increased both self-efficacy and physical activity, the inclusion of some recognised behaviour change techniques was associated with smaller combined effect sizes of interventions on self-efficacy and/or physical activity. As demonstrated by the evidence presented in this chapter, physical activity and healthy eating in older adults can be influenced by a wide range of factors that may not be experienced in other population groups. It is possible that some of these factors may influence the effectiveness of currently used behaviour change interventions. Understanding better how factors associated with aging moderate the impact of behaviour change interventions on physical activity and healthy eating in older adults will be central to the continuing development of interventions that are effective across the lifespan and through old age.

Conclusion

This chapter has provided a summary of the role of physical activity and healthy eating in promoting positive aging. Overall the evidence presented in this chapter suggests that older adults can benefit considerably from interventions to promote physical activity and healthy eating. However, there is a need for a greater focus on older adults by behaviour change researchers and practitioners to maximise this benefit and ensure that interventions are effectively tailored to the needs and preferences of this group. While many benefits to health for older adults can be inferred from the evidence presented in this chapter, there may well be one further benefit. Attributing illness to old age and thus, as aging is inevitable, seeing illness as uncontrollable is associated with higher mortality rates in older adults (Stewart et al., 2012). Additionally, perceived control of future age-related decline – and other psychosocial factors such as attitudes towards aging and mood – have been discussed as a potential mediator of exercise interventions effects on cognitive outcomes (Stock, Clifford, Hogervorst, 2012). Promoting the idea amongst older adults that engaging in physical activity and healthy eating can positively influence their health and well-being may give this population a greater sense of control over their own health with consequent psychological, as well as physical, health benefits.

References

Alemu, E., & Varnam, R. (2012). Awareness of vitamin D deficiency among at-risk patients. *BMC, Research Notes*, 5, 17.

Ball, K., Crawford, D., Timperio, A., & Salmon, J. (2010). Eating Behaviours and the Food Environment. In A. A. Lake, T. G. Townshend, and S. Alvanides (Eds.), *Obesogenic environments: Complexities, perceptions and objective measures* (pp. 149–163). Oxford: Wiley-Blackwell. doi:10.1002/9781118786611.ch10

Bandura, A. (1997). *Self-efficacy: The exercise of control*. New York: WH Freeman and Company.

Bandura, A. (1998). Health promotion from the perspective of social cognitive theory. *Psychology and Health*, 13, 623–649.

Barnes, D. E., Santos-Modesitt, W., Poelke, G., Kramer, A. F., Castro, C., Middleton, L. E., & Yaffe, K. (2013). The Mental Activity and eXercise (MAX) trial: A randomized controlled trial to enhance cognitive function in older adults. *JAMA Internal Medicine*, 173(9), 797–804.

Bell, N. H. (1995). Vitamin D metabolism, aging, and bone loss. *Journal of Clinical Endocrinology & Metabolism*, 80, 1051.

Berger, U., Der, G., Mutrie, N., & Hannah, M. K. (2005). The impact of retirement on physical activity. *Ageing and Society*, 25, 181–195.

Beydoun, M. A., Beydoun, H. A., Gamaldo, A. A., Teel, A., Zonderman, A. B., & Wang, Y. (2014). Epidemiologic studies of modifiable factors associated with cognition and dementia: Systematic review and meta-analysis. *BMC Public Health*, 14, 643.

Boyd, R., & Stevens, J. A. (2009). Falls and fear of falling: Burden, beliefs and behaviours. *Age and Ageing*, 38, 423–428.

Brown, W. J., McLaughlin, D., Leung, J., McCaul, K. A., Flicker, L., Almeida, O. P., Hankey, G. J., Lopez, D., & Dobson, A. J. (2012). Physical activity and all-cause mortality in older women and men. *British Journal of Sports Medicine*, 46, 664–668.

Buman, M. P., Giacobbi Jr, P. R., Dzierzewski, J. M., McCrae, C. S., Roberts, B. L., & Marsiske, M. (2011). Peer volunteers improve long-term maintenance of physical activity with older adults: A randomized controlled trial. *Journal of Physical Activity & Health*, 8, S257–S266.

Christakos, S., Dhawan, P., Porta, A., Mady, L. J., & Seth, T. (2011). Vitamin D and intestinal calcium absorption. *Molecular and Cellular Endocrinology*, 347, 25–29.

Chung, S., Domino, M. E., Stearns, S. C., & Popkin, B. M. (2009). Retirement and physical activity: Analyses by occupation and wealth. *American Journal of Preventive Medicine*, 36, 422–428.

Clifford, A., Bandelow, S., & Hogervorst, E. (2009). The effects of physical exercise on cognitive function in the elderly: A review. In Q. Gariépy and R. Ménard (Eds.), *Handbook of cognitive aging: Causes, processes and effects* (pp. 109–150). New York: Nova Science Publishers, Inc.

Clifford, A., Stock, J., Bandelow, S., Rahardjo, T. B., & Hogervorst, E. (2013). Alzheimer's disease and dementia: A midlife approach to treatment is needed. In Atta-ur-Rahman (Ed.), *Frontiers in clinical drug research – Alzheimer disorders* (1st ed., Vol. 1, pp. 217–242). Bentham Science Publishers.

Committee on Medical Aspects of the Food Nutrition Policy. (1998). Nutrition and bone health: With particular reference to calcium and vitamin D. Report of the Subgroup on Bone Health, Working Group on the Nutritional Status of the Population. *Reports on Health and Social Subjects*, 49, 1–24.

Cotter, K. A., & Lachman, M. E. (2010). Psychosocial and behavioural contributors to health: Age-related increases in physical disability are reduced by physical fitness. *Psychology and Health*, 25, 805–820.

Dawson-Hughes, B. (2008). Serum 25-hydroxyvitamin D and functional outcomes in the elderly. *The American Journal of Clinical Nutrition*, 88(2), 537S–540S.

Elavsky, S., McAuley, E., Motl, R. W., Konopack, J. F., Marquez, D. X., Hu, L., Jerome, G. J., & Diener, E. (2005). Physical activity enhances long-term quality of life in older adults: Efficacy, esteem, and affective influences. *Annals of Behavioral Medicine*, 30(2), 138–145.

Féart, C., Samieri, C., Rondeau, V., Amieva, H., Portet, F., Dartigues, J. F., Scarmeas, N., & Barberger-Gateau, P. (2009). Adherence to a Mediterranean diet, cognitive decline, and risk of dementia. *JAMA*, 302(6), 638–648.

Finch, S., Doyle, W., & Lowe, C. (1998). National diet and nutrition survey: People aged 65 years and over. *Report of the diet and nutrition survey* (Vol. 1). London: The Stationery Office.

Floegel, T. A., Giacobbi, P. R., Dzierzewski, J. M., Aiken-Morgan, A. T., Roberts, B., McCrae, C. S., Marsiske, M., & Buman, M. P. (2015). Intervention markers of physical activity maintenance in older adults. *American Journal of Health Behavior*, 39, 487–499.

Frank, M. R., Heiby, E. M., & Lee, J. H. (2007). Assessment of determinants of compliance to twelve health behaviors: Psychometric evaluation of the health behavior schedule ii 1. *Psychological Reports*, 100, 1281–1297.

Gardner, B., Bruijn, G. J. de, & Lally, P. (2011). A systematic review and meta-analysis of applications of the self-report habit index to nutrition and physical activity behaviours. *Annals of Behavioral Medicine*, 42, 174–187.

Graves, K. (2003). Social cognitive theory and cancer patients' quality of life: A meta-analysis of psychosocial intervention components. *Health Psychology*, 22, 210–219.

Harvey, I. S., & Alexander, K. (2012). Perceived social support and preventive health behavioral outcomes among older women. *Journal of Cross-Cultural Gerontology*, 27, 275–290.

Hausdorff, J. M., Rios, D. A., & Edelberg, H. K. (2001). Gait variability and fall risk in community-living older adults: A 1-year prospective study. *Archives of Physical Medicine and Rehabilitation*, 82, 1050–1056.

Jak, A. J. (2011). The impact of physical and mental activity on cognitive aging. In M-C. Pardon and M. W. Bondi (Eds.), *Behavioral neurobiology of aging* (pp. 273–291). Berlin, Heidelberg: Springer.

James, W. P. T., Jackson-Leach, R., & Rigby, N. (2010). An international perspective on obesity and obesogenic environments. In A. A. Lake, T. G. Townshend, and S. Alvanides (Eds.), *Obesogenic environments: Complexities, perceptions and objective measures* (pp. 1–9). Oxford: Wiley-Blackwell.

Johnson, B. T., Scott-Sheldon, L. A., & Carey, M. P. (2010). Meta-synthesis of health behavior change meta-analyses. *American Journal of Public Health*, 100, 2193.

Kanoski, S. E., & Davidson, T. L. (2011). Western diet consumption and cognitive impairment: Links to hippocampal dysfunction and obesity. *Physiology & Behavior*, 103, 59–68.

Kendig, H., Browning, C. J., Thomas, S. A., & Wells, Y. (2014). Health, lifestyle, and gender influences on aging well: An Australian longitudinal analysis to guide health promotion. *Frontiers in Public Health*, Article 70, 1–9.

Kramer, A. F., & Erickson, K. I. (2007). Capitalizing on cortical plasticity: Influence of physical activity on cognition and brain function. *Trends in Cognitive Sciences*, 11(8), 342–348.

Lally, P., Van Jaarsveld, C. H., Potts, H. W., & Wardle, J. (2010). How are habits formed: Modelling habit formation in the real world. *European Journal of Social Psychology*, 40, 998–1009.

Lautenschlager, N. T., & Cox, K. L. (2013). Commentary. *JAMA Internal Medicine*, 173(9), 805–806.

Locher, J. L., Bales, C. W., Ellis, A. C., Lawrence, J. C., Newton, L., Ritchie, C. S., Roth, D. L., Buys, D. L., & Vickers, K. S. (2011). A theoretically based behavioral nutrition intervention for community elders at high risk: The B-NICE randomized controlled clinical trial. *Journal of Nutrition in Gerontology and Geriatrics*, 30(4), 384–402.

Locher, J. L., Vickers, K. S., Buys, D. R., Ellis, A., Lawrence, J. C., Newton, L. E., Roth, D. L., Ritchie, C. S., & Bales, C. W. (2013). A randomized controlled trial of a theoretically-based behavioral nutrition intervention for community elders: Lessons learned from the Behavioral Nutrition Intervention for Community Elders Study. *Journal of the Academy of Nutrition and Dietetics*, 113, 1675–1682.

Luchsinger, J. A., & Gustafson, D. R. (2009). Adiposity and Alzheimer's disease. *Current Opinion in Clinical Nutrition and Metabolic Care*, 12(1), 15.

McIntosh, W. A., Shifflett, P. A., & Picou, J. S. (1989). Social support, stressful events, strain, dietary intake, and the elderly. *Medical Care*, 27, 140–153.

Mein, G. K., Shipley, M. J., Hillsdon, M., Ellison, G. T., & Marmot, M. G. (2005). Work, retirement and physical activity: Cross-sectional analyses from the Whitehall II study. *The European Journal of Public Health*, 15(3), 317–322.

Michie, S., Ashford, S., Sniehotta, F. F., Dombrowski, S. U., Bishop, A., & French, D. P. (2011). A refined taxonomy of behaviour change techniques to help people change their physical activity and healthy eating behaviours: The CALO-RE taxonomy. *Psychology & Health*, 26, 1479–1498.

Miller, D. I., Taler, V., Davidson, P. S. R. R., & Messier, C. (2012). Measuring the impact of exercise on cognitive aging: Methodological issues. *Neurobiology of Aging*, 33(3), 622, e29–e43.

Milligan, W., Bridges, C., & Christides, T. (2012). Audit of vitamin D intake in a nursing home (NH) for the elderly mentally infirm (EMI). *Proceedings of the Nutrition Society*, 71, E233.

Milte, C. M., Thorpe, M. G., Crawford, D., Ball, K., & McNaughton, S. A. (2015). Associations of diet quality with health-related quality of life in older Australian men and women. *Experimental Gerontology*, 64, 8–16.

Norton, S., Matthews, F. E., Barnes, D. E., Yaffe, K., Brayne, C. (2014). Potential for primary prevention of Alzheimer's disease: An analysis of population-based data. *The Lancet Neurology*, 13, 788–794.

Owen, N., Healy, G. N., Matthews, C. E., & Dunstan, D. W. (2010). Too much sitting: The population-health science of sedentary behavior. *Exercise and Sport Sciences Reviews*, 38, 105.

Peel, N. M., McClure, R. J., & Bartlett, H. P. (2005). Behavioral determinants of healthy aging. *American Journal of Preventive Medicine*, 28, 298–304.

Procter-Gray, E., Leveille, S. G., Hannan, M. T., Cheng, J., Kane, K., & Li, W. (2015). Variations in community prevalence and determinants of recreational and utilitarian walking in older age. *Journal of Aging Research*, 2015, 382703.

Pruchno, R., Wilson-Genderson, M., & Gupta, A. K. (2014). Neighborhood food environment and obesity in community-dwelling older adults: Individual and neighborhood effects. *American Journal of Public Health*, 104(5), 924–929.

Reelick, M. F., Iersel, M. B. van, Kessels, R. P., & Rikkert, M. G. (2009). The influence of fear of falling on gait and balance in older people. *Age & Ageing*, 38, 435–440.

Rejeski, W. J., & Mihalko, S. L. (2001). Physical activity and quality of life in older adults. *The Journals of Gerontology Series A: Biological Sciences and Medical Sciences*, 56, S23–S35.

Salazar, J. A., Poon, I., & Nair, M. (2007). Clinical consequences of polypharmacy in elderly: Expect the unexpected, think the unthinkable. *Expert Opinion on Drug Safety*, 6, 695–704.

Scientific Advisory Committee on Nutrition (SACN). (2007). *Update on vitamin D: Position statement by the Scientific Advisory Committee on Nutrition*. www.sacn.gov.uk/dfs/sacn_position_vitamin_d_2007_05_07.pdf

Scuffham, P., Chaplin, S., & Legood, R. (2003). Incidence and costs of unintentional falls in older people in the United Kingdom. *Journal of Epidemiology & Community Health*, 57, 740–744.

Shaw, B. A., & Spokane, L. S. (2008). Examining the association between education level and physical activity changes during early old age. *Journal of Aging and Health*, 20(7), 767–787.

Stewart, J., Crockett, R., Gritton, J., Stubbs, B., & Pascoe, A. (2014). Ageing at home? Meeting housing, health and social needs. *Journal of Integrated Care*, 22, 242–252.

Stewart, T. L., Chipperfield, J. G., Perry, R. P., & Weiner, B. (2012). Attributing illness to 'old age:' Consequences of a self-directed stereotype for health and mortality. *Psychology & Health*, 27, 881–897.

Stock, J., Clifford, A., & Hogervorst, E. (2012). Exercise interventions to improve cognitive performance in older adults – potential psychological mediators to explain variation in findings. *European Neurological Review*, 7(2), 107–112.

Touvier, M., Bertrais, S., Charreire, H., Vergnaud, A. C., Hercberg, S., & Oppert, J. M. (2010). Changes in leisure-time physical activity and sedentary behaviour at retirement: A prospective study in middle-aged French subjects. *International Journal of Behavioral Nutrition and Physical Activity*, 7, 1186.

Vesnaver, E., & Keller, H. H. (2011). Social influences and eating behavior in later life: A review. *Journal of Nutrition in Gerontology and Geriatrics*, 30, 2–23.

Whalley, L. J. Deary, I. J., Starr, J. M., Wahle, K. W., Rance, K. E., Bourne, V. J. & Fox, H. C. (2008). n – 3 Fatty acid erythrocyte membrane content, APOE ε4, and cognitive variation: An observational follow-up study in late adulthood. *The American Journal of Clinical Nutrition*, 87(2), 449–454.

Wilcox, S., Castro, C., King, A. C., Housemann, R., & Brownson, R. C. (2000). Determinants of leisure time physical activity in rural compared with urban older and ethnically diverse women in the United States. *Journal of Epidemiology and Community Health*, 54(9), 667–672.
Wise, J. (2014). NICE advises certain groups to take daily vitamin D supplement. *British Medical Journal*, 348, g3349.
Zamboni, M., Mazzali, G., Zoico, E., Harris, T. B., Meigs, J. B., Di Francesco, V., Fantin, V., Bissoli, L., & Bosello, O. (2005). Health consequences of obesity in the elderly: A review of four unresolved questions. *International Journal of Obesity*, 29, 1011–1029.

12

SEXUAL HEALTH FOR OLDER ADULTS

Geraldine Anthony

This chapter discusses:

- The effect of normal aging on sexual health
- The effect of disabling medical conditions on sexual health
- Safe sex awareness in older adults

Introduction

Whatever your age or gender the need for intimacy is a fundamental human desire. It is commonly believed that sexual desires diminish with age. Because sexuality tends to be a private matter, it is discussed less than any other element of aging. However, the good news for most healthy older adults is that pleasure and interest do not diminish with age. Not only does having a love life enhance your relationships, it can help keep you younger for longer. Most people are sexually active throughout their lives, with or without a partner. Some feel greater sexual freedom in their later years. It is also important to be aware that some men and women are content not to be sexually active. Getting older can present challenges for those wanting to continue to be sexually active. Issues related to physical changes, mental changes and social life can interfere with this. However, while aging involves a normal slowing response, the benefits of getting older can add a new dimension to intimacy not present during one's youthful years. Older adults are often more confident and relaxed about their bodies and they are less influenced by the pressure society places on beauty and perfection. Another positive factor is that some older adults feel a new lease of life once their children have flown the nest and responsibilities at work for some are reduced and mortgages are paid, resulting in less financial pressure and more time to devote to each other. In any case the process of aging can affect intimacy in both genders. Normal age-related changes (for example, menopause in women and the increased incidence of prostate cancer in men) may complicate issues with comfort and intimacy. Other medical conditions (for example, diabetes, arthritis, dementia) together with the side effects of some drugs used to control these chronic conditions can cause additional problems including emotional changes which can be further exacerbated with depression, low self-esteem and poor physical health. Although there is a low risk of pregnancy in sexual activity in older adults, maintaining safe practice is paramount.

The effect of normal aging on sexual health

There are currently over 23.6 million people over the age of 50 years, which accounts for over a third of the total UK population (Mid-2014 Population Estimates UK Office of National Statistics, 2015). Physical body changes evolve over time and from around the age of 50 years and upwards, both men and women begin to notice changes, including change in their sexual behaviour. Sexual health is often ignored in this group for two reasons: firstly, the assumption that they are no longer sexually active and secondly, people are too embarrassed to discuss it or seek advice. Although the incidence of sexual dysfunction increases with age, this appears to be due primarily to health problems, medications and the lack of available partners rather than to age itself (Deacon, Minichiello and Plummer, 1995). There are several factors that may interfere with developing and maintaining an intimate relationship, which may include divorce, separation, bereavement, living alone, menopause, impotence, cancer (e.g. ovarian, cervical and prostrate) and medical disorders (e.g. diabetes, arthritis, cognitive impairment and dementia), which are discussed below.

Sexual changes in women

Menopause is a normal part of a woman's aging process. Most women experience menopause around age 50; the usual age range is between 45 to 55. With menopause the ovaries cease to produce the hormones oestrogen and progesterone. Women may or may not know they have gone through menopause after they have had no periods for about one year. With the change in these hormones, other changes occur which include the vaginal walls becoming thinner, dryer and less elastic. Sometimes sex can become painful as a result of these changes. In addition, other common changes include symptoms such as hot flushes, moodiness, headaches, trouble sleeping, lower sex drive, decrease in breast tissue and the increased risk of osteoporosis. Some women may also feel urinary system changes (e.g. frequency and urgency of urination and increased risk of urinary infections). There may also be the additional loss of tone in the pelvic floor muscles, resulting in the vagina, uterus or urinary bladder falling out of position (prolapse). As mentioned above, these are normal physical changes which can be managed. Hormone Replacement Therapy (HRT) with oestrogen or progesterone, alone or combined, may help menopause symptoms such as hot flushes, vaginal dryness and pain during intercourse. As with all medication there are risks; HRT is not always suitable for every woman. The risks and benefits of HRT should be discussed on an individual basis with your doctor/specialist nurse. Due to some or all of the above, sexual problems are amongst the most frequently presented health concerns for women attending menopause clinics. There are several lubricants (e.g. Vagifem and other water-based lubricants such as KY Jelly) to help manage painful intercourse. Topical oestrogen creams can also be used to help thicken the vagina walls and increase moisture and sensitivity. Very few studies have been conducted on the menopause transition and sexual dysfunction; one reason for this is due to the effects of aging on menopause, as the hormonal changes of menopause take place over a variable period of time. Also of interest is that menopause can present at an earlier age, such as surgical menopause when a hysterectomy is performed in cases where cancer or menstrual problems are identified, such as heavy bleeding and uterine cancer.

Cervical health is also important. In the United Kingdom, cervical screening to detect pre-cancerous changes is offered to women from the ages of 25–65. The human papillomavirus is present in 99 per cent of cervical cancers. Cervical screening is one of the best screening tools used to detect changes in cervical cells and older adults are not discharged from screening until the age of 65. Any form of cancer – whether it is cervical, ovarian or uterine – can have a physiological effect on any woman and this is no less than in women as older adults.

Sexual changes in men

In the United Kingdom, one in 10 men are impotent and, as men get older, problems become much more common. Men beyond their 50s may find that their sex drive is minimally affected (although health problems, certain medicines or relationship/work stress can lower sex drive). Since the 1990s, there has been increasing recognition and documentation that erectile dysfunction (ED) is a common problem. There are no universally agreed criteria for how consistent the problem has to be and for what duration it needs to be present to fulfil the definition. A period of persistence of longer than three months has been suggested as a reasonable clinical guideline. Increasing awareness of effective treatment strategies on behalf of patients, effective advertising by drug companies and acknowledgement by healthcare providers that screening may help identify cardiovascular and other medical risks have led to higher rates of reporting, diagnosis and treatment of ED. Thyroid problems, diabetes and alcohol can have an effect on ED that may need to be investigated and treated. Several studies have looked at the prevalence of ED. The Massachusetts Male Aging Study reported a prevalence of 52 per cent and that ED is increasingly prevalent with age. At age 40, approximately 40 per cent of men are affected. The rate increases to nearly 70 per cent in men aged 70 years. The prevalence of complete ED increases from 5 per cent to 15 per cent as age increases from 40 to 70 years.

Prostate cancer

Prostate cancer is the most common malignancy amongst older men and is the second leading malignancy in the Western world (Crawford, 2003). The incidence of prostate cancer has increased at a steady pace over the last decade (Crawford, 2003; Jemal et al., 2007). Between 2000 and 2050, the number of men aged 65 years and over with prostate cancer is expected to increase four-fold worldwide. By 2030, the percentage of men older than 65 years with prostate cancer will rise to 19.6 per cent of the population compared with a lower incidence of 12.4 per cent of the population in 2000 (Crawford, 2003; Jemal et al., 2007). The good news is incidence of deaths from prostate cancer has decreased over the last decade, probably as a result of improved screening and diagnosis, improved treatments and better risk assessment to guide therapy.

Prostate cancer can affect sexual activity in three ways: the mind, the body and in relationships. Treatment for prostate cancer can cause a variety of side effects and any of these can affect sexual activity. The effects depend on the type of treatment. Many men feel very low after they have been told they have cancer and may not be interested in sexual activity. The treatment itself can cause erectile dysfunction and very often men have to wait until treatment is complete and they are feeling back to normal before embarking on resuming sexual activity. Radiotherapy to the prostate, having the actual surgery, having testicles removed and hormone therapy, including their side effects, can affect impotence. The effects on sexual activity can be difficult for men and side effects can affect them in different ways. Partner support and understanding is vital at this stage and everyone reacts to cancer in different ways. Counselling and support from doctors and nurses in this specialist field is available for those who need professional support and advice.

The effect of disabling medical conditions on sexual health

Not only does the aging body experience problems with sexual function, the likelihood of developing other medical health problems also increases in older adults. Very often sexual problems are mainly due to physical limitations, side effects of medication and simply lack of energy. The degree of restriction can vary from very minor to more restrictive depending on the severity, for example, of diabetes, arthritis, cancer, stroke and other serious illnesses. This may have an impact for one or both partners depending on if they have one or more disabilities, which can therefore make it difficult to provide an effective intervention and advice. Regardless of the type of treatment or advice, any problems encountered need to be discussed in the first instance. Age-related factors and health changes are rarely discussed, as often older adults are embarrassed to discuss sexual issues with health professionals. The most common aging medical conditions but not all will be discussed below. It is important to have some understanding of how these age-related medical conditions affect us so we know how best to manage these.

Diabetes

Diabetes and sexuality are related and may affect sexual activity in older adults of both sexes. However, this depends largely on the severity of the disease together with the age of onset. In addition, diabetes in men can lead to hardening and narrowing of the blood vessels, which can affect the erectile tissue of the penis. In older women, changes may be more subtle, with reduced blood flow causing the vagina to be dry. This can be further complicated in women with diabetes who have higher levels of sugar (glucose) in vaginal secretions, which means they are more likely to have vaginal yeast infections, which cause itching and irritation and make sex uncomfortable or undesirable. Women who do not have diabetes can have similar symptoms with vaginal yeast infections; however older adults with diabetes may not seek professional help and are less likely to discuss problems with their health professionals, particularly if their symptoms affect sexual activity (Lindau et al., 2010).

Arthritis

There are an estimated nine million older adults in the United Kingdom suffering from arthritis (Arthritis Research UK 2016) and it is one of the most common diseases in the United States. There are several kinds of arthritis, each with different signs and symptoms. Older adults most often have osteoarthritis (OA), rheumatoid arthritis (RA) or gout. People often think of arthritis as painful and having stiff joints. The pain and swelling may last only for a short time and is very uncomfortable, whereas other types may be less painful. Osteoarthritis is the most common type of arthritis in older adults and symptoms can range from mild pain to pain that never stops. This can be disabling, particularly if it is present in the hips, knees and back. Rheumatoid arthritis, an autoimmune disorder that makes the body attack itself, can cause pain and stiffness that may last for hours and people often feel tired. RA tends to affect more women than men. Gout is another form of arthritis that tends to affect the big toe but other joints can also be affected. The swelling causes the skin to pull tight around the joint and can appear very red or purple and very tender to touch. Certain food can lead to an attack of gout (for example, liver, dried beans, peas, anchovies and gravy) and this can be further exacerbated by being overweight, alcohol and some medication.

Along with taking prescribed medication, exercise and diet can also help. Daily exercise such as dancing and swimming can improve movement of joints, weight training for strengthening exercises and simply walking can lessen swelling in the joints and improve mobility, together with preventing weight gain to stay fit and healthy.

There are a number of ways that having an arthritic disorder can affect sexual activity. A person's mood can be affected by having arthritis with the additional discomfort of painful swollen joints affecting one's self-confidence, as well as the affected painful joints having to be moved into a comfortable position. This reduced mobility and the additional fatigue can reduce sexual desire. For some people with arthritis, pain can vary from day to day, so it may be beneficial to make the most of the opportunity of the pain-free days. Some of the medication (for example, steroids) can sometimes reduce sexual desire but overall most drugs used to treat arthritis are unlikely to affect sexual activity.

Dementia

Dementia causes many changes in people's lives. Some people with dementia show increased interest in sex, but they may not be able to judge what appropriate sexual behaviour is and in some instances where new relationships are formed there may be issues with consent. People with severe dementia may not recognise their partner but still want sexual contact. Having dementia does not mean the end of a happy sex life. Adaptions can be made to help cope with dementia and the provision of comfort and support, such as by cuddles, talking and supporting each other. People with dementia can have unpredictable sexual feelings and, depending on the area of the brain affected and the medication, their mood and memory changes frequently. Partners can struggle to cope with these constant changes and get upset, angry and very often frustrated, as this is difficult to cope with. By simply having a diagnosis of dementia, this does not always mean that someone does not have the mental capacity to make a decision; however they may not always understand the implications of those decisions. It is also important for families and health professionals to be aware and make sure people with dementia are not at risk of suspected sexual abuse. Sexual abuse is a criminal offence and needs to be prevented in this vulnerable group of people.

Depression

Feeling good at any age is important to a person's general health and well-being. Depression in older adults often presents itself, such as after retirement or the death of a partner, which may result in loneliness and often isolation, which can have serious effects on health. There are lots of other factors, such as the health problems mentioned above, which can result in restricted mobility, living alone, having no sense of purpose and loss of identity. Prescription medications which are taken to control various medical conditions (for example, stroke, heart disease, diabetes, cancer, dementia, Alzheimer's, etc.) often have side effects which have symptoms of depression. These side effects can affect anybody regardless of age; however older adults have an increased risk of developing symptoms of depression if they are taking a lot of medication for multiple medical conditions, together with the fact that they are more sensitive to drugs because of their age and the body's reduced efficiency at metabolising and processing them. Rather than dwell on symptoms of depression, it is important to focus on ways to avoid or reduce these. Diet, exercise and socialising are also important. Healthy eating and managing weight is good for everyone and in particular for older adults to promote healthy living. Older adults should do at least 150 minutes of physical activity a week where possible and be as physically active as their condition and abilities allow. Safe exercise can boost mood. Improved self-esteem is a key psychological benefit of regular physical activity. When you exercise, your body releases chemicals called endorphins which trigger a positive feeling in the body similar to that of morphine.

Another benefit is that endorphins can also act as an analgesic, which helps with pain and also produces a sedative effect. Spending time with others and participating in activities with people with similar interests is also important to help lift depression. It's a myth to think that older adults can't learn new skills. Trying new activities is beneficial if people can't maintain hobbies they had when they were younger. There are lots of ways (for example, Skype, FaceTime and computer skills) which older adults can easily learn and are taught at most local libraries to help keep in contact with old friends, make new ones and have fun. Growing old allows people to do things they did not have time to do before.

Safe sex awareness in older adults

Awareness of safe sex

The population of the world is living longer and sexuality is one of the most important quality-of-life issues for older adults who are healthier than previous generations. In addition to the normal changes as well as the effect of medical conditions and their associated medications, sexual health also needs to be addressed in order to improve quality of life and allow older adults to enjoy living. Regardless of age, anyone starting a new relationship should discuss safe sex. Whether a person is male or female, heterosexual, lesbian, gay, bisexual or transgender, it is just as important for older as it is for younger adults that safe sex is practiced (Ace, 2002). People of all ages who are sexually active are at risk of sexually transmitted diseases (STDs) and STDs in older adults are increasing. Many people with STDs do not have any symptoms and, despite the fact that people feel healthy, it is still important to get tested. As with all age groups, any unusual discharge, itchiness, discomfort, blisters, sores, spots or lumps around the genitals or anal region should be checked by a GP or at a genitourinary medicine (GUM) clinic. The focus for sexual health is geared towards the younger population and many of our older adults may have missed the boat when safe sex and prevention of STDs was introduced in the United Kingdom in the 1980s following the discovery of HIV/AIDS. Recent research shows that the rates of STDs is continuing to rise in older adults over the age of 50 years with diseases such as syphilis, gonorrhoea, chlamydial infection, genital herpes, Hepatitis B, genital warts and trichomonas (Age UK, 2015).

Our current population of over-50s grew up after the contraceptive pill was introduced, which gave women the freedom to control their own fertility. The focus then was in preventing pregnancy and awareness of condom use and the prevention of STDs were poor (Family Planning Association, 2010). STDs in older adults worldwide in the over-50s have more than doubled over the last decade and the reasons are unclear. One reason in men may be the improvement in treatment for erectile dysfunction, making sex possible for older men. Another reason may be due to the low rate of condom use amongst older adults who no longer think they have to worry about pregnancy and may not think they are at risk of STDs. Having reviewed the literature for this chapter, the focus on research has been on STDs in teens and younger adults, which are plentiful, but very little on why rates are increasing amongst older adults. Possible reasons for the incidence of STDs in older adults could be that the increase in divorce and separation rates have affected their sexual behaviour, lack of safe sex awareness and reluctance to seek help and advice.

Divorce and separation

In the United Kingdom, there is a steady increase in divorce and remarriage rates. The divorce rate in the over 60-years-old age group has doubled from 1990 to present (UK Office of National Statistics, 2015). The reasons identified include the increasing life expectancy, with men living a further 26 years and similarly in women than they were in 1991. Another factor is the increase in the female population in the labour market, which has risen from 53 per cent in 1971 to 66 per cent and rising in 2012. This means that women have become more financially independent and are more likely to have built up their own pensions and can support themselves. The International Longevity Centre in the United Kingdom (ILC-UK) is expressing concern that a growing divorce rate in old age could contribute to increasing isolation and a greater need for formal care. In the new report dubbed 'The rise (and rise) of the silver separator', ILC-UK found that from 1990 to 2012, the divorce rate for both genders aged 60 or above has risen by over 85 per cent and the rate continues to rise (Bamford et al., 2015). Based on these current rates by age, the total number of people over the age of 60 will increase from 15,700 in 2012 to over 22,000 by 2037 – a 41 per cent rise – by 2037, which means that almost one in every 10 people experiencing divorce will be aged over 60. With the increase in the rates of divorce and separation in older adults, there is an increase in sexual activity with new partners.

Sexually transmitted diseases (STDs)

A recent study conducted by Schick et al. (2010) on health risks and sexual intimacy has shown that 85 per cent aged over 50 years old were sexually active and 68 per cent did not use any contraception or barrier protection. The introduction and availability of the drug Viagra has afforded older men the opportunity to be sexually active again (Kingsberg, 2002). In addition, similar findings have been reported in relation to gay, lesbian, and bisexual older adults (Age Concern England, 2002). Diagnosed STDs have increased substantially in the United Kingdom since the 1990s (Nicoll et al., 2001) and throughout the last decade to the end of 2012, emphasising the importance of sustained public health programmes to identify, treat and reduce morbidity and mortality to prevent further transmission of STDs. There are several strategies in the United Kingdom, such as the National Strategy for Sexual Health & HIV in England (2001), the Action Plan for Improving Sexual Health In Scotland (2005) and a similar strategy in Wales which is called the Strategic Framework for Promoting Sexual Health in Wales (2001) (Kinghorn, 2001). The focus on all these strategies is to reduce the risk of STDs and is focused mainly for adolescents and younger adults.

The sex life of older adults has long been ignored and poorly researched and is only really getting attention in light of the current staggering statistics that STDs, in line with divorce and separation rates in the United Kingdom and United States, have doubled in the last decade. The increase is seen in cases of chlamydia, HIV and syphilis. The best way to avoid STDs is to practise safe sex (for example, wearing a condom). Many older people who experience single or relationship changes do not feel the need to use protection with new partners and are increasingly at risk of contracting STDs. The cultural shift to meeting new partners is much easier with the advent of Internet dating and ease of international travel.

Another STD known as Human Immunodeficiency Virus (HIV), for which there currently is no cure and no vaccine to prevent from becoming infected, is on the increase. In older adults, if HIV is suspected, it is extremely important that they are tested as early as possible because without treatment they are more likely to develop late stage HIV infection faster than in younger people. Untreated older adults are more likely to die compared to younger people. Condom use is paramount and medication for heart disease, depression, high blood pressure, Alzheimer's disease and arthritis can all effect antiretroviral treatments. Erectile dysfunction problems in men with HIV can also occur from nerve damage and HIV medication.

Barriers to seeking help for older adults

Older adults making midlife changes who go back to dating again, who probably never used condoms when they were younger, are unaware of the risk of contracting STDs. Older adults may not perceive themselves to be at risk for contracting STDs and HIV/AIDS, believing that such diseases are likely to affect only young people. In addition, older adults experience stigma associated with STDs and are less likely than younger adults to disclose symptoms to health professionals. Such stigma is commonly associated with feelings of shame, guilt, negative self-image and fear, along with the embarrassment to ask for advice, seek screening and treatment as required.

Many older adults feel unable to ask for help and support at their GP practice for several reasons which include GP attitudes towards later-life sexuality, shame/embarrassment and fear, perceived sexual problems as 'not serious' and lack of knowledge about appropriate services (Gott and Hinchliff, 2003). In contrast, a more recent study by Gott et al. (2004) surveyed GPs and practice nurses, where it was identified that GPs were concerned about their own knowledge and expertise in this area and fears of opening a 'floodgate' and their own personal embarrassment when discussing sexual health issues with older adults. The barriers identified by practice nurses were similar and included lack of time, lack of training and concerns about not being able to cope with the issues raised by older adults. This area warrants further attention if sexual health management in primary care policy recommendations is to be met.

Conclusion

Many people want and need to be closer as they get older and still have fun, and this includes the desire to continue to have sex. It is important that older adults are comfortable with discussing any physical changes that normal aging brings with their doctor or health professional if it affects intimacy. Sexual health in older adults has not received much research attention in recent years despite the statistics which show that people are living longer and the rate of STDs has doubled in the last decade. More older adults than ever before are attending genitourinary clinics for sexually transmitted infections and diseases. Sexual healthcare policy, health education, and healthcare communities need to be improved to include older adult sexual health behaviour to the same level as they address sexual health needs of adolescents. The rising number of divorces amongst the over-60s is something that policymakers, charities and services providers should factor in when considering sexual health for older adults. The views of older people who are forming increasingly larger proportions of the aging population due to increased life expectancy are not represented. However, in recent years there has been a change in policymakers' wishes to understand the sexual needs of older people, as demonstrated by the UK NATSAL studies. Getting regular exercise, eating healthy foods and staying involved in activities with friends and loved ones can help the aging process go more smoothly and to maintain safe sexual health. Age brings intelligence, experience, wisdom and beauty, so what are we so scared of? Older adults who have a positive view of aging stay active and healthier longer. Regardless of age, gender or sexual orientation, intimacy and safe sexual activity can continue as long as one chooses and is a fundamental human desire.

References

Age Concern England. (2002). *Age concern England issues facing older lesbians, gay men, and bisexuals*. Policy Position Paper 15, Age Concern England.

Age UK. (2017). www.ageuk.org.uk/latest-news/archive/rise-in-stis-among-over-50s/ (accessed March 23, 2017).

Arthritis UK website. (2016). www.arthritisresearchuk.org (accessed May 4, 2017).

Crawford, E. D. (2003). Epidemiology of prostate cancer. *Urology*, 62(6 Suppl. 1), 3–12.

Deacon, S., Minichiello, V., and Plummer, D. (1995). Sexuality and older people: Revisiting the assumptions. *Educational Gerontology: An International Quarterly*, 21(5), 497–513.

Family Planning Association. (2010). www.fpa.org.uk/ (accessed May 4, 2017).

Franklin, B., & Creighton, H. (2014). *The rise and rise of the silver seperator.* International Longevity Centre. http://www.ilcuk.org.uk/images/uploads/publication-pdfs/The_rise_and_rise_of_the_silver_separator.pdf, (accessed May 4, 2017).

Gott, M., Galena, E., Hibchliff, S., and Elford, H. (2004). "Opening a can of worms": GP and practice nurse barriers to talking about sexual health in primary care. *Family Practice*, 21(5), 528–535.

Gott, M., and Hinchliff, S. (2003). Barriers to seeking treatment for sexual problems in primary care: A qualitative study with older people. *Family Practice*, 20, 690–695.

Jemal, A., Siegel, R., Ward, E., Murray, T., Xu, J., and Thun, M. J. (2007). Cancer statistics, 2007. *CA: A Cancer Journal for Clinicians*, 57(1), 43–66.

Kinghorn, G. (2001). A sexual health and HIV strategy for England: This ambitious strategy could, if properly resourced, greatly improve sexual health. *British Medical Journal*, 323(7307), 243.

Kingsberg, S. A. (2002). The impact of aging on sexual function in women and their partners. *Archives of Sexual Behaviour*, 31(5), 431–437.

Lindau, S. T., Tang, H., Gomero, A., Vable, A., Elbert, S., Huang, E. S., Drum, M. L., Qato, D. M., Marschalll, H., and Chin, M. D. (2010). Sexuality Among Middle Age and Older Adults with Diagnosed and Undiagnosed Diabetes: A National, Population-Based Study. *Diabetes Care*, 33(10), 2202–2210, October.

Nicoll, A., Hughes, G., Donnelly, M., Livingstone, S., De Angelis, D., Fenton, K., and Catchpole, M. (2001). Assessing the impact of national anti-HIV sexual health campaigns: Trends in the transmission of HIV and other sexually transmitted infections in England. *Sexually Transmitted Infections*, 77(4), 242–247.

Schick, V., Herbenick, D., Reece, M., Sanders, S. A., Dodge, B., Middlestadt, S. E., and Fortenberry, J. D. (2010). Sexual behaviors, condom use, and sexual health of Americans over 50: Implications for sexual health promotion for older adults. *The Journal of Sexual Medicine*, 7(s5), 315–329.

UK Office for National Statistics. (2016). *Mid-2015 population estimates*. www.ons.gov.uk/peoplepopulationandcommunity/populationandmigration/populationestimates (accessed May 4, 2017).

13
COGNITIVE AGING

Nelson A. Roque and Walter R. Boot

This chapter discusses:

- Age-related changes in cognition
- Mechanisms of age-related cognitive decline
- Intervention studies to improve cognition later in life
- Designing for aging

Learning outcomes

In this chapter you will learn how to:

- Describe basic age-related changes in cognition and theories of cognitive aging
- Describe various intervention approaches that have been explored to combat age-related cognitive decline
- Discuss evidence for the efficacy of different methods to boost cognitive performance
- Describe how age impacts technology use and the potential of technology to support the independence of older adults

Introduction

As we age, we can all expect to experience some degree of cognitive decline. Large longitudinal studies find that age is associated with slower and less accurate performance of a variety of laboratory tasks tapping different aspects of cognition. Alongside these declines, some cognitive skills are preserved or even improve later in life. For the abilities that do decline, the implication of these declines extend beyond the laboratory: perceptual and cognitive declines measured by these tasks are associated with difficulty performing the everyday activities required for independent living. These activities, referred to as Instrumental Activities of Daily Living (IADLs), include driving, meal preparation, medication adherence, and shopping. When an individual's cognitive abilities decline enough to interfere with the performance of these important tasks, he or she is at risk of losing their independence and may need to transition from their own home to an environment that provides daily assistance and support (e.g., assisted living facility).

Understanding cognitive decline and how these declines impact everyday living and independence is growing increasingly important as many countries in the world undergo the processes of population aging. Declining birth rates, in conjunction with increasing life expectancy, is causing a demographic shift in more- and less-developed nations that will lead to a greater proportion of older individuals in the population and relatively fewer younger individuals (United Nations, 2013). This represents a major challenge. The economic and societal costs of supporting the needs of a rapidly expanding older adult population, especially if this population is experiencing cognitive decline, will grow substantially over the next few decades, and there will be fewer younger individuals to support these costs and provide care. By better understanding age-related declines we are better able to design solutions to counter their effect on independence (e.g., through technological solutions that support the performance of everyday activities), and we may also be able to design interventions to slow or reverse cognitive aging.

The aim of this chapter is to provide a basic characterization of *normative* age-related perceptual and cognitive declines informed by the literature. These are declines that most of us can expect to experience. Non-normative cognitive changes (e.g., Alzheimer's disease and other forms of dementia, see Chapter 10) will not be a primary focus. After characterizing basic age-related changes, we will discuss theories of cognitive aging and summarize some of the changes to the nervous system thought to play a role in declining perceptual and cognitive abilities. Finally, we conclude with a discussion of proposed methods to prevent, reduce, or reverse cognitive aging, or lessen their impact on independence.

Age-related changes

Overview

Cross-sectional and longitudinal studies, in which different age groups are compared to one another, or one group of individuals is measured multiple times over the course of many years, provide strong evidence for age-related differences and changes in cognition. These studies demonstrate that declines later in life are not restricted to one or two domains of cognitive functioning (e.g., memory), but instead indicate that a variety of abilities show declines with advancing age (Ball et al., 2002; Park et al., 2002; Schaie, Willis & Caskie, 2004; Nyberg et al., 2010). While measuring and quantifying age-related changes in cognition might seem like a straightforward endeavor, there are a number of challenges associated with doing so. For example, factors associated with age, but not the aging process itself, may partly drive differences in cognitive performance. These factors include general health and the environment and educational system an individual was exposed to during development (e.g., see the Flynn Effect for an example of a cohort difference in cognition; Fox & Mitchum, 2013). When comparing the cognition of groups of people of different ages, one needs to be mindful that variables other than age likely contribute to observed performance differences and this method of studying cognitive aging can overestimate or underestimate age-related declines. This is not a problem in longitudinal studies in which the cognition of the same group of individuals is measured multiple times over many years. However, longitudinal studies can underestimate the effect of age as a result of performance benefits from multiple test administrations (Salthouse, 2014). Retest benefits have the potential to mask or lessen the appearance of cognitive declines over time. Issues of cross-generation generalizability are a concern as well. If you were to follow a sample of individuals and measure their cognition for 50 years, other future generations may age in ways that are different from the sample you studied. Despite these methodological challenges there is a convergence of evidence from multiple types of studies confirming that as we age we can expect to experience fairly broad declines in cognitive ability.

When does age-related cognitive decline begin? While this may again seem like a simple question, there is disagreement among cognitive aging researchers. This relates to whether one believes cross-sectional or longitudinal data provide a more valid answer. Salthouse (2009) argues that declines can be observed starting as early as one's twenties or thirties, based largely on cross-sectional data in which the cognitive abilities of individuals of different ages are compared. Longitudinal data, however, often indicate that declines may not be observed until the age of 60 or later (Nilsson et al., 2009). While there is disagreement regarding exactly when cognitive aging begins, it is clear that cognition later in life (e.g., 70s and beyond) is often worse than cognition in early adulthood. Next we describe some of the most commonly observed changes (and lack of changes) as a function of advancing age.

Memory

One of the most commonly reported complaints of older adults is forgetfulness, and data indicate clear age-related changes in memory. It is important to note, however, that there are multiple forms of memory (e.g., short-term, long-term, working memory), with some forms of memory being more susceptible to age-related decline than others. This next section defines different types of memory and the impact of age on each. Distinctions between memory systems relate to how long information is stored and available for recall and the type of information that is processed and retained by these systems.

Long-term versus short-term versus working memory

Time course can be used to differentiate among different types of memory systems. Relatively long-lasting memories (e.g., home phone number, the capital of France) are considered to be supported by long-term memory systems. The capacity of long-term memory is practically unlimited and these memories can persist for a lifetime. In contrast, short-term memory systems hold relatively small amounts of information temporarily while it is needed and afterward this information quickly fades. For example, when following a new recipe one might read the next two or three steps and retain these steps in memory until they are performed. Similar to this type of short-term memory, working memory allows for the temporary storage and manipulation of information to complete a task or solve a problem (Baddeley, 2012). For example, while calculating the total cost of a purchase, one might add the cost of two items and store this information temporarily until the cost of a third item is added to it. Thus, the defining characteristic of working memory is the transformation and updating of information temporarily stored in short-term memory. Another way to differentiate among several memory systems is by whether the content of the memories can be consciously recalled or not. Those that can be consciously recalled with details are said to be stored by declarative memory systems, while those that cannot be recalled consciously (e.g., procedural skills such as how to ride a bike) are said to be non-declarative. These broad classifications of memory systems are used to help organize memory findings below.

Semantic memory

Semantic memory is a form of long-term memory that refers to our knowledge of facts about the world, including vocabulary. When you are asked to recall the name of your high school, the capital city of a country, or the definition of a word, you are relying on your semantic memory. Our knowledge and vocabulary are also referred to as crystalized intelligence (Cattell, 1963). This construct, measured by the knowledge accumulated over time, has been extensively studied with most findings pointing in the same direction – aging has little effect on crystalized intelligence. Most of the literature on this subject finds that the function of this system is largely stable across the adult lifespan, with some studies finding mild improvement across the lifespan (Bowles & Salthouse, 2008; Park et al., 2002). As we age, we accumulate more knowledge about the world, and it is thought that this increase in knowledge can to some degree offset declines in other abilities.

Episodic memory

This memory system can be thought of as related to your personal story, told from your own perspective, mainly focusing on events connected to places, people, and things you have encountered and the factual information you have stored about them. Reminiscing with friends and family about past vacations you have taken together, the sights you saw, and the food you ate will make use of the episodic memory system. Considerable age-related deficits in episodic memory are observed, but the magnitude of age-related change depends on the nature of the task and the particular processing phase being studied (storage, maintenance, or retrieval of information). Deficits may largely be accounted for by shallower encoding of new episodic memories (Persson & Nyberg, 2008). Episodic memory encompasses source memory, remembering not just the information from an episode but the context in which this information was learned (e.g., who told you something). Evidence suggests that source memory may be particularly sensitive to age (Schacter et al., 1991).

Prospective memory

Prospective memory refers to remembering to complete some intention in the future. For example, you may need to remember to take a medication this evening with dinner, or you may need to remember to leave by 1pm for a doctor's appointment to be there on time. In a meta-analysis of prospective memory studies, it was found that on laboratory tasks of both time-based prospective memory (remembering to perform a task at a specific time) and event-based prospective memory (remembering to perform a task after a specific event), younger adults outperformed older adults. However, with more naturalistic tasks, older adults may show an advantage compared to younger adults (Henry et al., 2004).

Implicit memory

Implicit (non-declarative) memories encompass the non-conscious learning of information. For example, we can sometimes pick up on regularities in our environment and respond appropriately largely in a way that is automatic and without awareness. This type of memory includes procedural memory or memory for complex motor sequences (e.g., how to ride a bike). It is difficult to consciously express the steps involved in these complex motor sequences and these actions can often be carried out with little attention to the task. This type of memory appears to be relatively spared with respect to age-related decline (though see Ward, Berry & Shanks, 2013 for a more nuanced discussion).

Working memory

To solve various problems we need to temporarily store information in mind so that it can be manipulated, compared, and integrated with other information. This ability is referred to as working memory. Accumulated evidence suggests that age is associated with significant declines in working memory capacity (Bopp and Verhaeghen, 2005) and that performance declines in working memory tasks are greater than for tasks in which information simply needs to be remembered and recalled (without information needing to be manipulated or updated). This is consistent with a more general pattern of age-related decline in which deficits are more likely to be observed in more complex, effortful tasks involving more cognitive operations.

Attention

Our ability to efficiently navigate the complex environments we encounter daily is a result of our attention system prioritizing information relevant to our goals for subsequent processing, while filtering out information irrelevant to our goals. Without attention we would be overwhelmed by the amount of information in our environment. Although attention is commonly referred to as a unitary construct, it can also be conceptualized as a multi-faceted construct that includes divided attention, sustained attention, and selective attention. Attention in general can be thought of as the control of the amount of cognitive resources allocated to one stimulus or another, or one task or another.

Divided attention

When you are performing two (or more) tasks at once, you are said to be tapping your divided attention capacity (your attention is split across tasks or stimuli). The capacity for effectively performing simultaneous tasks has been found to be reduced with increasing age, over and above the decrement in performance expected from general age-related slowing (Verhaeghen & Cerella, 2002). In a number of measures, older adults are found to be able to divide their attention between multiple objects in the environment less efficiently compared to younger adults (Trick, Perl and Sethi, 2005).

Sustained attention

The ability to maintain attention on a task for a long period of time can be referred to as vigilance, alertness, or sustained attention. One common task used to measure sustained attention is the sustained-attention-to-response task (SART), in which participants are asked to respond to all items that appear on screen except for one for an extended period of time (Robertson et al., 1997). Using this task, researchers have found an age-related decline in sustained attention, with a moderate to large effect size (McAvinue et al., 2012).

Selective attention

The ability to focus on one goal (i.e., searching for a target within a visual scene) while ignoring distracting information irrelevant to that goal is best characterized as selective attention. Similar to divided attention, selective attention has been found to decline overall as a function of age, resulting in less search efficiency (Madden, 2007).

Executive control

Our ability to manage and control our cognitive processes can be referred to as executive control. A brief review of the age-related effects observed across these areas of research is presented in the sections below.

Inhibition

Our ability to limit the influence of task-irrelevant information taps directly into the construct of inhibition. This construct has been considered by some to be largely responsible for explaining age-related declines in cognitive function. One paradigm used to measure inhibition is the antisaccade task (Munoz & Everling, 2004), in which observers are asked to look in the opposite direction of the stimulus that is presented on the screen (to the left or right of a fixation cross). There is evidence that age-related declines in the frontostriatal systems may be contributing to a reduced capacity to voluntarily suppress an eye movement towards the target amongst older adults compared to younger adults (Sweeney et al., 2001). The evidence for age differences in inhibition is mixed, with an early meta-analysis on measuring inhibitory control mechanisms using the Stroop task (Stroop, 1935) finding no age differences in inhibition (Verhaeghen & De Meersman, 1998), compared to a large-scale study looking at the Stroop task that found age differences not attributed to general slowing (Troyer, Leach & Strauss, 2006).

Task-switching and dual-tasking

As we go through our day we often find ourselves shifting our attention from one goal to the next. Our ability to update our goals and responses depending on the current task we confront is an aspect of executive control. This is often measured in the laboratory using task-switching paradigms in which, depending on a cue, a different task needs to be performed. Switching between tasks often invokes a greater cost for older adults compared to younger adults (Wasylyshyn, Verhaeghen & Sliwinski, 2011). Similarly, dual-tasking (performing two tasks simultaneously) is another executive control function indicative of cognitive flexibility. In most dual-task paradigms, performance on a dual-task condition is compared to a single task condition (on latency and accuracy) in order to understand to what extent each task competes for the same resources. A meta-analysis on the subject of dual-task performance found evidence for a difference in performance between younger and older adults on dual-task latency, but a lack of an age-related decline in dual-task accuracy (Verhaeghen et al., 2003).

Reasoning, problem-solving

When faced with a complex situation, our ability to understand the problem-space, consider options, and ultimately inform a decision is reasoning or problem-solving. A meta-analysis looking at age differences in everyday problem-solving and decision-making effectiveness found a moderate decline in this construct with increased age (Thornton & Dumke, 2005). In general, fluid intelligence, our ability to reason and detect patterns, declines with advancing age (Staff, Hogan and Whalley, 2014).

Language comprehension

Our ability to understand language is crucial to our daily living (e.g. understanding medication instructions, reading road signs) and also for our ability to interact in social environments. Language comprehension includes both spoken and written language, as each is attributed to a different subset of component sensory inputs (e.g. reliance on audition for spoken language and reliance of vision for comprehension of written language). The relationship between language comprehension and aging is not well understood, as the literature on the topic is quite mixed, with some finding that comprehension abilities are relatively stable (Baltes, Staudinger & Lindeberger, 1999) while others argue that working memory is a strong predictor of a decline that is evident (Daneman & Merikle, 1996).

Processing speed

A general characteristic of the aging process is a slowing of cognitive operations (processing speed), which has been proposed by some as the primary factor behind most age-related cognitive declines (Salthouse, 1996b). Visual processing speed has received much attention recently, with clear evidence that visual information is processed more slowly by older adults (Owsley, 2013).

Impact on everyday tasks

In the previous sections we have described numerous age-related changes in the performance of mostly abstract laboratory tasks. However, of greater significance is the effect that cognitive changes may have on the performance of important everyday tasks such as driving and medication adherence. Available evidence does indicate a relationship between cognitive decline measured by laboratory-based measures of cognition and everyday difficulties. For example, performance on a measure of visual processing speed, the Useful Field of View test, has been consistently associated with increased crash risk among older drivers (Clay et al., 2005). As another example, Gross et al. (2011) examined the relationship between various cognitive measures in a large older adult sample and the performance of simulated everyday activities (e.g., interpreting a medication label, balancing a checkbook). Laboratory measures of processing speed, memory, and reasoning ability all contributed uniquely in terms of predicting the speed and accuracy of performance of important everyday tasks. Reasoning ability accounted for the most variance. However, memory performance was the best predictor of changes in everyday ability over a five-year period. These are among many examples of observed relationships between laboratory measures and tasks vital for living independently. This pattern suggests that measures typically used to study cognitive aging have real-world relevance and that age-related changes in these measures are meaningful.

Now that we have characterized basic cognitive changes and the implication of these changes for everyday living, we next turn to what might underlie these changes. First, we discuss several theories of cognitive aging, then we turn our attention to biological changes that might explain why cognition changes with age.

Models of cognitive aging and biological changes

There are several competing theories regarding the processes that underlie age-related cognitive decline. These models must account for the pervasiveness of cognitive decline (i.e., age is associated with declines of not just one or a few cognitive abilities, but many), and also the fact that in many cases age is associated with greater performance deficits for more complex tasks (Salthouse, 1996a, 1996b). To account for these data, and the fact that age-related differences in cognitive abilities such as working memory largely disappear once processing speed is statistically controlled for, Salthouse proposed a processing-speed theory of cognitive aging. This account posits that slowing in basic information processing is the primary factor underlying age-related cognitive decline and has pervasive effects on cognition. By this account, the implication for simple information processing tasks is clear (e.g., older adults will be slower when performing a simple choice reaction time task in which they have to respond with a keypress to whether the letter X or O appears). However, the performance of more complex tasks and decisions should suffer more because they involve a greater number of operations that are each slowed. Further, in speeded tasks involving several cognitive steps, earlier initial operations may not be completed by the time their output is needed for later processing and decision stages, resulting in both slower and less accurate performance. Delays in information transmission can also result in information being decayed or lost by the time it is needed. Degraded or lost information can account for poorer performance by older adults even on tasks that do not have a strong speeded component. Transmission delays are consistent with age-associated demylenization – a loss of the protective coating around neuron axons that help speed neural signals.

Other models account for broad declines through mechanisms other than processing speed. Similar to the processing speed account, these models propose that age is associated with a decline in some fundamental resource or ability crucial to the performance of many different tasks. Older adults may have a smaller pool of cognitive resources overall to allocate to tasks (e.g., Craik & Byrd, 1982). For relatively simple and automatic processes, age-related changes may be absent or minimal because the pool of cognitive resources is sufficient for these tasks. However, for more complex tasks and tasks that require effortful processing, age-related declines are more pronounced. This "pool of resources" might be conceptualized as working memory, attention, or executive functioning; related cognitive processes fundamental to the performance of a variety of tasks. Others have conceptualized inhibitory deficits as a primary factor responsible for age-related cognitive decline (e.g., Hasher & Zacks, 1988). As mentioned previously, strong differences in inhibitory control can be observed across the lifespan. Without the ability to inhibit irrelevant information performance across a range of tasks is expected to suffer, and it may be difficult for older adults to select and maintain goals because failures of inhibition can result in irrelevant information entering working memory.

Cognitive declines are related to a variety of changes that occur in the brain as we age. The Scaffolding Theory of Aging (STAC) suggests that these changes impact cognitive functioning, but that a variety of neural and behavioral compensatory mechanisms may counteract these effects (Park & Reuter-Lorenz, 2009). This framework is important because it both explains why cognition changes with age, but also potential mechanisms through which these changes can be minimized or countered. Some of these are adaptive mechanisms of the brain, and others involve lifestyle choices and intervention.

One of the more salient changes is brain atrophy, which has been observed in a number of structural magnetic resonance imaging (MRI) studies. Cross-sectionally, in a sample that ranged from 59–85 years of age, Resnick and colleagues (2000) found that increased age was associated with decreased grey and white matter volume. Longitudinally over a five-year period, Raz and colleagues (2005) observed in a sample of healthy older adults pervasive declines in brain volume. A thinning of the cortex can also be observed as a function of age (Lemaitre et al., 2012). This atrophy may be less related to a decline in the number of neurons than to the size of neurons and the number of connections between them (Burke & Barnes, 2006). Some of this evidence suggests a "last-in, first-out" pattern of decline, such that the areas of the brain that reach maturity latest during development (e.g., frontal areas critical for working memory, inhibition, and executive control) are most sensitive to age. This is consistent with notable changes in the abilities supported by these regions with age. In addition to these structural changes, at the smaller scale, age is associated with less efficient neural transmission, partly through a decline in neurotransmitter receptors and decreased neurotransmitter synthesis.

Age is also associated with changes in functional brain activation as well. One pattern that has been observed is a pattern of dedifferentiation (e.g., Carp et al., 2011). That is, while younger adults recruit specific brain regions to perform different tasks, older adults may recruit broad and overlapping regions to perform the same tasks. Another pattern that has been often observed is one of "contralateral recruitment." Younger adults may recruit a brain region within one hemisphere to perform a task, with older adults recruiting that region and the region within the opposite hemisphere to perform the same task (Cabeza, 2002). This recruitment may be compensatory, allowing better performance by pooling processing resources across hemispheres.

Cognitive interventions

It is clear that age is associated with declines in our ability to remember, reason, juggle multiple tasks, inhibit responses, respond quickly, and more. Can anything be done to prevent, reduce, or reverse age-related cognitive decline? If so, this would allow older adults to maintain their independence longer and reduce the societal costs of supporting and caring for individuals experiencing age-related declines that interfere with independent living. Longitudinal and intervention studies have suggested a number of factors related to maintaining cognition later in life (Hertzog et al., 2008).

Cognitive engagement

Large-scale longitudinal studies find that the number of cognitively engaging activities an older adult engages in is associated with less-steep cognitive decline years later (e.g., Wilson, Barners & Bennett, 2003). Other studies find that the greater amount of education one has, the less severe cognitive decline one can expect to experience (e.g., Albert et al., 1995). These results are broadly consistent with a "use-it-or-lose-it" hypothesis that makes the analogy that the brain is like a muscle. With regular exercise a muscle gets stronger, and without exercise it will atrophy. Due to the non-experimental nature of these investigations, numerous other factors might explain observed relationships between activity, education, and cognition; however these data are suggestive that cognitive stimulation may serve to preserve cognitive functioning later in life.

Brain training programs are intended to provide cognitive exercise and have been proposed as a means to reverse age-related cognitive decline. There are a multitude of products on the market with the aim of improving cognition. Most of these products are computer-based activities or digital games. However, the efficacy of such interventions is uncertain at this time. A consensus statement, organized by the Stanford Longevity Center and signed by 70 scientists, recently stated that there is little convincing evidence that such interventions can meaningfully improve the cognition of older adults (http://longevity3.stanford.edu/blog/2014/10/15/the-consensus-on-the-brain-training-industry-from-the-scientific-community/). A counter-consensus statement released a few months later, signed by 127 scientists and practitioners, claimed that the evidence was clear that brain training can make a meaningful difference in people's lives (www.cognitivetrainingdata.org/). While there is disagreement among scientists at this point regarding the benefits of brain training programs, both groups of scientists appear to agree that some marketing claims of brain training products go beyond the evidence and are frequently exaggerated.

The Advanced Cognitive Training for Independent and Vital Elderly (ACTIVE) clinical trial was the largest and most rigorous test of the efficacy of brain training with a sample of 2,832 participants who were randomly assigned to receive brain training focused on reasoning, memory, or processing speed, or who were assigned to a control group that received no training. Participants were followed for 10 years and a variety of primary and secondary outcome measures were collected that tapped aspects of cognition, well-being, and independence (see Tennstedt & Unverzagt, 2013 for a summary). Immediately after training, reports indicated little generalizable benefit of cognitive training. Participants improved on the trained tasks but improvements did not transfer to other tasks, including simulated everyday tasks. Five and 10 years post-training, however, there were improvements in self-reported ability to perform everyday tasks relative to the passive control group. Some evidence also suggested a reduction in at-fault crashes for some of the training groups, especially the processing speed group. However, this reduction in at-fault crash rate is somewhat difficult to interpret in light of a substantial increase in not-at-fault crashes relative to the control group. While proponents of brain training effects point to the ACTIVE trial as supporting general benefits of cognitive training, those skeptical of these effects note that the clearest pattern observed was one of specificity: participants mostly improved on the tasks they trained on. They also note a variety of methodological weaknesses (including the reliance of a passive control group that might not control for placebo effects and the reliance on subjective measures) cast doubt upon whether effects might generalize to a broader population.

Physical exercise

Even if physical exercise had no effect on cognition, it is something that most people should engage in due to the host of associated health benefits. However, longitudinal studies suggest that individuals who engage in frequent physical activities tend to age more gracefully compared to more sedentary individuals with respect to cognition. For example, Yaffe and colleagues (2001) observed in a large sample of older women that higher baseline levels of physical activity predicted less cognitive decline six to eight years later. Research with mice and rats also finds that experimental manipulations of exercise (e.g., the introduction of a running wheel into the living environment) can improve memory and result in a number of positive benefits to brain health (e.g., increased number of hippocampal cells; Van Praag et al., 2005).

Human intervention work appears to confirm the positive cognitive benefits of physical exercise, especially aerobic exercise. Benefits are supported by several meta-analyses of physical fitness intervention studies (e.g., Colcombe & Kramer, 2003; Smith et al., 2010). These intervention studies often have sedentary older adults participate in a walking intervention (aerobic) or a stretching and toning intervention (non-aerobic) several times a week for six months to a year. Positive cognitive benefits – including benefits to measures of executive control, memory, and processing speed – are frequently observed for the aerobic group relative to the non-aerobic control group.

A variety of changes to the brain appear to be linked to physical fitness and aerobic exercise. For example, Colcombe and colleagues (2006) asked older adults to participate in a six-month intervention that involved either aerobic or non-aerobic exercise and measures of brain structure were collected before and after this period. Older adults assigned to the aerobic intervention demonstrated significant increases in grey and white matter volume compared to the non-aerobic control group. Changes were observed in frontal regions associated with attention, executive control, and memory, some of the same cognitive processes observed to improve in other intervention studies. Erickson and colleagues (2011) performed a similar intervention, with the intervention lasting one year. This study found that aerobic exercise increased the volume of the hippocampus, a brain structure critical to memory formation. Further, this study found that volume changes were associated with increased levels of brain-derived neurotrophic factor (BDNF), a protein that promotes the survival of neurons and encourages the growth of neurons and synapses. Within the animal literature, increased aerobic fitness is linked to angiogenesis (proliferation of new blood vessels), neurogenesis (new cells), and increased levels of neuroprotective chemicals (Voss, Nagamatsu, Liu-Ambrose, & Kramer, 2011).

Overall, evidence from a variety of types of studies (longitudinal, intervention, human, animal, behavioral, neuroimaging) converge to provide evidence for the cognitive benefits of aerobic fitness. Unlike cognitive engagement interventions (i.e., brain training), the problem of wasted "opportunity cost" does not appear to apply. An older adult spending time on brain training software package that doesn't produce the intended benefit is likely wasting his or her time. However, even if exercise had no cognitive benefits (though evidence supports the fact that it does), being more active is good for overall health and is a good investment in terms of time.

Nutrition

Evidence also points to a potential role of proper nutrition in promoting healthy cognitive aging. Much of this work has focused on the consumption of antioxidants, substances that protect against cellular damage by neutralizing reactive molecules known as free-radicals. For example, in a large longitudinal study, Morris and colleagues (2002) examined the potential role of two antioxidants in maintaining cognitive functioning late in life: vitamins E and C. Dietary intake from a large sample of older adults was assessed and cognitive measures were collected at baseline and again about three years later. Individuals who consumed more vitamin E (but not C) experienced less steep cognitive decline across assessment points. Other studies have examined diet type, with a focus on the effects of a Mediterranean diet (MD). A Mediterranean diet includes fish, fruits, vegetable, nuts, cereals, and legumes, and is generally low in saturated fat, red meat, and processed meat. MD foods tend to be high in antioxidants and part of an MD also includes a moderate amount of alcohol consumption. In a longitudinal study of over 500 older adults, MD was associated with better cognition (executive functioning) and a more Western diet was associated with steeper cognitive decline (visuospatial ability, Gardener et al., 2014; see Morris et al., 2015 for additional evidence for the cognitive benefits of a MD-style diet).

The number of large-scale human randomized controlled trials examining the effect of diet on late-life cognition is smaller compared to cognitive engagement and physical exercise trials. Some animal work, specifically with dogs, suggests that a diet rich in antioxidants can reduce age-related cognitive decline (Cotman et al., 2002). A recent clinical trial in which participants were randomly assigned to a MD diet that either included nuts or olive oil, or a control diet, suggested some modest cognitive benefits over a four-year period (Valls-Pedret et al., 2015). Another study that explored the effect of a different antioxidant (vitamin B), however, found no benefit (van der Zwaluw et al., 2014). At this point, there is not enough data from large randomized controlled trials to recommend the adoption of specific dietary habits with the sole purpose of improving cognition; however initial results are positive and there are likely to be health benefits in general from adopting a diet that included less processed and red meats.

Social support

Finally, some studies find that social connections or social activities may have protective effects against cognitive aging, though currently there is a dearth of intervention data linking social activities and support to reduced age-related cognitive decline. A more active social life does appear to be associated with less-steep decline. For example, Bassuk and colleagues (1999) found that in a sample of about 3,000 older adults, social activities and number of social contacts predicted cognitive decline over a 12-year period. The social measure used in this study included whether or not a spouse was present in the household, the number of face-to-face contacts with friends and family members, the number of non-face-to-face contacts (e.g., letters, phone calls), church attendance, and participation in clubs and gatherings. Greater social activity participation has also been linked to better processing speed later in life, an ability thought to underlie age-related performance declines generally (Lövdén, Ghisletta & Lindenberger, 2005). Consistent with this observation, reports of loneliness are related to declines in memory, spatial ability, perceptual speed, and transition to Alzheimer's disease (Wilson et al., 2007). In general, remaining socially engaged and maintaining social connections has been suggested as one means to maintain cognitive health.

Like all cross-sectional or longitudinal studies a variety of confounds and alternative explanations might account for the relationship between social activity and cognition. Only intervention studies can provide evidence for a causal link, but few interventions have explored this issue. Some preliminary evidence for a causal link comes from studies involving the Experience Corps program. This is a program that gets older adults more socially involved by having them volunteer in inner city schools. Older adults read to students, help them learn to read, and also perform library activities such as recommending age-appropriate books. Early evidence suggests some cognitive benefits (Carlson et al., 2008) and brain benefits (Carlson et al., 2015). Some early evidence also suggests that social activities such as digital photography and quilting classes may confer some cognitive benefits (Park et al., 2014). An interesting future direction is whether technology-based social interactions may be beneficial as well (Czaja et al., 2015). More evidence is required before we might recommend face-to-face and digital social contact as a means to improve cognition.

Cognitive intervention summary

A variety of activities and lifestyle factors have been suggested to prevent, reduce, or reverse age-related cognitive decline. The efficacy of brain training programs is controversial. The most compelling evidence at this point is associated with physical fitness interventions. Aerobic exercise appears to improve cognition in animal and human intervention studies. Numerous plausible mechanisms have been explored to explain this effect, with exercise being associated with positive changes in brain structure, function, and neurochemistry. In addition to cognitive health, exercise is associated with general health benefits as well, making it a safe bet with respect to time investment. Evidence for the efficacy of short-term nutrition and social interventions is still accumulating. Rather than thinking about this in terms of "interventions," perhaps a better way to think about addressing cognitive aging is in terms of accumulating a lifetime of enriching experiences, including maintaining a healthy diet, engaging in physical activity, forming meaningful social connections, and participating in stimulating activities over the course of decades, starting early in life. This is in contrast with "get smart quick" approaches, in which older adults might engage in shorter-term exercise or brain training interventions later in life.

Implications for design and training

As perceptual and cognitive abilities decline, older adults may experience difficulty using products and technologies that do not take these declines into account during the design process. This may in part contribute to the observed "digital divide" in which newer technologies tend to be adopted more slowly by older adults compared to younger adults. For example, older adults lag substantially in terms of smartphone adoption. In 2015, while 64 percent of all Americans 18 years of age or older owned a smartphone (71 percent across European samples), only 27 percent of Americans 65 years of age or older did (comparable to smartphone penetration statistics from Europe at 34 percent) (Smith, 2015; *The smartphone generation gap: over 55? There is no app for that*, 2013). While 86 percent of all adults used the Internet in 2013, only 59 percent of seniors 65 years of age or older did (Smith, 2014). This is unfortunate, as information and communication technologies (ICTs) have the potential to help older adults remain independent despite age-related perceptual and cognitive declines (Charness & Boot, 2009). Technology can serve as "environmental support," compensating for the effects of age (Morrow & Rogers, 2008). For example, digital calendar systems might support prospective memory (e.g., remembering appointments) and medication adherence might be assisted by electronic pill dispensers with alarm reminders. In other words, these devices can serve as "cognitive prosthesis." Technology may especially benefit older adults at risk for social isolation (e.g., older adults who live alone, rural older adults, older adults who can no longer drive). ICT has the potential to allow these individuals to better connect to friends, family, and local and national resources. Telehealth technologies that facilitate the delivery of healthcare without the patient having to leave the home may also be especially valuable to older adults. However, without good design and training, benefits may not be realized. Technological solutions to benefit independence are only viable if individuals of all ages can use them.

Why are older adults more reluctant to adopt new technologies? Cognition likely plays a role. This is consistent with research finding that fluid and crystalized intelligence are associated with technology use (Czaja et al., 2006). In this large sample, data also supported the potential of attitudinal barriers, with computer anxiety being a significant predictor of technology use. Human factors and design issues also contribute to technology use and adoption (Fisk et al., 2009). Poor design for aging includes devices with small, low contrast text and buttons, as well as complex navigation menus that place high demands on working memory. Design should also consider the diversity of technology experience individuals of different ages bring to a piece of technology. Not all users will have the same mental model of how to use a device. By designing well for older adults, they too will be able to access the benefits of technology, especially technology that might assist them with the performance of everyday tasks important for independence. In general, a device designed well for an older adult is easier for younger adults to use as well. Another important factor to consider is training. Older adults may need as much as twice the amount of time to master a new piece of technology compared to younger adults (Charness et al., 2001), and the preferences and needs of older learners may differ significantly from younger learners (Czaja & Sharit, 2012). By taking these factors into account, technology can serve as a more direct method (compared to "brain training") to support older adults experiencing age-related cognitive declines.

Conclusions

This chapter introduced the issue of cognitive aging and why it is an important topic of investigation. Due to population aging the number of older adults in the world will be greater than ever before. Understanding cognitive aging, and methods to address it, is a crucial challenge that we face. The declines we can expect to experience are many, and these declines have clear implications for independence. However, not all cognitive abilities decline. As we age we continue to maintain, and even grow, our knowledge about the world, which may help us manage declines in other areas of cognition.

The evidence that brain training interventions, or any short-term intervention (with perhaps the exception of aerobic fitness training), can meaningfully improve cognition is controversial at this point. Overall, not enough is known at this point to recommend specific brain training programs. An active, engaged, and stimulating lifestyle over many years is most likely a much more promising approach compared to "get smart quick" approaches. Physical exercise and healthy eating are associated with a number of general health benefits, and thus they are likely to be worth the investment even if they had no cognitive benefit.

Technology has the potential to help older adults live independently by offsetting the effect of age-related cognitive decline. However, this solution depends on designing technology that is usable by all. In the near future, it is likely that automation and robotics will play a greater role in supporting older adults. For example, autonomous vehicles might soon provide safe and accessible transportation for an aging population.

References

Albert, M. S., Jones, K., Savage, C. R., Berkman, L., Seeman, T., Blazer, D., & Rowe, J. W. (1995). Predictors of cognitive change in older persons: MacArthur studies of successful aging. *Psychology and Aging*, 10(4), 578–589.

Baddeley, A. (2012). Working memory: Theories, models, and controversies. *Annual Review of Psychology*, 63, 1–29.

Ball, K., Berch, D. B., Helmers, K. F., Jobe, J. B., Leveck, M. D., Marsiske, M., . . . Active Study Group. (2002). Effects of cognitive training interventions with older adults: A randomized controlled trial. *JAMA*, 288(18), 2271–2281.

Baltes, P. B., Staudinger, U. M., & Lindenberger, U. (1999). Lifespan psychology: Theory and application to intellectual functioning. *Annual Review of Psychology*, 50, 471–507.

Bassuk, S. S., Glass, T. A., & Berkman, L. F. (1999). Social disengagement and incident cognitive decline in community-dwelling elderly persons. *Annals of Internal Medicine*, 131(3), 165–173.

Bopp, K. L., & Verhaeghen, P. (2005). Aging and verbal memory span: A meta-analysis. *The Journals of Gerontology Series B: Psychological Sciences and Social Sciences*, 60(5), P223–P233.

Bowles, R. P., & Salthouse, T. A. (2008). Vocabulary test format and differential relations to age. *Psychology and Aging*, 23(2), 366.

Burke, S. N., & Barnes, C. A. (2006). Neural plasticity in the ageing brain. *Nature Reviews Neuroscience*, 7(1), 30–40.

Cabeza, R. (2002). Hemispheric asymmetry reduction in older adults: The HAROLD model. *Psychology and Aging*, 17(1), 85–100.

Carlson, M. C., Kuo, J. H., Chuang, Y. F., Varma, V. R., Harris, G., Albert, M. S., . . . Fried, L. P. (2015). Impact of the Baltimore experience corps trial on cortical and hippocampal volumes. *Alzheimer's & Dementia*, 11(11), 1340–1348.

Carlson, M. C., Saczynski, J. S., Rebok, G. W., Seeman, T., Glass, T. A., McGill, S., . . . Fried, L. P. (2008). Exploring the effects of an "everyday" activity program on executive function and memory in older adults: Experience Corps®. *The Gerontologist*, 48(6), 793–801.

Carp, J., Park, J., Hebrank, A., Park, D. C., & Polk, T. A. (2011). Age-related neural dedifferentiation in the motor system. *PloS one*, 6(12), e29411.

Cattell, R. B. (1963). Theory of fluid and crystallized intelligence: A critical experiment. *Journal of Educational Psychology*, 54(1), 1.

Charness, N., & Boot, W. R. (2009). Aging and information technology use: Potential and barriers. *Current Directions in Psychological Science*, 18, 253–258.

Charness, N., Kelley, C. L., Bosman, E. A., & Mottram, M. (2001). Word-processing training and retraining: Effects of adult age, experience, and interface. *Psychology and Aging*, 16(1), 110–127.

Clay, O. J., Wadley, V. G., Edwards, J. D., Roth, D. L., Roenker, D. L., & Ball, K. K. (2005). Cumulative meta-analysis of the relationship between useful field of view and driving performance in older adults: Current and future implications. *Optometry & Vision Science*, 82(8), 724–731.

Colcombe, S. J., Erickson, K. I., Scalf, P. E., Kim, J. S., Prakash, R., McAuley, E., Elavsky, S., Marquez, D. X., Hu, L., & Kramer, A. F. (2006). Aerobic exercise training increases brain volume in aging humans. *The Journals of Gerontology Series A: Biological Sciences and Medical Sciences*, 61(11), 1166–1170.

Colcombe, S., & Kramer, A. F. (2003). Fitness effects on the cognitive function of older adults: a meta-analytic study. *Psychological Science*, 14(2), 125–130.

Cotman, C.W., Head, E., Muggenburg, B. A., Zicker, S., & Milgram, N.W. (2002). Brain aging in the canine: A diet enriched in antioxidants reduces cognitive dysfunction. *Neurobiology of Aging*, 23(5), 809–818.

Craik, F.I.M., & Byrd, M. (1982). Aging and cognitive deficits. In F.I.M. Craik and S. E. Trehub (Eds.), *Aging and cognitive processes* (pp. 191–211). New York: Springer.

Czaja, S. J., Boot, W. R., Charness, N., Rogers, W. A., Sharit, J., Fisk, A. D., . . . Nair, S. N. (2015). The personalized reminder information and social management system (PRISM) trial: Rationale, methods and baseline characteristics. *Contemporary Clinical Trials*, 40, 35–46.

Czaja, S. J., Charness, N., Fisk, A. D., Hertzog, C., Nair, S. N., Rogers, W. A., & Sharit, J. (2006). Factors predicting the use of technology: Findings from the Center for Research and Education on Aging and Technology Enhancement (CREATE). *Psychology and Aging*, 21(2), 333–352.

Czaja, S. J., & Sharit, J. (2012). *Designing training and instructional programs for older adults*. Florida: CRC Press.

Daneman, M., & Merikle, P. M. (1996). Working memory and language comprehension: A meta-analysis. *Psychonomic Bulletin & Review*, 3(4), 422–433.

Erickson, K. I., Voss, M. W., Prakash, R. S., Basak, C., Szabo, A., Chaddock, L., Kim, J. S., Heo, S., Alves, H., White, S. M., & Wojcicki, T. R. (2011). Exercise training increases size of hippocampus and improves memory. *Proceedings of the National Academy of Sciences*, 108(7), 3017–3022.

Fisk, A. D., Rogers, W. A., Charness, N., Czaja, S. J., & Sharit, J. (2009). *Designing for older adults: Principles and creative human factors approaches*. Florida: CRC Press.

Fox, M. C., & Mitchum, A. L. (2013). A knowledge-based theory of rising scores on "culture-free" tests. *Journal of Experimental Psychology: General*, 142(3), 979–1000.

Gardener, S. L., Rainey-Smith, S. R., Barnes, M. B., Sohrabi, H. R., Weinborn, M., Lim, Y.Y., . . . Martins, R. N. (2014). Dietary patterns and cognitive decline in an Australian study of ageing. *Molecular Psychiatry*, 20, 860–866.

Gross, A. L., Rebok, G.W., Unverzagt, F.W., Willis, S. L., & Brandt, J. (2011). Cognitive predictors of everyday functioning in older adults: Results from the ACTIVE Cognitive Intervention Trial. *The Journals of Gerontology Series B: Psychological Sciences and Social Sciences*, 66(5), 557–566.

Hasher, L., & Zacks, R. T. (1988). Working memory, comprehension, and aging: A review and a new view. *The Psychology of Learning and Motivation*, 22, 193–225.

Henry, J. D., MacLeod, M. S., Phillips, L. H., & Crawford, J. R. (2004). A meta-analytic review of prospective memory and aging. *Psychology and Aging*, 19(1), 27–39.

Hertzog, C., Kramer, A. F., Wilson, R. S., & Lindenberger, U. (2008). Enrichment effects on adult cognitive development can the functional capacity of older adults be preserved and enhanced? *Psychological Science in the Public Interest*, 9(1), 1–65.

Lemaitre, H., Goldman, A. L., Sambataro, F., Verchinski, B. A., Meyer-Lindenberg, A., Weinberger, D. R., & Mattay, V. S. (2012). Normal age-related brain morphometric changes: Nonuniformity across cortical thickness, surface area and gray matter volume? *Neurobiology of Aging*, 33(3), 617-e1.

Lövdén, M., Ghisletta, P., & Lindenberger, U. (2005). Social participation attenuates decline in perceptual speed in old and very old age. *Psychology and Aging*, 20(3), 423–434.

McAvinue, L. P., Habekost, T., Johnson, K. A., Kyllingsbæk, S., Vangkilde, S., Bundesen, C., & Robertson, I. H. (2012). Sustained attention, attentional selectivity, and attentional capacity across the lifespan. *Attention, Perception, & Psychophysics*, 74(8), 1570–1582.

Madden, D. J. (2007). Aging and visual attention. *Current Directions in Psychological Science*, 16(2), 70–74.

Morris, M. C., Evans, D. A., Bienias, J. L., Tangney, C. C., Bennett, D. A., Aggarwal, N., . . . Scherr, P. A. (2002). Dietary intake of antioxidant nutrients and the risk of incident Alzheimer disease in a biracial community study. *JAMA*, 287(24), 3230–3237.

Morris, M. C., Tangney, C. C., Wang, Y., Sacks, F. M., Barnes, L. L., Bennett, D. A., & Aggarwal, N. T. (2015). MIND diet slows cognitive decline with aging. *Alzheimer's & Dementia*, 11(9), 1015–1022.

Morrow, D. G., & Rogers, W. A. (2008). Environmental support: An integrative framework. Human Factors: *The Journal of the Human Factors and Ergonomics Society*, 50(4), 589–613.

Munoz, D. P., & Everling, S. (2004). Look away: The anti-saccade task and the voluntary control of eye movement. *Nature Reviews Neuroscience*, 5(3), 218–228.

Nilsson, L. G., Sternäng, O., Rönnlund, M., & Nyberg, L. (2009). Challenging the notion of an early-onset of cognitive decline. *Neurobiology of Aging*, 30(4), 521–524.

Nyberg, L., Salami, A., Andersson, M., Eriksson, J., Kalpouzos, G., Kauppi, K., . . . Nilsson, L. G. (2010). Longitudinal evidence for diminished frontal cortex function in aging. *Proceedings of the National Academy of Sciences*, 107(52), 22682–22686.

Owsley, C. (2013). Visual processing speed. *Vision Research*, 90, 52–56.

Park, D. C., Lautenschlager, G., Hedden, T., Davidson, N. S., Smith, A. D., & Smith, P. K. (2002). Models of visuospatial and verbal memory across the adult life span. *Psychology and Aging*, 17(2), 299.

Park, D. C., Lodi-Smith, J., Drew, L., Haber, S., Hebrank, A., Bischof, G. N., & Aamodt, W. (2014). The impact of sustained engagement on cognitive function in older adults the synapse project. *Psychological Science*, 25(1), 103–112.

Park, D. C., & Reuter-Lorenz, P. (2009). The adaptive brain: Aging and neurocognitive scaffolding. *Annual Review of Psychology*, 60, 173–196.

Persson, J., & Nyberg, L. (2008). Structure – function correlates of episodic memory in aging. *Handbook of Behavioral Neuroscience*, 18, 521–634.

Raz, N., Lindenberger, U., Rodrigue, K. M., Kennedy, K. M., Head, D., Williamson, A., Dahle, C., Gerstorf, D., & Acker, J. D. (2005). Regional brain changes in aging healthy adults: general trends, individual differences and modifiers. *Cerebral Cortex*, 15(11), 1676–1689.

Resnick, S. M., Goldszal, A. F., Davatzikos, C., Golski, S., Kraut, M. A., Metter, E. J., Bryan, R. N., & Zonderman, A. B. (2000). One-year age changes in MRI brain volumes in older adults. *Cerebral Cortex*, 10(5), 464–472.

Robertson, I. H., Manly, T., Andrade, J., Baddeley, B. T., & Yiend, J. (1997). Oops!: performance correlates of everyday attentional failures in traumatic brain injured and normal subjects. *Neuropsychologia*, 35(6), 747–758.

Salthouse, T. A. (1996a). Constraints on theories of cognitive aging. *Psychonomic Bulletin & Review*, 3(3), 287–299.

Salthouse, T. A. (1996b). The processing-speed theory of adult age differences in cognition. *Psychological Review*, 103(3), 403–428.

Salthouse, T. A. (2009). When does age-related cognitive decline begin? *Neurobiology of Aging*, 30(4), 507–514.

Salthouse, T. A. (2014). Why are there different age relations in cross-sectional and longitudinal comparisons of cognitive functioning? *Current Directions in Psychological Science*, 23(4), 252–256.

Schacter, D. L., Kaszniak, A. W., Kihlstrom, J. F., & Valdiserri, M. (1991). The relation between source memory and aging. *Psychology and Aging*, 6(4), 559–568.

Schaie, K. W., Willis, S. L., & Caskie, G. I. (2004). The Seattle longitudinal study: Relationship between personality and cognition. *Aging Neuropsychology and Cognition*, 11(2–3), 304–324.

The smartphone generation gap: Over 55? There is no app for that. (2013). Deloitte. www2.deloitte.com/content/dam/Deloitte/global/Documents/Technology-Media-Telecommunications/gx-tmt-2014prediction-smartphone.pdf

Smith, A. (2014). *Older adults and technology use.* Pew Research Center. www.pewinternet.org/2014/04/03/older-adults-and-technology-use/ (accessed May 4, 2017).

Smith, L. (2015). *The smartphone difference.* Pew Research Center. www.pewinternet.org/2015/04/01/us-smartphone-use-in-2015/ (accessed May 4, 2017).

Smith, P. J., Blumenthal, J. A., Hoffman, B. M., Cooper, H., Strauman, T. A., Welsh-Bohmer, K., . . . Sherwood, A. (2010). Aerobic exercise and neurocognitive performance: A meta-analytic review of randomized controlled trials. *Psychosomatic Medicine*, 72(3), 239.

Staff, R. T., Hogan, M. J., & Whalley, L. J. (2014). Aging trajectories of fluid intelligence in late life: The influence of age, practice and childhood IQ on Raven's Progressive Matrices. *Intelligence*, 47, 194–201.

Stroop, J. R. (1935). Studies of interference in serial verbal reactions. *Journal of Experimental Psychology*, 18(6), 643.

Sweeney, J. A., Rosano, C., Berman, R. A., & Luna, B. (2001). Inhibitory control of attention declines more than working memory during normal aging. *Neurobiology of Aging*, 22(1), 39–47.

Tennstedt, S. L., & Unverzagt, F. W. (2013). The ACTIVE study: Study overview and major findings. *Journal of Aging and Health*, 25(8 Suppl.), 3S–20S.

Thornton, W. J., & Dumke, H. A. (2005). Age differences in everyday problem-solving and decision-making effectiveness: A meta-analytic review. *Psychology and Aging*, 20(1), 85.

Trick, L. M., Perl, T., & Sethi, N. (2005). Age-related differences in multiple-object tracking. *The Journals of Gerontology Series B: Psychological Sciences and Social Sciences*, 60(2), P102–P105.

Troyer, A. K., Leach, L., & Strauss, E. (2006). Aging and response inhibition: Normative data for the Victoria Stroop Test. *Aging, Neuropsychology, and Cognition*, 13(1), 20–35.

United Nations, Department of Economic and Social Affairs, Population Division. (2013). *World population ageing 2013.* New York: United Nations publication.

Valls-Pedret, C., Sala-Vila, A., Serra-Mir, M., Corella, D., Torre, R. de la, Martínez-González, M. Á., . . . Ros, E. (2015). Mediterranean diet and age-related cognitive decline: A randomized clinical trial. *JAMA Internal Medicine*, 175(7), 1094–1103.

Van Praag, H., Shubert, T., Zhao, C., & Gage, F. H. (2005). Exercise enhances learning and hippocampal neurogenesis in aged mice. *The Journal of Neuroscience*, 25(38), 8680–8685.

Verhaeghen, P., & Cerella, J. (2002). Aging, executive control, and attention: A review of meta-analyses. *Neuroscience & Biobehavioral Reviews*, 26(7), 849–857.

Verhaeghen, P., & De Meersman, L. (1998). Aging and the Stroop effect: A meta-analysis. *Psychology and Aging*, 13(1), 120.

Verhaeghen, P., Steitz, D. W., Sliwinski, M. J., & Cerella, J. (2003). Aging and dual-task performance: A meta-analysis. *Psychology and Aging*, 18(3), 443.

Voss, M. W., Nagamatsu, L. S., Liu-Ambrose, T., & Kramer, A. F. (2011). Exercise, brain, and cognition across the life span. *Journal of Applied Physiology*, 111(5), 1505–1513.

Ward, E. V., Berry, C. J., & Shanks, D. R. (2013). Age effects on explicit and implicit memory. *Frontiers in Psychology*, 4, 639.

Wasylyshyn, C., Verhaeghen, P., & Sliwinski, M. J. (2011). Aging and task switching: A meta-analysis. *Psychology and Aging*, 26(1), 15.

Wilson, R. S., Barnes, L. L., & Bennett, D. A. (2003). Assessment of lifetime participation in cognitively stimulating activities. *Journal of Clinical and Experimental Neuropsychology*, 25(5), 634–642.

Wilson, R. S., Krueger, K. R., Arnold, S. E., Schneider, J. A., Kelly, J. F., Barnes, L. L., . . . Bennett, D. A. (2007). Loneliness and risk of Alzheimer disease. *Archives of General Psychiatry*, 64(2), 234–240.

Yaffe, K., Barnes, D., Nevitt, M., Lui, L. Y., & Covinsky, K. (2001). A prospective study of physical activity and cognitive decline in elderly women: Women who walk. *Archives of Internal Medicine*, 161(14), 1703–1708.

Zwaluw, N. L. van der, Dhonukshe-Rutten, R. A., Wijngaarden, J. P. van, Brouwer-Brolsma, E. M., Rest, O. van de, In't Veld, P. H., . . . Groot, L. C. de. (2014). Results of 2-year vitamin B treatment on cognitive performance Secondary data from an RCT. *Neurology*, 83(23), 2158–2166.

14
ENVIRONMENT, HOUSING, HEALTH, AND SOCIAL CARE

Jill Stewart, Ann Pascoe, Elaine Wiersma and Hilde Verbeek

This chapter discusses:

- Aging in place, housing condition and adaptations
- Responses to loneliness, isolation, and dementia
- Purpose-designed residential accommodation
- Sensitivity in integrating a portfolio of services to support more independent living

Learning outcomes

In this chapter you will learn how to:

- Apply positive solutions to suitably repair or improve housing conditions and more closely meet the changing needs of a person staying in their own home
- Integrate evidence-based housing, health and social care needs to help prevent home accident and illness and encourage independence for as long as possible
- Develop appropriate initiatives for providing housing and care interventions across a range of settings, taking service users' views into consideration
- Inform the development of enhanced residential care opportunities and availability
- Apply evidence-based approaches to contributing positively to quality of life across housing sectors

Introduction

Life expectancy continues to rise internationally (Rutherford, 2012; Salomon et al., 2012) and policy and practice need to recognise this as a future for us all that is 'unavoidable' (Coleman, 2001). Since population aging is predicted to continue to rise, particularly in wealthier countries, it needs to become a global priority. This situation is complex, as with population aging comes a change in disease patterns such as increasing numbers of those with dementia as well as increasing frailty, loneliness, and isolation. As we age beyond 60 years, we become increasingly vulnerable to domestic health and safety hazards and, at the age of over 85 years, we are likely to need home care (Rutherford, 2012). We need to find new and viable ways for providing quality housing, health and social care services into the future as our older population increasingly outnumbers our younger population (International Housing Partnership, 2013).

The living environment is key to well-being and quality of life as we age and our housing, health, and social care needs change. The University of Greenwich Centre for Positive Ageing, Environment, Housing, Health, and Social Care cluster has sought to further understand and analyse the living environment – both of the physical individual homes (regardless of tenure) and of how an older person and where applicable their carer can live fuller lives within their community, particularly as they become less mobile and with onset of dementia.

Deciding how to resource older people's changing needs, their housing, health, and social care both now and in the future are complex, at times controversial, and can be ideologically driven (see for example Care and Repair publications including Adams and Ellison, 2009; Adams and Ellison, 2010; and the International Housing Partnership, 2013). It also relies on the organisational relationships between housing, health, and social care services in different international settings. There is evidence to show that it is cost effective to invest in housing to prevent knock-on costs to health and social care services and this has influenced government policy (Heywood and Turner, 2007), but options for funding can be highly challenging to access (O'Connor, Age UK, 2014).

There are gaps in evidence around issues of aging in place and the policy and personal dilemmas this presents are rarely factored into front-line services either individually or in partnership. Providing evidenced solutions requires greater research and evaluation to ensure dignity as we all age. We need to move from people fitting services, to services fitting around each unique scenario presented. There is a need for more research on each part of the service package on offer, but also on how effectively services can operate together in developing their 'offers' to service commissioners. Additionally, we need to identify ways in which older adults can retain their autonomy, independence, mobility, and social interaction.

In this chapter we consider the complex relationships of environment, housing, health, and social care and the importance of local amenities, community, and services. We explore how more effective integrated services can help address inequalities for older people (see for example Marmot et al., 2010), for those aging in their own homes and carrying personal responsibility for its maintenance and adaptation, and we explore more specialist and purpose-built residential care homes with aging already factored into the design. We also explore the wider community and how we can better utilise existing social capital in addressing loneliness and isolation and extending this more widely into dementia-friendly communities. We look at meaningful activities to address declining health, frailty, loneliness, and isolation, as these areas risk being overlooked.

The housing, well-being, health, and safety relationship

Housing and health: aging in place

Housing conditions affect health across the life course, but can be more pronounced where residents 'age in place' and, through lack of routine maintenance, housing can fall into disrepair (even decline), which can affect the health and safety of residents. This can become particularly pronounced with older people who risk suffering both health and safety ill effects, aggravated by growing frailty and illness episodes.

Most people age in their own homes, rather than in purpose-built residential care environments. More of us will age in place in private sector housing and we spend the majority of our time in our older lives within our home environments. Sustaining independence in our living environments is therefore key to our health, safety, and quality of life. Interventions need to focus in prevention on areas of greatest risk; but to focus here, we first need evidence of what works well, and why.

There is a growing body of evidence into how we age in place and how we might make provision for funding both ongoing maintenance and repair needs, but also adaptation needs. England and Wales have a long history since the Second World War of private sector housing renewal grants to help preserve the nation's housing stock. This was successful in, for example, provision of standard amenities in older housing stock (e.g. internal toilet, hot water supply), but there was never a requirement to evaluate health gain arising from interventions. These grants were cut in 2011 and, like many other countries, owners now hold responsibility for funding repairs. Many however find themselves equity rich and revenue poor and accessing equity for home owners generally require private sector fund release, which is sometimes problematic.

Most people wish to remain in their own homes for as long as possible. It is generally better for health and more cost effective than a residential care home setting, but in some cases can no longer be maintained for a range of reasons. Some organisations offer Home Improvement Agencies with multiple referral options for various health, social care, and other support to help older and other vulnerable people to remain in their homes for longer, as well as offer advice on alternative housing options that may be suitable for older residents. Care and Repair in the United Kingdom has taken a pioneering role since the later 1970s – see Box 14.1. Table 14.1 summarises key housing, health and safety issues facing an aging population.

Box 14.1 Care and Repair schemes

Since the start of systematic collection of data about housing conditions in the 1960s, older people have been consistently over-represented in poor housing in the United Kingdom, particularly those in old age (75–84) and the oldest old (those aged over 85). Following the shift to owner occupation amongst lower income groups, and the large-scale improvement of social housing under the labour government, low-income owner-occupiers in substandard homes outnumber those in poor rented accommodation.

From the end of the Second World War the UK government intervened to improve private sector stock condition, but the system of home improvement grants of the 1970s largely failed to reach older people. During the late 1970s and early 1980s a charity sector initiative emerged which supported older home owners who needed practical and financial help in order to organise essential home repairs and adaptations, as well as to access grants.

These 'Care and Repair' schemes were based on a philosophy of enabling older people to live where they chose – most often the current mainstream home. This was in contrast to much of the thinking of the time – that is, that older people should move to specialist housing. It also challenged the large-scale housing regeneration approach as the householder decided on the scale of work that they wished to have done to their home. Care and Repair offered impartial housing, finance and care advice, and support to low-income older people, helping them find the money from grants/loans where needed for essential repairs and adaptations, combined with technical services to advise on what building work was needed, prepare plans and quotes, manage the selection of builders, and supervise work to completion.

From small charity projects in the late 1970s and early 1980s, these local schemes (now generically referred to as 'Home Improvement Agencies' or HIAs) gradually became part of mainstream local housing provision during the 1990s and 2000s. Many started to employ their own 'handyperson' staff to carry out small repairs and minor works at low cost or created hardship funds to pay for small jobs. Today they are increasingly operated by local authorities and, since the cessation of national government home repair grants, many focus more on provision of home adaptations (e.g. to adapt bathrooms, install stair lifts), where means-tested grants are still available.

The most important aspect of Care and Repair projects has been their cross-cutting approach which straddles housing, health, and social care. Much of the building work improves the health and safety of the older occupant (e.g. upgrading heating, removing hazards, and caseworkers also check incomes, broker access to other care and support services, and generally improve the wider living conditions of the older person). A growing number also assist older people to move to more suitable accommodation if that is their chosen option.

See a film about local Care and Repair cases on the Care and Repair homepage (scroll down to the end of website page) at http://careandrepair-england.org.uk/.

With thanks to Sue Adams OBE (sueadams@careandrepair-england.org.uk) Chief Executive, Care and Repair England

Table 14.1 Summary of key housing, health, and safety issues facing an aging population

Poor-quality housing	Poor state of repair, inadequate facilities and amenities (e.g. external WC, no hot water supply) leading to possible health and safety concerns
Domestic accidents	More accidents (including fatalities) than other environments; closely correlates to physical housing standard (e.g. vulnerability by age); fire safety, etc.
Meeting changing needs and housing adaptations	Suitability of housing into old age, other changing needs, e.g. disability or ill health, safe access, and mobility around the home, dementia, greater risk of domestic accident, etc.
Security; fear of crime and anti-social behaviour	Fear of crime (not necessarily actual crime), but can induce stress and affect emotional health
Cold and damp; fuel poverty	Main reason for 'non decent housing' – linked to low income, poor-quality housing, inadequate heating and insulation leading to respiratory disease, accident, discomfort, stress, hypothermia, etc.; also sustainability and unnecessary waste of energy resource; particularly problematic for older people who spend longer periods at home and benefit from higher temperatures, so heating costs are higher
Indoor air quality; pollutants, etc.	Poor quality can cause ill health or death, e.g. carbon monoxide poisoning, radon, asbestos, etc.
Community – social capital and social cohesion	Integration with local community; support networks; access to health, welfare and services; empowerment; capacity; loneliness and isolation
Noise pollution (e.g. air, road or rail traffic; neighbours)	Can cause or aggravate tension, stress, depression – particular issues for those with dementia
Pest invasion (e.g. rats, mice, cockroaches, ants)	May result from lack of routine cleaning, may go unnoticed

Table adapted from Stewart (2005)

The Housing Health and Safety Rating System (HHSRS) for England and Wales has received international recognition in that it provides an evidence-based, dynamic system to assess hazards and risks and to prioritise interventions. Cold homes and falls are recorded as priority areas and interventions are therefore prioritised here (for example, see Building Research Establishment, 2008 and 2011). The HHSRS also rates hazard and risk by vulnerability, so older people can be catered for and it is possible to scrutinise wider data based on age for further analysis; although this does not tend to be done routinely, it is becoming more commonplace as a 'life course' approach is increasingly adopted (Stewart and Dhesi, 2016).

Some health and safety issues become particularly acute as we age, notably cold homes and fall hazards, and cold homes can contribute to risk of domestic fall, which we discuss later. In England, some local authorities are currently piloting hospital discharge services (Department of Energy and Climate Change, 2015) and exploring what could be improved or adapted in the home environment to prevent a return to hospital (such as installation of better heating systems and thermal insulation) but also more effective rehabilitation. At the time of writing, this remains in early stages but there is a focus on cold homes, known to contribute to a range of physical and emotional ill health, including stroke, hypothermia, and respiratory disease, as well as improved emotional well-being. Evidence from New Zealand provides compelling evidence of rapid cost returns and positive health effects arising from retrofitting heating and insulation (Chapman et al., 2009) and evidence from England indicates the early stages of a range of partners working together can help deliver 'warmer homes on prescription' (Gentoo, 2014).

Home safety: slips, trips, and falls

Risk to safety in the homes can increase as we age; things once taken for granted, such as, steps to front door, level surfaces, access to kitchen cupboards can all present new risk with aging due to a decline in mobility, increasing frailty, and visual impairment.

Some 30 per cent of all over-65s fall each year and this percentage rises with age (National Health Service, 2015; Center for Disease Prevention and Control, 2015; Australian and New Zealand Falls Prevention Society, 2015). Much intervention activity focuses falls prevention in the home around a medical model, which may risk missing a wider focus on holistic service provision around sustaining independence and combating loneliness, which can also be contributory factors. Older people fall at home for a range of reasons as they become less mobile and more frail. Kitchen cupboards that may once have been easily accessible now may prove too high or too low. Activities of daily living, such as cleaning, getting in and out of the bath, and preparing meals may become high risk when they previously were not. This may be aggravated by non-level surfaces, tripping hazards, slippery floor coverings or unnoticed accidental spillages, with which risk increases with age.

An international study reviewing interventions for preventing falls in older people living in the community (Gillespie et al., 2012) sought to assess the effects of interventions designed to reduce risks. It reiterates that older people are more likely to fall for a range of reasons and up to 30 per cent may fall each year; that falls prevention interventions are difficult for people living in the community; that group and home-based exercise programmes focusing on strength and balance can help; individual multi-factorial risk assessments and referrals require further investigation; home safety interventions appear to be effective; vitamin supplements can help but some medications and medical conditions can increase risk; and, finally, there is inconclusive evidence that educational materials alone are of use.

Demand for services is usually complex, as service providers try to prevent crisis interventions and maintain independence, choice, and control in the home through personalised and joined up services. There are economic, physical, and mental health arguments to intervene to help prevent falls, with costs to health and social care services as well as loss of mobility and the loneliness and social isolation this can cause. However, there is limited evidence of what works effectively and it has been difficult to look comparatively at different systems and approaches which tend to be erratic. Responses are both proactive and reactive, combining falls prevention with rehabilitation (e.g. physiotherapy) and appropriate housing adaptations.

Preventative considerations include who is most at risk, whether there is a history of falls, which interventions best reduce risk, how can people themselves become more proactive, how fit for purpose are local initiatives and what evidence do we have around what works best. A telling fact is that falls are easy to quantify, but loneliness is not; we need to ensure that we are supporting all areas where health and safety is at risk, not just those easily subscribing to a medical model.

Housing for our whole lifetime?

International policy needs to be able to cater for population aging. As more of us will live into old age and extreme old age in our own homes, it is likely that we will need to take earlier responsibility for our own housing, health, and social care futures by planning when we are younger and before we have health crises and our incomes are in decline.

There is real need for us all to think about our housing and what we can do to make it more appropriate for us as we age, but also for the wider population's future use. A useful exercise is to look at our own homes now and ask ourselves, in 20, 30 or 40 years' time, do we think that we will be able to get easily in and out? Will we be able to manage the stairs? Will we need a level access shower, wider doorways, better fire safety detection and management, assistive technologies, plug sockets situated high up the walls or more accessible kitchen units? However, we probably do not really want to think about these things or about our own aging and mortality. But these things are important and a policy shift needs to ensure that, where possible, people are able to make more informed decisions based on good local advice and support about what may be available, but also what would not be available. This is already happening in some parts of England: in Bristol, for example, Care and Repair have pioneered Home Independence Centres (see www.wecr.org.uk/home-independence-centres), where people are able to more actively shop and make choices about what aids and adaptations they would like as they age.

This is not of course to say that making active choices is an option for all and therefore the need for creative and well-resourced integrated local services which meet needs, add value, and improve quality of life for our aging population remains paramount. For an example, see Islington's award winning SHINE scheme in Box 14.2.

Box 14.2 An innovative multi-agency referral scheme

For older people or their carers, trying to find and identify helpful available services and other forms of support can be problematic but the London Borough of Islington's SHINE referral pathway is addressing this.

SHINE (the Seasonal Health Interventions Network – www.islington.gov.uk/services/parks-environment/sustainability/energy-services/Pages/shine.aspx) is a proactive and innovative multi-agency single point of access referral pathway that co-ordinates health interventions across some

130 teams across almost 90 different organisations, including housing, environmental health, medical doctors, social workers, mental health, health and social care, and financial advice. Interventions are able to tackle poor housing as well as to help improve quality of life in tackling loneliness and isolation.

In 2014, SHINE saw almost 2500 people and these received more than 11,000 focused interventions. There has been an emphasis on 'making every contact count' a bit more, and SHINE was awarded an Ashden Award for Fuel Poverty in 2015 for its innovative and multi-agency approach – see www.ashden.org/winners/Islington15.

The Dementia Navigator Services also enables access to SHINE, which helps support those with a new diagnosis of dementia and their carers: www.candi.nhs.uk/services/dementia-navigator-service. This service helps assess needs and develop a plan of support such as attending day centres, social services support, help with housing issues, and relevant signposting elsewhere.

Single point of access intervention hubs like SHINE are models of practice demonstrating that effective permanently joined up integrated care and collaborative efforts between social care, healthcare, and public health practitioners can strengthen preventative health interventions.

With thanks to Ellis Tuner, Principal Environmental Health Officer and Toby Morgan, Seasonal Health and Affordable Warmth Advisor, London Borough of Islington

Homelike residential care environments

Policy principles aim to enable older people to remain at home for as long as possible, although this is not always feasible as care needs increase. Older people are at risk of developing multimorbidity, having a poor physical and/or mental health status. Dementia in particular has a large impact on ability to live within the local community. Dementia is characterised by a global cognitive deterioration (e.g. decline in memory functioning and language perception), decline in the performance of daily activities, and behavioural and psychological symptoms (BPSD), such as agitation, depression, and apathy. It is caused by various diseases and conditions, all affecting the brain. Support networks of professional and informal caregivers are essential to support people with dementia living at home in their community successfully. In addition, environmental design has an important influence in supporting people with dementia. Research has provided design guidelines to make local neighbourhoods more 'dementia-friendly', focusing on six elements: familiarity, legibility, distinctiveness, accessibility, comfort, and safety (Mitchel and Burton, 2010). For example, the legibility of their environment is important for people with dementia to help them understand where they are and identify which way they need to go, which may prevent and alleviate spatial disorientation, confusion, and anxiety.

When care needs can no longer be met sufficiently within home and community care services, residential care providing 24-hour supervision becomes necessary. A variety of residential care services are available along the continuum of long-term care, ranging from very sheltered housing and extra care housing schemes that are mainly supported through community services (e.g. Darton et al., 2012) to group homes, small-scale living facilities, and more traditional nursing homes. Traditionally, residential care was based on a medical model and focusing on residents' disease, deficit, and underlying pathology. However, over the last few decades a paradigm shift has emerged regarding care models.

Nowadays, residential care should be as homelike as possible. Person-centred models of care are prominent, in which emphasis is put on support of residents' autonomy and overall well-being. Older people should be enabled to continue their lifestyle as before admission to a residential or nursing care setting. Furthermore, environmental design should support autonomy, privacy, personal identity, and socialisation (e.g. Fleming and Purandare, 2010). Instead of big hospital or hotel-like surroundings with a complex organisation, small settings that resemble an archetypical home situation were suggested to support people with dementia. Current theory, with Lawton's ecological model on supportive environments being highly influential (Lawton and Nahemow, 1973), stresses that a match is needed between the person's needs, his/her abilities, and environmental demands to elicit adequate behaviour in people with dementia. This is also referred to as person/environment fit. If environmental demands exceed people's ability to cope, they will have more difficulty to maintain adequate behaviour. These principles have important implications for care environments, especially for people with dementia, as they experience diminished physical and/or mental disabilities due to their illness, increasing the environment's influence on their behaviour and general well-being.

Adopting cultural change

It has proven to be very difficult to adopt the cultural change towards a homelike, person-centred care approach in existing traditional residential care settings. A main reason for this is that the care environment often does not correspond with the new therapeutic goals. As a result, new initiatives have been developed that provide health, social, and nursing care in a small-scale and homelike environment (Verbeek et al., 2009). Radical changes have been made in comparison with traditional residential settings such as nursing homes, with changes in the organisational, physical, and social environment.

Purpose-built settings could be located within the community, with residents having their own flat, or could exist at a large-scale nursing home. For example, building features could resemble a homelike environment with archetype symbols such as a kitchen, dining room, living room, and a laundry area. The social environment within small-scale, homelike settings resembles a family-like structure, in which residents form a group (maximum of eight to 10 residents). Nursing staff are part of the household, whereas in traditional large-scale nursing homes many fellow residents and staff reside at one unit together (usually around 30). The organisational structure dictates the daily routines for residents living in large-scale nursing homes, such as when to get out of bed in the morning and when to have their lunch or dinner in the evening. In small-scale, homelike environments, residents and family caregivers have a large influence on their daily life and decide together with nursing staff what is the best fit with residents' needs and preferences. Furthermore, nursing staff have integrated tasks, meaning that they are not only responsible for medical and nursing care, but also organise activities and perform household tasks. In traditional homes, there is a large task differentiation: many functions and specific staff for nutrition assistance, personal care, activities, household, etc. Many similar concepts have been developed worldwide, such as Green Houses® in the United States, group homes in Japan, and group living in Sweden (Verbeek et al., 2009). New initiatives include green care farms, in which agricultural activities are combined with care (see Box 14.3). Originally being developed for day care only, in the Netherlands 24-hour green care farms are now increasing to provide 24-hour residential dementia care as well.

Research into experiences of residents and family caregivers with small-homelike care environments show mainly positive experiences (e.g. van Zadelhoff et al., 2011; Verbeek et al., 2012). Small-scale, homelike care settings created structural opportunities for individualised care and attention to the residents' personal needs. Residents themselves expressed being at home because they could maintain their personal characteristics and felt connected and united. Family caregivers enjoyed the personal contact and attention from nursing staff, not only with the residents but also with family caregivers themselves. They appreciated the focus on freedom in making one's own choices and felt a strong sense of involvement. Furthermore, nursing staff felt they could spend more time with residents, which could be related to the broadening of their tasks. In small-scale, homelike care environments, nursing staff not only interact with residents during standard nursing care moments, but also encourage residents to participate in daily activities. These household chores may serve as a handle for undertaking meaningful activities and provide opportunity for reciprocity. Negative aspects were mentioned as well (e.g. Verbeek et al., 2012). In some settings family caregivers indicated a lack of amenities and general facilities such as a restaurant. Furthermore, nursing staff worked alone a lot and some missed a team to discuss difficulties and share responsibility.

Although experiences with small-scale, homelike care environments are mainly positive, this does not necessarily result in positive effects for residents, family caregivers, and nursing staff. Several studies have been conducted comparing small-scale, homelike care environments with traditional settings and they found mixed results. Overall, no effects were found for quality of life and behavioural outcomes (e.g. agitation, depression) for residents (Verbeek et al., 2010; de Rooij et al., 2012; te Boekhorst et al., 2009). Positive effects included less use of physical restraints and more social interaction (Verbeek et al., 2014; te Boekhorst et al., 2009). Nursing staff reported different job characteristics, such as increased autonomy and perceived social support (Willemse et al., 2014). However, effects on job satisfaction and motivation remain unclear.

The working mechanisms of small-scale, homelike care environments on outcomes remain unclear. As a result, many changes are currently implemented in practice without knowledge on which and how these are most effective. The main focus in research and practice has often been on physical aspects of the environment, such as (group) size, location, and design features of an archetypical home (e.g. kitchen, doorbell, and furniture). This is understandable, since physical aspects are most visible and easy to measure, and therefore provide a clear distinction with traditional nursing homes. However, social environmental and organisational aspects are of vital importance as well to create supporting surroundings in dementia care.

Box 14.3 Green care farms for people with dementia

Green care farms are an innovative form of small-scale, homelike care environments in the Netherlands. At a green care farm, agricultural activities are combined with care. One initiative is a dairy farm, which provided day care activities for people with dementia since 2005. The owners are a couple, of whom the husband is the farmer and the wife is responsible for care management. She is a nurse by background and has previously worked in traditional nursing home care. Since the opening of the green care farm for day care activities, the owners have received many questions from their clients about why they couldn't stay at the farm as care needs increased and admission to a nursing home was inevitable. In the Netherlands, the level of care needed is determined by a standardised assessment procedure, carried out by government agency. Admission to a nursing home setting is based on this assessment and the families' preferences. The farmer and his wife wanted to expand their caring activities and have therefore established two small-scale, homelike settings for 20 people with dementia at their farm. The official opening was in March 2013. Two homes for eight people with dementia were established downstairs and four apartments were created upstairs.

Activities at the green care farm include domestic chores (e.g. peeling potatoes, cooking, growing own vegetables, getting milk at the dairy farm) or involve animals and outdoor activities (e.g. sowing, feeding the cattle such as sheep, chickens, dog, and cat). If you would like to take a look, please visit www.academischewerkplaatsouderenzorg.nl/node/10802 and watch the film (English subtitles).

Combatting loneliness and isolation

Older people can feel lonely in both urban and rural settings and services that can help provide welcoming social activities can provide a real boost; for example, see Islington's Claremont project – connecting with older people to tackle loneliness (www.claremont-project.org/). The issue of connecting is also key for those with dementia who are already in a residential care home. It is of course possible to be in the middle of a crowd and to feel lonely and this must be especially true for those with dementia, who may struggle with memory recall and communication. Age Exchange have carried out innovative work to enhance quality of life, as illustrated in Box 14.4.

Box 14.4 Reminiscence Arts in Dementia: Impact on Quality of Life (RADIQL): a project aiming to bring about service change in dementia care

Age Exchange are leaders in the field of reminiscence and arts, working to combat loneliness in older people. In 2012, the charity initiated RADIQL, a research study to investigate how their creative intervention could improve health outcomes for people in care homes with low, severe, and end-of-life dementia, and ultimately improve social care delivery.

Independent researchers Royal Holloway University of London and Simetrica found measurable increases in well-being and quality of life. Following a 26, 1-hour weekly intervention, participants' levels of well-being (mood and engagement) were statistically significant, improving by 42 per cent and positive behaviour by 25 per cent in comparison to the control group.

The programme and services include a group and 1–1 bedside mixed structured relationship-centred psycho-social Reminiscence Arts intervention, workforce training, and seminars. Based upon a standardised framework, it is personalised to the culture, interests, previous occupation, cognitive and functional abilities, and preferences of the individual. It is delivered through a variety of different art forms including visual arts, music, drama, dance, movement, singing, words, and craft. Promoting communication, social inclusion, pleasure, and cognitive stimulation, it incorporates relationship-centred engagement within a social context with memory (embodied and sensory as well as spoken) that connects people to their past, the present, the social space, and to others.

The evaluation and cost-effectiveness analysis is enabling Age Exchange to develop a conceptual and pedagogic framework for social care workforce, art practitioners, and intervention for care homes for people with dementia.

With thanks to Belinda Sosinowicz MA, MSc, Art and Wellbeing Coordinator, Age Exchange

The challenge of rural communities: changing demographics and services

Rural communities are often described as isolated by virtue of their geographic location. The perceptions of the "rural idyll" are as places where social networks are strong are common, despite scholars who have critiqued these ideas (Cloke, 2006; Skinner et al., 2008). In fact, relationships amongst community members are complex and rural communities are heterogeneous; as such, a "one-size-fits-all model" does not represent the realities and complexities of rural and remote communities.

In many countries, the demographics of rural communities are changing significantly. Many rural communities are also aging communities; as economic and social changes occur, younger people tend to leave the communities, often related to economic opportunities, while seniors remain (Hanlon and Halseth, 2005). As such, rural populations tend to age faster than urban regions (Dandy and Bollman, 2008) and have a higher proportion of older people.

In rural communities, health and social services are often limited (Hanlon and Halseth, 2005; Innes et al., 2005; Morgan, Innes and Kosteniuk, 2011). The lower health status of rural, remote, and northern residents in comparison with urban counterparts, the lack of accessible health resources, inadequate diagnostic and treatment services, and limitations on home care are all significant issues in rural communities (Cook et al., 2007; Hayes, 2006; Ministerial Advisory Council on Rural Health, 2002). Particular health needs are not often met by available health-care services in rural areas and have been described as inadequate (Hanlon and Halseth, 2005; Leipert and Reutter, 2005). DiGregorio, Ferguson and Wiersma (2015) outlined the limitations of health and social care services at various stages along the dementia journey in northern Ontario, Canada, including lack of awareness and understanding of dementia, health service providers with limited understanding of dementia, and limited services to support people living with dementia in rural communities.

Studies of loneliness have looked at the differences between emotional and social isolation and perceptions of loneliness. As defined by de Jong Gierveld (1998), "Loneliness is a situation experienced by the individual as one where there is an unpleasant or inadmissible lack of (quality of) certain relationships" (p. 73–74) and is related to how people perceive their relationships. De Jong Gierveld (1998) has outlined dimensions of loneliness, including feelings associated with absence of intimate attachment; time perspective (loneliness as a long-term or short-term situation, changeable, and treatable); and different emotional aspects including sadness, shame, and guilt (p. 74). Based on these dimensions, geographic isolation does not necessarily translate into social isolation.

Loneliness and social isolation are common for people living with dementia and care partners (Alzheimer's Society, 2013). A report by the Alzheimer's Society of England, Wales, and Northern Ireland found that nearly two-thirds of people with dementia surveyed who lived alone reported feeling lonely. Relationships often change and a third of those surveyed said that they lost friends following a diagnosis. For care partners and other family members of people living with dementia, loneliness and changes in relationships are also common (Alzheimer's Society, 2013).

Dementia-friendly communities: inclusion and a culture of caring

A key characteristic of a dementia-friendly community, or a dementia-capable community, is a community that is inclusive of people with dementia and enables people living with dementia to have choice and control over their lives, as well as to remain independent for as long as possible(Lin and Lewis, 2015; Prior, 2012; Wiersma and Denton, 2016). Dementia-friendly communities also involve accessible physical environments and local facilities, appropriate support services, strong social networks, inclusion in local groups, and awareness of dementia (Prior, 2012; Wiersma and Denton, 2016).

While scholars have questioned the stereotypes of strong social networks in rural communities (Cloke, 2006), other research has demonstrated the importance of social networks within rural communities (Wiersma and Denton, 2016). While this is not to say that social networks are strong in every community (indeed, we know that rural communities are heterogeneous), some research has demonstrated how social networks become safety nets in the absence of formal services (Wiersma and Denton, 2016). Some rural community members have very strong informal bonds (DiGregorio, Ferguson and Wiersma, 2015), where community members often look out for and support people living with dementia and their families, including checking up on them, bringing them home if they are wandering, including them in social activities, helping with errands, shovelling snow, and other tasks (Wiersma and Denton, 2016). It is these communities that truly demonstrate what it means to be dementia-friendly. In light of limited health and social services as well as family members who have often moved away, the community has, and can, become the safety net. Essentially, dementia-friendly is about inclusion and a culture of caring – see Box 14.5.

Box 14.5 "I didn't sign up for this": caring for a partner with vascular dementia

Many who live with and care for someone who develops dementia report feeling very alone with their situation because many other people simply do not understand what they are faced with.

What dementia families really want is simply to live an ordinary life, doing ordinary things. The more that people with dementia can be supported in socially inclusive communities, rather than being side-lined into dementia ghettos, the better for all concerned.

With the vision that strong and knowledgeable inclusive communities are vital to improving the well-being and quality of life for dementia families, I founded – working with strategic partners such as NHS, local authority, voluntary groups and Alzheimer organisations – one of the first rural dementia-friendly communities in Scotland.

Key to our success was involving people with dementia and their carers from the outset, allowing them to be directly involved in all major decision-making, especially at Board level. We also connected with other communities and learnt a lot by working with other dementia-friendly initiatives, not just in Scotland, but in the rest of the United Kingdom and worldwide.

It is very clear that professionals generally support dementia families only during crises and that it is our rural community that provides the day-to-day interventions that allow dementia families to self-manage. Some examples include:

- by providing transport to regular fun activities at the community centre; not only does the person with dementia have access to new horizons, but the carer is also given a much-needed regular break;
- by supporting people with dementia to continue their hobbies/interests (e.g. golf, swimming, walking, music, photography, art, etc.), not only are issues of loneliness reduced, but the body and mind are made to work;

- by supporting carers to continue their caring roles despite temporary incapacity (e.g. supporting a carer who fell and broke her hand/ribs with food preparation, driving and other activities, the person with dementia can continue to live at home).

There is no doubt in my mind that without our dementia-friendly community supporting us in what essentially is preventative work, stigma around dementia would have kept us withdrawn from society, less likely to get involved in activities and therefore terribly alone.

Conclusions

We all need to be more proactive in our future housing options and listen to what older people are saying now about the needs and options they would find helpful and the better integration of available services so that individualised interventions can be offered. Most of us live in our own homes and this is likely to increase internationally; with this comes more responsibility for maintenance, repair, and adaptation. Some residential care homes can provide a purpose-designed environment that offers appropriate accommodation for aging people, including specific needs arising from dementia. Finally, there is evidence of ill-health effects of loneliness and isolation: it is here that we also need to focus our efforts so that we can increasingly live in decent housing accommodation and enjoy our quality of life now and into the future.

References

Adams, S., and Ellison, M. (2009). *Time to adapt: Home adaptations for older people. The increase in need and future of state provision*. Nottingham: Care and Repair England.

Adams, S., and Ellison, M. (2010). *A perfect storm: An ageing population, low income home ownership and decay of older housing*. Nottingham: Care and Repair England.

Alzheimer's Society. (2013). *Dementia 2013: The hidden voice of loneliness*. www.alzheimers.org.uk/site/scripts/download_info.php?fileID=1677 (accessed August 27, 2015).

Australian and New Zealand Falls Prevention Society. (2015). *The problem and prevalence with falls*. www.anzfallsprevention.org/info/ (accessed July 25, 2015).

Boekhorst, S. te, Depla, M. F., Lange, J. de, Pot, A. M., and Eefsting, J. A. (2009). The effects of group living homes on older people with dementia: A comparison with traditional nursing home care. *International Journal of Geriatric Psychiatry*, 24(9), 970–978.

Building Research Establishment. (2008). *Good housing leads to good health: A toolkit for environmental health practitioners*. London: Chartered Institute of Environmental Health. www.cieh.org/uploadedFiles/Core/Policy/Housing/Good_Housing_Leads_to_Good_Health_2008.pdf

Building Research Establishment. (2011). *Health costs of cold dwellings*. Hertfordshire: Building Research establishment. www.foe.co.uk/sites/default/files/downloads/warm_homes_nhs_costs.pdf

Center for Disease Prevention and Control. (2015). *Older adult falls: Get the facts*. www.cdc.gov/home andrecreationalsafety/falls/adultfalls.html (accessed July 25, 2015).

Chapman, R., Howden-Chapman, P., Viggers, H., O'Dea, D., and Kennedy, M. (2009). Retrofitting houses with insulation: A cost-benefit analysis of a randomised community trial. *Journal of Epidemiology and Community Health*, 63(4), 271–277.

Cloke, P. (2006). Conceptualizing rurality. In P. Cloke, T. Marsden, and P. H. Mooney (Eds.), *Handbook of rural studies* (pp. 18–28). Thousand Oaks, CA: Sage.

Coleman, D. (2001). *Population Ageing: An unavoidable future*. Working Paper Series no. 7, August 2001, University of Oxford, Oxford Centre for Population and Migration Studies.

Cook, C. C., Martin, P., Yearns, M., and Damhorst, M. L. (2007). Attachment to "place" and coping with losses in changed communities: A paradox for aging adults. *Family and Consumer Sciences Research Journal*, 35(3), 201–214.

Dandy, K., and Bollman, D. (2008). Seniors in rural Canada. *Rural and Small Town Canada Analysis Bulletin*, 7(8), December. www.statcan.gc.ca/pub/21-006-x/21006-x2007008-eng.pdf (accessed March 13, 2015).

Darton, R., Bäumker, T., Callaghan, L., Holder, J., Netten, A. and Towers, A. M. (2012). The relationship between building design and residents' quality of life in extra care housing schemes. *Health and Social Care in the Community*, 20(1), 87–96.

de Rooij, A. H., Luijkx, K. G., Schaafsma, J., Declercq, A. G., Emmerink, P. M., Schols, J. M. (2012). Quality of life of residents with dementia in traditional versus small-scale long-term care settings: a quasi-experimental study. *International Journal of Nursing Studies*, 49(8), 931–940.

Department of Energy and Climate Change. (2015). *The heat is on to ensure warmer, healthy homes for everyone.* www.gov.uk/government/news/the-heat-is-on-to-ensure-warmer-healthy-homes-for-everyone (accessed July 25, 2015).

DiGregorio, D., Ferguson, S., and Wiersma, E. (2015). The dementia journey in rural northern Ontario. *Canadian Journal on Aging*, 34(1) 100–112.

Dupuis, S. L., Wiersma, E. C., and Loiselle, L. (2012). Pathologizing behaviour: Meanings of behaviors in dementia care. *Journal of Aging Studies*, 26(2), 163–173.

Fleming, R. and Purandare, N. (2010). Long-term care for people with dementia: environmental design guidelines. *International Psychogeriatrics*, 22(7), 1084–1096.

Gentoo Group. (2014). *Boiler on prescription.* www.gentoogroup.com/media/123772/Boiler-on-Prescription-Report-The-story-so-far.pdf?guest=1421113453224987 (accessed July 25, 2015).

Gillespie, L. D., Robertson, M. C., Gillespie, W. J., Sherrington, C., Gates, S., Clemson, L. M., and Lamb, S. E. (2012). Interventions for preventing falls in older people living in the community. *Cochrane Database of Systematic Reviews*, 2012(9). Art. ID. CD007146. doi:10.1002/14651858.CD007146.pub3. www.bhfactive.org.uk/userfiles/Documents/Cochranereviewfalls.pdf (accessed July 25, 2015)

Hanlon, N., and Halseth, G. (2005). The greying of resource communities in northern British Columbia: Implications for health care delivery in already-underserviced communities. *The Canadian Geographer*, 49(1), 1–24.

Hayes, P. A. (2006). Home is where their health is: Rethinking perspectives of informal and formal care by older rural Appalachian women who live alone. *Qualitative Health Research*, 16(2), 282–297.

Heywood, F. S., and Turner, L. (2007). *Better outcomes, lower costs: Implications for health and social care budgets of investment in housing adaptations, improvements and equipment – A review of the evidence.* Bristol: HM Government Office for Disability Issues and University of Bristol.

Innes, A., Blackstock, K., Mason, A., Smith, A., and Cox, S. (2005). Dementia care provision in rural Scotland: Service users' and carers' experiences. *Health and Social Care in the Community*, 13(4), 354–365.

International Housing Partnership. (2013). *Fit for the Future: Meeting the challenge of housing and ageing population.* Australia, Canada: IHP.

Jong Gierveld, J. de. (1998). A review of loneliness: Concept and definitions, determinants and consequences. *Reviews in Clinical Gerontology*, 8, 73–80.

Lawton, M. P., & Nahemow, L. (1973). Ecology and the aging process. In C. Eisdorfer & M. P. Lawton (Eds.), *The psychology of adult development and aging* (pp. 619–674). Washington, DC: American Psychological Association.

Leipert, B. D., and Reutter, L. (2005). Developing resilience: How women maintain their health in northern geographically isolated settings. *Qualitative Health Research*, 15(1), 49–65.

Lin, S.Y., and Lewis, F. M. (2015). Dementia friendly, dementia capable, and dementia positive: Concepts to prepare for the future. *The Gerontologist*, 55(2), 237–244.

Marmot, M. G., Allen, J., Goldblatt, P., Boyce, T., McNeish, D., Grady, M., and Geddes, I. (2010). *Fair society, healthy lives: Strategic review of health inequalities in England post-2010.* London: The Marmot Review.

Ministerial Advisory Council on Rural Health. (2002). *Rural health in rural hands: Strategic directions for rural, remote, northern, and aboriginal communities.* http://publications.gc.ca/collections/Collection/H39-657-2002E.pdf (accessed August 27, 2015).

Mitchel, L. & Burton E. (2010). Designing Dementia-Friendly Neighbourhoods: Helping People with Dementia to Get Out and About. *Journal of Integrated Care*, 18(6), 12–19.

Morgan, D., Innes, A., and Kosteniuk, J. (2011). Dementia care in rural and remote settings: A systematic review of formal or paid care. *Maturitas*, 68, 17–33.

National Health Service. (2015). *Fall prevention*. www.nhs.uk/conditions/falls/Pages/Introduction.aspx (accessed July 25, 2015).

O'Connor, S. (2014). *Care in crisis: What's next for social care*. London: AgeUK.

Prior, P. (2012). *Knowing the foundations of dementia friendly communities for the North East*. www.phine.org.uk/uploads/doc/vid_16756_Dementia_Friendly_Communities_Report_Final.pdf (accessed December 3, 2010).

Rutherford, T. (2012). *Population ageing: Statistics. Commons library standard note SN3229*. London: House of Commons.

Salomon, J., Wang H., Freeman, M. K., Vos, T., Flaxman, A. D., Lopez, A. D. and Murray, C.J.L. (2012). Healthy life expectancy for 187 countries, 1990–2010: A systematic analysis for the Global Burden Disease Study 2010. *The Lancet*, 380(9859), 2144–2162.

Skinner, M. W., Rosenberg, M. W., Lovell, S. A., Dunn, J. R., Everitt, J. C., Hanlon, N., and Rathwell, T. A. (2008). Services for seniors in small-town Canada: The paradox of community. *Canadian Journal of Nursing Research*, 40(1), 80–101.

Stewart, J. (2005). A review of UK housing policy: Ideology and public health. *Public Health*, 119(6), 525–534.

Stewart, J. and Dhesi, S. (2016). Affordable warmth: housing strategies for older people, *Housing, Care and Support*, 19(1), 23–31.

Van Zadelhoff, G. G., Verbeek, H., Widdershoven, G. A. M., Rossum, E. van, and Abma, T. (2011). Good care in group home living for people with dementia. Experiences of residents, family and nursing staff. *Journal of Clinical Nursing*, 17, 2490–2500.

Verbeek, H., van Rossum, E., Zwakhalen, S. M., Kempen, G. I., & Hamers, J. P. (2009). Small, homelike care environments for older people with dementia: a literature review. *International Psychogeriatrics*, 21(02), 252–264.

Verbeek, H., Zwakhalen, S. M. G., Rossum, E. van, Ambergen, T., Kempen, G. I. J. M., and Hamers, J. P. H. (2010). Dementia care redesigned: A quasi-experimental study into the effects of small-scale living facilities on residents, their family caregivers and staff. *Journal of the American Medical Directors Association*, 11, 662–670.

Verbeek, H., Zwakhalen, S. M. G., Rossum, E. van, Ambergen, T., Kempen, G. I. J. M., and Hamers, J. P. H. (2014). Effects of small-scale, home-like facilities in dementia care on residents' behavior, and use of physical restraints and psychotropic drugs: A quasi-experimental study. *International Psychogeriatrics*, 26(4), 657–668.

Verbeek, H., Zwakhalen, S. M. G., Rossum, E. van, Kempen, G. I. J. M., and Hamers, J. P. H. (2012). Small-scale, homelike facilities in dementia care: A process evaluation into the experiences of family caregivers and nursing staff. *International Journal of Nursing Studies*, 49, 21–29.

Wiersma, E. C., and Denton, A. (2016). From social network to safety net: Dementia friendly communities in rural northern Ontario. *Dementia*, 15(1), 51–68.

Willemse, B. M., Depla, M. F., Smit, D., and Pot, A. M. (2014). The relationship between small-scale nursing home care for people with dementia and staff's perceived job characteristics. *International Psychogeriatrics*, 26(5), 805–816.

Further reading and websites

Age Exchange (uses reminiscence arts to unlock creativity) www.age-exchange.org.uk/

Age UK Health and Wellbeing www.ageuk.org.uk/professional-resources-home/services-and-practice/health-and-wellbeing/falls-prevention-resources/

Alzheimer's Society www.alzheimers.org.uk/?gclid=COGt9cfu1sMCFWKWtAodTQoA2A –

Alzheimer's Society on Dementia Friendly Communities http://alzheimers.org.uk/site/scripts/documents_info.php?documentID=1843

Campaign to End Loneliness www.campaigntoendloneliness.org/threat-to-health/

Care and Repair England (aging well at home) www.careandrepair-england.org.uk

Crawley Dementia Friendly Communities www.youtube.com/watch?v=rNRohfabB7A

Dementia Action Alliance www.dementiaaction.org.uk/

Dementia Service Development Centre, University of Stirling http://dementia.stir.ac.uk/information/dementia-research

Housing Learning and Improvement Network www.housinglin.org.uk/Topics/browse/HousingandDementia/

Islington Claremont project – connecting with older people to tackle loneliness www.claremont-project.org/ –

Local Government Association – creating dementia friendly communities www.local.gov.uk/aging-well/what-makes/-/journal_content/56/10180/3489659/ARTICLE

National Housing Federation 'Dementia: finding housing solutions' www.housing.org.uk/publications/browse/dementia-finding-housing-solutions/

University of Greenwich Centre for Positive Ageing, see in particular the Environment, Housing, Health and Social Care Cluster http://enterprise.gre.ac.uk/expertise/groups/centre-for-positive-ageing

WHO on aging and the lifecourse, useful fact sheets available and regular updates on news stories www.who.int/ageing/en/

15
SOCIAL LIVES, SOCIAL ENGAGEMENT, AND WORK

Eshtar Hamid, Joanna Malone and Jennifer Stock

Learning outcomes

- To understand the relationship between social engagement and health and well-being in later life
- To understand the impact of specific factors on this relationship, such as types and quality of social engagement and gender differences
- To gain insight into social engagement patterns in later life across different cultures, including traditional family structures and filial piety in Asian cultures; and societal changes in this context
- To understand the role of social groups for identity and well-being in older adults
- To gain insight into the benefits of work and volunteering for increased social interaction and well-being

Introduction

The transition into later life is associated with numerous changes, including social lives and social engagement. It is important to consider these changes and transitions because evidence suggests that changes in social lives can impact on health and well-being. Evidence also suggests that these relationships are moderated by gender and also vary across cultures and societies. This chapter discusses this evidence and also provides an international perspective on social lives in later life, including insights into traditional family structures and the concept of 'filial piety' in Asian cultures, as well as societal changes in this context. Additionally, this chapter discusses the role of social groups in social identity within society and the beneficial effect of this on well-being. And finally, the benefits of work and volunteering for increased social interaction and well-being is also discussed.

Social engagement patterns in later life

Social roles in later life are significantly affected by life events and changes occurring in later-life transitions. Accordingly, this can lead to loss of social relationships and a reduction in social network size due to many key events such as retirement from work, the death of a partner or friends, and poor health, which can result in the restriction of physical activities such as hobbies (Shaw et al., 2007). To gain insight into the significance of social role changes with aging due to events in later life, a study by Burn et al. (2016) examined major social changes occurring in the lives of females aged 45–55 as they transitioned to 'older age'. One of the most prominent findings of this study relates to household composition; it was found that participants who have no children living with them at home often experienced a negative impact on their social activities. On the other hand, there was evidence of compensation through the emerging of a new social role by engaging in volunteerism and grandparenthood; minding grandchildren at this stage was reported as a source of daily activity, especially when it helps to fill the gap left by retirement or reduced working hours. Subsequently, there was a notable decline in the social lives of participants as they approached the transition into later life, despite the fact that there was some evidence of compensation in the high rate of volunteering and minding grandchildren (Burn et al., 2016).

Within the context of the social interaction of older people, there is a growing body of evidence which suggests that maintaining high levels of social engagement has a crucial impact on the physical and cognitive health of older adults. Based on 'Social Integration Theory', which highlights that integration into social structures can have an impact on individual's health, Cohen (2004) pointed out that social integration is a predictor of our physical health. This has been examined through the impact on individuals who participate in a social network whereby social control and peer pressure within the network influences their health behaviour – for example, in the way they eat and exercise. A number of studies linked social relations to cognitive health; for example, Cohen (2004) explained that being socially connected is beneficial in the way it influences positive psychological status (e.g. identity, self-worth, and self-affect) and encourages health-promoting behaviours. However, most of this research did not examine social engagement over time from the differing perspectives of individuals; therefore examining the association between social engagement patterns and health outcomes over the life course is crucial (Thomas, 2011).

A study by Béland et al. (2005) found that social integration based on monthly attendance in community centre activities, public meetings, and religious services was related to cognitive functioning in older age. Those who had high levels of social integration experienced stable cognitive functioning over time, while those with low levels of social integration experienced deteriorating cognitive capability. In line with these findings, Thomas (2011) also found that maintaining high levels of social attachments through social engagement has a potentially protective effect on physical and cognitive functions.

Overview of social network patterns and mental health in later life

There is considerable variation in the types of social networks amongst older adults, such as network size. Fiori, Antonucci and Cortina (2006) have explored the implications of network typologies on the mental health of older adults, particularly the association between network types and depressive symptomatology. Their study identified five types of social networks: nonfamily-restricted, non-friends, family, diverse, and friends based on different sociodemographic variables, such as being married, contact with children, frequency in attending meetings and religious services, gender, and race. In this study, those with a nonfamily- restricted network have limited social ties compared with individuals in other networks. Members of this network were unlikely to be married or to have children, and if they did have children they had lower levels of contact with them. Findings from this study indicated a bi-directional influence of social network types on the mental health of older adults. In relation to mental health outcomes, individuals in diverse networks had the best outcome with less depressive symptoms compared to individuals in the restricted network, who had worse outcomes. From another perspective, the network size for older people decreases as they age; it becomes smaller but beneficial to their emotional well-being as the number of close contacts within the network remains stable. At this stage, according to 'Socioemotional Selectivity Theory' highlighted by English and Carstensen (2014), older people focus more on the emotional exchange and interaction with close network members.

Social network types have practical implications because they correlate with adverse mental health outcomes; thus they would have an impact on the planning of health and social care services based on different group needs (Fiori, Antonucci and Cortina, 2006). In addition to social network type, others attempt the categorisation of different groups of older adults according to social engagement activities, which has largely contributed to design public health interventions (Croezen et al., 2009). In particular, older adults were grouped according to types of social engagement activities, sociodemographics, and health. Most prominently, Croezen et al. (2009) described five clusters of older adults according to their participation in different social activities such as caregiving, leisure, and other productive activities. Findings from this study indicated that clusters of caregivers reported worse mental health outcomes compared to other clusters of leisure and productive activities who had good self-perceived physical and mental health. This suggests that the type or quality of social connections rather than simply the quantity may be important to consider.

Relationship quality and psychological well-being

Social networks are an integral structure of a person's social relationships. Social network integration will influence mental well-being through different functional properties such as the amount and type of social relations, frequency of contact, social participation, and quality of the relationship (Smith and Christakis, 2008). The quality of relationships has been examined in many studies relating to mental health outcomes, in particular depression. Good-quality social relationships can be considered a source of social support such as emotional, informational, and physical support (Teo, Choi and Valesteine, 2013).

A recent study by Santini et al. (2016) assessed different aspects of relationship quality amongst older men and women with a variety of network members (spouse, children, other family members, and friends) in addition to the association between social network integration and depression symptoms. Findings from this study highlighted gender differences in relation to the quality of relationships and perceived social support. Social support from children and friends had a buffering effect to depressive symptoms in both genders. On the other hand, lack of support from children increases the risk of depression in women. In men, spousal support and good-quality social network integration was found to be protective against depressive symptoms. In general, poor-quality relationships and social isolation increased the feeling of loneliness, which may result in adverse mental health outcomes (Santini et al., 2016).

Social support approaches to health and well-being

While social support is one of the crucial components of social relations, it represents the subjective aspects of social relations. Social ties on the other hand are viewed as the objective aspect of social relations in terms of other indicators such as marital status, frequency of contact with children, and friends. Both conceptions of social relations found to have an indicative psychological impact in many large population-based studies (Sugisawa et al., 2002). In light of this, Okabayashi and Hougham (2014) found that increased contact with adult children in addition to good-quality spousal relationships seem to be a crucial source of social support amongst older people. Marital activities, such as conversations, were found to have an impact on a spouse's tendency to have depressive symptoms. Frequent and good-quality conversations between husbands and wives were found to be equally beneficial for both. Additionally, in the relationships between aging parents with their adult children, gender roles have cultural differences which can shape the impact of social interaction on psychological well-being. For instance, in Japan, women with more children were found to have a low risk of depression compared to those with a lesser number. This finding could be explained by the traditional gender roles in Japan, whereby older women have a stronger family commitment in addition to tight bonds with their adult children (Okabayashi and Hougham, 2014).

As already discussed, people experience aging in a number of different ways and much of this is culturally specific. Cross-cultural understandings of age can be influenced, not only by gender, but by underlying social forces such as religious teachings, reciprocity, relationships, and bonds within society. The following section briefly sheds light on some of the more social consequences of an aging society, with a discussion of older individuals in Asia.

International perspective on social relationships in later life

Increasing aging populations across the world have a number of implications for everyday life and society more widely, including relationships, family structures, health and social care provision, living arrangements, and much more. A report by the UN predicted that

> [b]etween 2015 and 2030, the number of people in the world aged 60 years or over is projected to grow by 56 per cent, from 901 million to 1.4 billion, and by 2050, the global population of older persons is projected to more than double its size in 2015, reaching nearly 2.1 billion.
>
> *(2015, p. 2)*

This aging population is particularly prevalent in a number of Asian countries and the UN report on World Population Ageing stated that, in 2015, 'Asia was home to 56 per cent of the global older population, and in 2030, Asia's share of the world's older persons is projected to increase to 60 per cent' (p. 12). But it cannot be assumed that perceptions and experiences of aging and older individuals is the same everywhere.

With increasing greying populations evident worldwide, the heterogeneous nature of older individuals can be seen and the position of and care of older individuals differs from society to society, as well as culture to culture, This section explores some key characteristics of the care of older adults in a handful of Asian societies. For example, a number of Asian cultures traditionally focus on ideas of filial piety, which stems from Confucian teachings about the reciprocal relationships and duties that are expected between children and their aging parents. Japan is an example of a society in which the ideas of filial piety still have a significant weighting on everyday life, something expressed by Takagi and Silverstein (2011, p. 1561), who suggest that '[a]s a fundamental norm in Japanese society, filial piety represents a culturally coercive force that requires adult children to acquiesce to the demands of their older parents'. Following these teachings, it was expected that the eldest son, his wife, and children live with his aging parents and care for them in their old age. This continued influence of filial piety is something also found in traditional Korean family structures, argue Yoon, Eun, and Park (2000), and the feelings of obligation and duty towards elders is still very persuasive for many. It can also be seen in China, as Gu and Liang (2000) highlight; filial piety emphasises the obligation children have to care for and respect their aging parents' wishes. Although many children look after their aging parents in Western societies too, the cultural roots and influence for this are very different.

Traditional family structures

As mentioned, the way in which family relationships were traditionally structured in a number of Asian societies is contrasted to many Western societies. Dore (1963) explains that, traditionally, within the Japanese family, there was a greater emphasis on the parent-child relationships rather than the conjugal bond of husband and wife, which is stressed within the 'Western family', which further illuminates the obligational relationships expected of children and their aging parents. The traditional family system in Japan is known as the *ie* and everyone in the *ie* had to conform to the duties and responsibilities expected of them. Through this family system the intergenerational duties and obligations for care were sustained through the family networks (Ronald and Alexy, 2011). Although the *ie* is no longer the legal family structure, its ideologies and implications can still be felt in many families today. Campbell and Ingersoll-Dayton (2013) highlight how the perceptions and relationships of family caregiving are different in Japan than in America, stating that, in Japan, caring for a family member is normally equated with living with that family member, whereas in America, it is equated with giving care to an aging parent but living separately from them, thus the expectations and implications of family relationships and care are perceived differently from culture to culture. This emphasis on family relationships and familial contracts can also be seen in China, where the family is seen as a form of social support and a social network built on reciprocal relationships (Gu and Liang, 2000). And the emphasis and importance of the family, in terms of support for older adults, is further enforced by the law in China:

> Only those without family support can be assisted by social welfare programs. According to the Marriage Law of 1981 and the Criminal Law of 1979, children have the duty and legal obligation to support and assist their aged parents, and violators are subject to criminal penalties.
>
> *(Gu and Liang, 2000, p. 83)*

Furthermore, an amendment of the Law of Protection of the Rights and Interests of the Elderly in 2013 stated that children have a duty to visit and care for their aging parents, highlighting the continuing influence of filial piety in modern Chinese society. The prevalence of this obligational relationship in law shows how it still has a huge cultural influence on people's everyday lives in China, despite many other societal changes.

Societal changes

The traditional *ie* family structure in Japan, as discussed earlier, comprised of a three-generational household. The three-generational household is an 'entirely concrete and tangible informal social security system that established exactly who will do what for the elderly when they become frail, bedridden or otherwise acutely needy', according to Hashimoto (2013, p. 20). The

Annual Report on the Aging Society (2015) put forward by the Japanese Cabinet Office reports that in 2014, 13.2 per cent of adults over 65 lived in a three-generation household (Cabinet Office, 2015). So, even though the tradition of children living with aging parents has fallen considerably, Tamiya et al. (2011) explain how compared with other developed countries, this traditional practice is still considered 'normal' in Japanese society. Yet, in recent years, demographic and societal changes in many Asian societies means that, although still informally influential, the traditional structures and obligational relationships that once were concrete are slowly breaking down. This declining three-generational household can be seen in Yoon, Eun, and Park's (2000) discussion of demographic changes in Korea. Although ideas of filial piety *(hyo)* in Korea still have influence over the care of older relatives, improved education means younger Korean individuals have higher levels of education than their forbearers. This education means more exposure to Western ideals, culture, and notions of individualism, which all have effects on the familial and social structures once overarching in Korea. Trends such as low fertility rates, women working for longer, late marriages, and no marriage at all add toward the demographic and societal changes apparent in countries such as Japan. Additionally, as Kawano (2010) explains, many older individuals continue to see themselves as psychologically independent and healthy and thus actively add towards the changing structures in traditional family caregiving. Thus we shouldn't just assume that 'older people' are passive to the societal changes and the changes in traditional caregiving; rather they can actively help shape it.

So although the cultural norms such as filial piety, obligational relationships, and age-based obligations, which have been apparent since Confucian teachings, still have an influence on everyday lives in a number of Asian societies, these traditions are not as widespread as they previously were. Also, despite the influence of traditional family structures not being as widespread as it was in the past, their impact can still be seen, as the comparison with Japan and America described above shows. Demographic and societal changes have been hugely influential in the decline of traditional caregiving situations; these changes have been brought about in a number of ways and are still actively shaping family relationships and caregiving environments worldwide, constantly changing and adapting with society and the world more widely. Yet when it comes to looking at age, the health of older adults, and the position of older adults in society, the continuing importance of cultural norms on social identity and relationships should not be overlooked.

Social groups, social identity, and well-being

Social groups for human beings tend to have a crucial role in shaping our social identity in terms of enhancing our psychological well-being and self-worth. According to 'Social Identity Theory', belonging to a certain social group is not just a peripheral part of our environment but it adds emotional and self-value to us as members of these groups and it has a central role to our health and well-being (Haslam et al., 2009). People often refer to different social entities in our lives – such as family, friends, neighbours, and community and religious groups – as groups from which they seek a sense of belonging and self-identity. Haslam et al. (2009) describe such groups to have a positive impact on shaping our social identity and providing us with a sense of belonging to a place, as well as providing stability and emotional support which would have positive consequences to our psychological well-being. The concept of social identity has been explored from the perspective of gender-based groups and their role in providing social support to older people in long-term residential care in addition to their role in enhancing cognitive ability. Gleibs et al. (2011) found that there are gender differences in these aspects (such as social identity and feelings of belonging) in particular for males more than females. Findings from this study highlight the significance of social engagement in social groups such as gentleman's clubs for men in relation to improving mental health outcomes. For women, they showed no significant changes and their well-being was maintained over the period of study. Finally, it was evident that there was no impact of gender-based groups on improving cognitive abilities for both men and women. Nevertheless, there were a few aspects which have not been examined by the authors, such as the impact of sexual orientation, race/ethnicity and cultural diversity on the social identity and well-being which needs further investigation in the future (Gleibs et al., 2011).

Work and psychological well-being

Continued work in later life has been well investigated in relation to mental health and the psychological well-being of older people. In this respect, older people who continue work after retirement were found to have less depressive symptoms than those who are fully retired (James and Spiro, 2007 p. 162). In line with these findings, other studies explored types of work which are particularly related to mental well-being of older adults. According to the findings, volunteerism seems to have a critical relation to the mental well-being of older retirees in terms of maintaining cognitive abilities and alleviating depressive symptoms (Schwingel, Niti and Tang, 2009). Full-time employment and volunteering represent a form of social interaction which is a fundamental component of healthy aging, as suggested by the 'successful aging model' described by Hao (2008). Therefore, what has been found in previous studies is in line with the 'activity theory', which defined successful aging as 'maintaining the activities and attitudes of middle age as far and as long as possible' (Havighurst, 2009, p. 309). Engaging in different types of productive and leisure activities was found to have an impact on reducing depression and improving quality of life of retirees and older employees. Such activities should be targeted by practitioners when designing intervention programmes for retirees to enhance their engagement in the community to achieve more successful aging (Potocnik and Sonnentag, 2013).

Occupation can be considered an integral component of socialisation, especially for older people, because of the significant role of positive aspects of work such as providing financial and social support. As occupation could play a critical role in successful aging, it is important to consider what predicts the possibility of continuing to work or starting to work in later life. A longitudinal study with a sample of men aged 55–80 found that social engagement and health status predicted employment in later life (Min et al., 2012). Therefore, social engagement is likely to increase the opportunities for working in older adults – and thus potentially improve their mental well-being.

Conclusion

This chapter discussed a range of evidence relating to various aspects of social engagement in later life, with the overall trend of studies suggesting that it is beneficial for the health and well-being of older adults. However, this relationship varies depending on a number of factors including gender, type, and quality of relationship. Additionally, some of the evidence discussed is limited to cross-sectional data and therefore causal inferences cannot be made. Further research utilising longitudinal study design is needed to determine this. Another limitation is the lack of generalisability for studies conducted within one culture. This chapter also discussed cultural differences and in particular the traditional family structures and attitudes towards aging in Asia, as part of which younger generations traditionally cared for their older relatives within the same household. However, due to societal changes, the frequency of this has decreased. This chapter has highlighted the importance of maintaining social engagement in later life and also demonstrated the numerous types of social interaction that can have a beneficial effect on health and well-being. As our population is aging, finding ways for individuals to maximise their physical and mental health is becoming increasingly important so they can age more positively.

References

Béland, F. S., Zunzunegui, M., Alvarado, A., Otero, A., and Del Ser, T. (2005). Trajectories of cognitive decline and social relations. *Journal of Gerontology: Psychological Science*, 60(6), 320–330.

Burn, K., Dennerstien, L., Browning, C., and Sezoeke, C. (2016). Patterns of social engagement in the transition to later life. *Elsevier*, 88, 90–95.

Cabinet Office. (2015). *The aging society: Current situation and implementation measures* (in English). www8.cao.go.jp/kourei/english/annualreport/2015/2015pdf_e.html

Campbell, R., and Ingersoll-Dayton, B. (2013). Variations in family caregiving in Japan and the US. In S. Long (Ed.), *Caring for the elderly in Japan and the U.S.* (pp. 231–247). London: Routledge.

Cohen, S. (2004). Social relationships and Health. *American Psychologist*, 59(8), 676–684.

Croezen, S., Haveman-Nies, A., Alvarado, V. J., and Van't Veer, C. P. (2009). Characterization of different groups of elderly according to social engagement activity patterns. *The Journal of Nutrition, Health & Aging*, 13(9), 776–781.

Dore, R. (1963). *City life in Japan: A study of a Tokyo ward.* London: Routledge.

English, T., and Carstensen, L. (2014). Selective narrowing of social networks across adulthood is associated with improved emotional experience in daily life. *International Journal of Behavioral Development*, 38(2), 194–202.

Fiori, K., Antonucci, T. C., and Cortina, K. (2006). Social network typologies and mental health among older adults. *Journal of Gerontology: Psychological Services*, 61B(1), 25–32.

Gleibs, I. H., Haslam, C., Jones, J. M., and Haslam, S. A. (2011). No country for old men? The role of 'Gentlemen's club' in promoting Social engagement and Psychological well-being in residential care. *Ageing and Mental Health*, 15(4), 456–466.

Gu, S., and Liang, J. (2000). China: Population aging and old age support. In V. L. Bengtson, K-D. Kim, G. C. Myers, and K-S. Eun (Eds.), *Aging in East and West: Families, states, and the elderly* (pp. 59–93). New York: Springer Publishing Company.

Hao, Y. (2008). Productive activities and psychological well-being among older adults. *Journal of Gerontology: Social Services*, 36B(2), 64–72.

Hashimoto, A. (2013). Cultural meanings of "security" in aging policies. In S. Long (Ed.), *Caring for the elderly in Japan and the U.S.* (pp. 19–27). London: Routledge.

Haslam, A., Jetten, J., Postmes, T., and Haslam, C. (2009). Social identity, health and well-being: An emerging agenda for Applied Psychology. *Applied Psychology: An International Review*, 58(1), 1–23.

Havighurst, R. J. (2009). Successful ageing. [e-book]. In R. H. Williams, C. Tibbitts, and W. Donohue (Eds.), *Process of ageing: Social and psychological perspectives* (Chapter: 16, pp. 299–311). New Brunswick, NJ: Transaction Publishers.

James, J. B., and Spiro, A. (2007). The impact of work on the psychological well-being of older American. [e-book] In J. James, P. Wink, and K. W. Schaie (Eds.), *The crown of life: Dynamics of the early post-retirement period* (Chapter: 8, pp. 153–165). New York: Springer.

Kawano, S. (2010). *Natures embrace: Japan's ageing urbanites and new death rites.* Honoluli, HI: University of Hawai'i Press.

Min, J., Lee, K., Park, J., and Cho, S. (2012). Social engagement, Health and Changes in Occupational status: Analysis of the Korean Longitudinal Study of Ageing (KLOSA). *PLOS ONE*, 7(10), 2–7.

Okabayashia, H., and Hougham, G. W. (2014). Gender differences of social interactions and their effects on subjective well-being among Japanese elders. *Ageing and Mental Health*, 18(1), 58–71.

Potocnik, K., and Sonnentag, S. (2013). A longitudinal study of wellbeing of older adults and retirees: The role of engaging in different types of activities. *Journal of Occupational and Organizational Psychology*, 86, 497–521.

Ronald, R., and Alexy, A. (2011). Continuity and change in Japanese homes and families. In R. Ronald and A. Alexy (Eds.), *Home and family in Japan: Continuity and transformation* (pp. 1–24). London: Routledge.

Santini, Z. I., Fiori, K. L., Feeney, J., and Tyrovolas, S. (2016). Social relationship, loneliness, and mental health among older men and women in Ireland: A perspective community-based study. *Journal of Affective Disorder*, 204, 59–69.

Schwingel, A., Niti, M. M., and Tang, C. (2009). Continued work employment and volunteerism and mental well-being of older adults: Singapore longitudinal study. *Age and Ageing*, 38, 531–537.

Shaw, A. B., Krause, N., Liang, J., and Bennett, J. (2007). Tracking changes in social relations throughout life. *Journal of Gerontology: Psychological Services*, 62(2), 90–99.

Smith, K. P., and Christakis, N. K. (2008). Social networks and health. *The Annual Review of Sociology*, 34, 405–429.

Sugisawa, H., Shibata, H., Hougham, G. W., and Liang, J. (2002). The impact of social ties on depressive symptoms in U.S. and Japanese elderly. *Journal of Social Issues*, 58(4), 785–804.

Takagi, E., and Silverstein, M. (2011). Purchasing piety? Co-residence of married children with their older parents in Japan. *Demography*, 48(4), 1559–1579.

Tamiya, N., Noguchi, H., Nishi, A., Reich, M., Ikegami, N., Hashimoto, H., Shibuya, K., Kawachi, I. and Campbell, J. C. (2011). 'Population ageing and wellbeing: lessons from Japan's long-term care insurance policy' *The Lancet,* 378(9797), 1183–1192.

Teo, A. R., Choi, H., and Valenstein, H. (2013). Social relationships and depression: A ten years follow up study of a nationally representative study. *PLOS ONE*, 8(1), 1–8.

Thomas, P. A. (2011). Trajectories of social engagement and limitations in later life. *Journal of Health and Social Behavior*, 52(4), 430–443.

United Nations, Department of Economic and Social Affairs, Population Division. (2015). *World population ageing 2015*. ST/ESA/SER.A/390.

Yoon, G., Eun, K-S., and Park, K-S. (2000). Korea: Demographic trends, sociocultural contexts, and public policy. In V. L. Bengtson, K-D. Kim, G. C. Myers, and K-S. Eun (Eds.), *Aging in East and West: Families, states, and the elderly* (pp. 121–113). New York: Springer Publishing Company.

16

DIGITAL TECHNOLOGIES AND AGING

Liz Bacon and Professor Lachlan MacKinnon

This chapter discusses:

- Smart homes technologies
- Acceptability issues
- Social, economic, political, environmental and privacy issues
- Assistive technologies for specific conditions
- Future directions for IT for positive aging

Introduction

There are numerous statistics available worldwide on the definition and the size of the aging population, but whether counted from the age of 55 or 60, there is one aspect researchers all agree on, which is that the volume of the aging population is increasing as enhanced healthcare is allowing people to live longer, and this is creating both a challenge and an opportunity for society. With information technology (IT) already woven into all aspects of life, it is unfathomable that it will not also play a major role in the lives of older adults going forward, in particular in the provision of increasing support for care at home and in the community, which is generally desired by older adults and also more cost effective for them and society in general.

IT has the capacity to provide a wide range of support to the aging population; however to respond appropriately to what is different about the aging population, we need to understand what changes come with age. These changes can be broadly categorised into the following areas: physical decline, cognitive decline, illness, and disabilities (Jia, Lu and Wajda, 2015). IT can provide support in all these areas including supporting physical treatments, enhanced quality of life, support for independent living, social interaction, and assisting in managing and providing care. This impacts almost every aspect of life, including human behaviour, personal issues, health and health services, environmental, economic, social challenges, and so on. This gerontology-informed technology is called gerontechnology, the success of which involves a multitude of physical, social, and mental issues.

There are many ways to classify the use of IT in aging, such as the work of Parra et al. (2013), who identified the following four main goals:

1 Prevention – for example, the use of fitness machines to stay active and brain games to keep mentally fit
2 Compensation – when a disease or ailment cannot be cured, IT can be used to reduce the impact of the decline or to replace a capability (e.g. use of a home control system); IT can be used on a personal level or in the environment to support or monitor the person
3 Care – to support or replace a carer such as a physician, nurse, or family member
4 Enhancement – to create new opportunities and enhance capabilities (e.g. use of social media to contact family or to find new learning or work opportunities)

Fahim et al. (2012) produced a gerontechnology matrix to show how five domains of human activity – "health & self-esteem", "housing & daily living", "mobility & transport", "communication & governance", and "work & leisure" – match the four goals identified above, showing how IT interventions have changed between 1990 and 2010. For example, in the goal of "Compensation", in the area of "communication & governance", in 1990 an IT intervention example was a hearing aid, but in 2010 it was a cochlear implant.

In each of the above four goals there are a wealth of applications covering "the full range of physical, cognitive and emotional functioning as well as the maintenance of individual independence, self-efficacy and dignity" (Fahim et al., 2012). These applications include alerting, monitoring, assisting, training, eLearning, physical and mental games, and communication/social applications (Parra et al., 2013). Chan et al. (2012) provide an excellent list of smart wearable systems, too extensive to repeat here, that can be used for monitoring health, which of course include a focus on support for the aging population.

One of the key challenges in referring to older adults is that they are not a homogenous group. "In studies of older adults, research design still often describes ages 55+ as the target group. This is controversial for several reasons. Life expectancy in western countries, as well as the number of healthy years, has increased significantly" (Taipale, 2014). It could be argued that many adults at the age of 55 have physically and mentally more in common with someone in their thirties than someone in their eighties, especially given that Väyrynen (2012) reports that statistics commonly show the age when some kind of support is required starts at around 75. That aside, in terms of the attitudes, preferences, and use of technology, these also vary tremendously between age groups (Intosalmi et al., 2013). For a more extensive discussion on the differences between age-related cohorts, the reader is referred to the paper by Fozard and Wahl (2012). However, we do need to recognise the heterogeneous nature of this very large group of citizens and a stratified or cohort model similar to that used to classify the general adult population might well be beneficial in targeting both the provision of services and technologies, as well as the activities and engagement of these citizens.

In terms of the scope of this chapter, it is very much focused on the four goals identified above. There are of course many fields which consider IT and the aging population such as psychology, human motion studies, ethnographic studies, policy-making reports, human-computer interaction, and technology-oriented reviews (Parra et al., 2013), and of course IT is extensively used in medical diagnosis. However, a discussion of all these areas is beyond the scope of this chapter.

In terms of the structure of the remainder of this chapter, it is difficult to disconnect the technologies from their actual use, as one technology may support the aging process in a number of ways. Technologies tend to fall into two key types: active and passive. Active technologies are where older adults are pro-active in engaging with technology, such as use of self-reporting tools in social media or an exercise app to help them keep fit. Passive technologies are where the older adults do not pro-actively engage but are monitored through software (e.g. video and tracking devices which may report directly to relatives and health professionals). Given a key focus of support for older adults in the future revolves around the smart home, or care home, which is also reflected by extensive research in the literature, a section of this chapter is devoted to discussion of this area and the technologies which can be used to support older adults at every stage. Other important areas to review are the context and external drivers for the use of IT to support aging, which include: acceptability; trustworthiness; and social, economic, political, and environmental issues. A final and important area to review is assistive technologies for specific conditions. Whilst not specific to the aging population, this tends to be the dominant group who they will support.

Smart homes technologies

The vast majority of older adults prefer to live in their own home as long as they can and although some live with families, there is an increasing tendency for people to live alone. It is therefore important that their home environment supports them in an age-friendly way and ensures as full a participation in life as possible, thus meeting one of the core needs of humans (Taipale, 2014). Smart homes can provide independence to the older adult which can, in turn, increase their well-being (Barlow, Bayer and Curry, 2006; Mynatt and Rogers, 2001; Nugent et al., 2008); given the growth in the older population, the demand for smart homes is set to increase (Peine, Rollwagen and Neven, 2014).

But what exactly is a smart home, which can also be referred to as a "smart house, home automation, domotique, intelligent home, adaptive home, and aware house" (Alam, Reaz and Ali, 2012)? The concept of a smart home is complex and brings together a number of fields such as "housing, technology, engineering, sociology, and healthcare in relation to robotics, sensors, telehealth, ergonomics, communications, social care and safety" (Morris et al., 2013). It generally refers to a connected home using "Information and Communication Technology (ICT) in the home to facilitate the interoperability of household products and services in a built entity" (Peine, 2008) and has the potential to offer increased comfort and more cost-effective healthcare, which also has the potential to impact on many pressing social issues. Smart homes can offer a range of technologies and services. Ehrenhard et al. (2014) discusses the definition of smart homes and defines a number of key research areas such as:

- Comfort (entertainment, heating, and lighting control)
- Security and safety (for monitoring inhabitants and intruders)
- Wellness monitoring (activity tracking, monitoring of falls and immobility)
- Intelligent energy usage (smart electricity metering and energy control)
- Healthcare which can overlap with the above (telemedicine)

The range of possible technologies in smart homes is extensive and is summarised here (Piau et al., 2014; Walsh, 2014; Bouchard et al., 2014):

- Monitoring and associated support/alerts for relatives and healthcare professionals – this is a huge area and depending on the number and variety of sensors in a house, they can provide a very rich data set, all activities logging date and time information for later analysis if needed. These sensors are not only useful for alerting and analysis but also to build behavioural profiles and psychological monitoring as shown by Walsh et al. (2014), who noted that "The number of light switch firings, for some locations, were associated significantly with anxiety", demonstrating that patterns of behaviour could be used to detect loneliness. Examples of monitors include: those to detect proximity and motion; measuring vital signs using multiple sensors such as wearable sensors; bed sensors to measure sleep patterns and bed-restlessness; blood pressure tests; recognition of breathing and heart problems; smart carpets with pressure sensors to detect falls, toilet use, gait tracking for speed, analysis, and even intelligent predictions of future falls; detection of cooking patterns using temperature sensors, water, and stove usage sensors; smart services for food preparation; phone records; contact switch sensors to detect door and window opening; usage sensors on medicine containers (i.e. smart pill boxes to remind people to take their medication; if the pill box hasn't been opened, a range of infrared, video, and audio sensors, to listen for audio alerts such as calls for help by residents, are activated); monitoring of socialisation habits including outings and visitors; RF localisation systems (worn by occupants); smart mailboxes (e.g. to alert if post has not been collected); automatic front door unlocking for residents; automatic blinds; an interactive mirror for communicating with residents (particularly for medication prompting); safety features such as gas shut off and water temperature sensors; flood detectors; gesture recognition; etc.

- Pro-active technologies such as robots for assistive support, mobility aids, and social use as companions (sometimes called socially assistive robots) and pet-like robots, which are a growth area – it is however important that these are able to retrieve sensory information from the environment in order to be context aware, giving them the potential to adapt over time, taking into account location, activity, preferences, and social situation, etc. Acceptance of companion robots is influenced by a number of factors such as "age, gender, education and technological experience, family status, and cultural background", but it also depends on how robots are advertised to the older adult (Flandorfer, 2012). Robots need to be able to be configured with user preferences; for example, even though someone might have fallen over, the person may prefer, in the first instance, to try to stand on their own as opposed to have a robot immediately call for help. Ethical principles which should govern the design of robots suggested by Amirabdollahian et al. (2013) were as follows, noting that of course there may be times when these are in tension with each other (for example, between privacy and safety):

    - Autonomy – being able to set goals in life and choose means
    - Independence – being able to implement one's goals without the permission, assistance, or material resources of others
    - Enablement – having or having access to means of realising goals and choices
    - Safety – being able readily to avoid pain or harm
    - Privacy – being able to pursue and realise one's goals and implement one's choices unobserved
    - Social connectedness – having regular contact with friends and loved ones and safe access to strangers one can choose to meet.

Despite the potential of smart home technology and the fact that the concept has been around for about 50 years, it has yet to take off in a significant way due to a number of factors such as cost, standards, and the explosion of sensors and products on the market. Interoperability of devices can also be a significant issue, although there are some consortia that are attempting to define standards and protocols for smart homes (Van de Kaa, Den Hartlog and De Vries, 2009). Smart homes are just one example of the Internet of Things (IoT) and they bring with them issues for debate such as whether these should be hosted in the local home or in the cloud – the latter having many benefits such as shared, cloud-based web services (Soliman et al., 2013); however reliability is noted as extremely important by many and therefore a permanent reliable Internet connection is a must (Ehrenhard et al., 2014). The number of sensors and constant new products on the market has also been identified as causing confusion. These must however be integrated in an intelligent and context-sensitive way, such as that described by Valero et al. (2014) in which they outline a framework for integrating multisensory hybrid reasoners to support personal autonomy in a smart home.

Acceptability issues

Portet et al. (2013) discuss the two major quality measures for success in smart homes technology. These are "acceptability (Usability, Affordability) and trustworthiness (Safety, Security, Reliability, Privacy)"; however these are general issues that apply to all technology for all age users and not just the technologies used in smart homes, although there are key factors in the development of smart homes for older adults and these may need to be different for older adults.

In terms of acceptability, Damant and Knapp (2015) define technology as including "both traditional and new forms of social media, along with technological advances in support such as robotics and telecare". They estimate, based on data from the Office for National Statistics that in the United Kingdom (ONS, 2015), "4.8 million people aged over 64 have never used the internet" although that number is decreasing annually. The aging population is typically educated by family and friends, and although third-sector organisations "work to improve the e-inclusion of vulnerable groups", the older generation are generally more reluctant than the general population to let it encroach on their lives, expressing more concerns about privacy, the elderly being an obvious target for fraud and identify theft, especially those with cognitive decline. Research by Wagner, Hassanein, and Head (2010) and Xie (2003) shows that attitudes towards ICT tend to become more negative as age increases; however Wagner, Hassanein and Head (2010) also identified gender differences in that men appeared to have less "computer-related anxiety". Dutton and Blank (2011), reporting on the Oxford Internet Survey (OxIS) in 2011, established that 73.2 per cent of women had never used the Internet compared to 56.3 per cent of men. Lee, Chen, and Hewitt (2011) reported that the main reasons given by women for a lack of engagement with the Internet were personal anxiety or stress, and limited self-confidence, in addition to other barriers such as computer virus problems. Czaja et al. (2006) also reported two main barriers for the acceptance of new technologies as low self-efficacy and high anxiety; however access, acceptance, and use are also impacted by education and/or prior experience with technology. Wagner, Hassanein, and Head (2010), showed that even when older adults do use the Internet, it is often for limited purposes such as to keep in touch with family, but also only when it does not interfere with their daily life (Selwyn, 2004). There is considerable research into acceptability issues by older adults; for example Renaud and van Biljon (2008) proposed a Senior Technology Acceptance Model (STAM) and discussed how to design for technology acceptance in the elderly, ensuring that the unique characteristics, capabilities, and limitations of the elderly are considered in technology acceptance.

In terms of usability, older adults can be affected by both cognitive decline and a decline in motor skills which can affect a person's ability to navigate and engage with the Internet (Hardhill and Olphert, 2012). With regard to cognitive decline, difficulties can be encountered with menu structures. For example, Gudur et al. (2013) demonstrated that, in general, older people (in common with all ages) tend to encounter more difficulty using nested/multi-layered menus compared with flat/broad interfaces as nested structures require more working memory, which tends to deteriorate with age. However, the physical screen size of a mobile can make flat menu structures more challenging to develop. In terms of physical decline, older adults can face challenges interacting with IT, such as due to tremors, arthritis, and deteriorating eyesight. However Mertens et al. (2012) reported a decrease in the error rate of older adults with hand tremors when using 'swabbing motions' on touchscreens, compared to tapping a screen or moving a pointer and clicking with a mouse. It should also be noted that "older people with and without previous computer experience place much more importance to words than icons in their everyday interactions with the web" (Parra et al., 2013).

Needing to be physically close to an alarm can sometimes be an issue and may restrict older adults with impaired mobility to certain areas within their own homes (Milligan, Roberts and Mort, 2011). One solution to this is the use of pendant alarms; however, some users have found them too bulky and awkward to wear (Walsh and Callan, 2011). A possible solution to both these problems is the use of audio, which can play a significant part in smart homes, such as calling for help if a physical interface is out of reach (Portet et al., 2013). Audio can also be used in the form of speech to remind residents of appointments. However, technology is not perfect and poor sound quality can cause problems for those with hearing impairments (Demeris, Doorenbos and Towle, 2009). Some redundancy in technology, communication methods, and data collected can prove useful not only to provide a choice regarding mode of interaction but data from multiple sources can also be used to detect and correct errors; for example, recognition of falls is still prone to false positives (Haux et al., 2014).

Telecare or remote health consultation systems have significant potential to reduce costs (e.g. the need for physical visits by healthcare professionals). However, some studies have shown that older adults can find the technology hard to use or 'inconvenient' or 'confusing' (Lai et al., 2010).

Social, economic, political, environmental, and privacy issues

Developments for the aging population can also be applicable in wider society and smart homes have the potential to contribute to "environmental, social and fiscal sustainability" (Ehrenhard et al., 2014). However, the aging population is a very heterogeneous group due to differences in health, wealth, lifestyle, education, living environment, and social connectedness (Jia, Lu and Wadja, 2015). Perceptions of affordability will impact use of ICT, with many viewing it as a "luxury" based on deep-rooted spending patterns and consumer habits. However, the first criteria for a smart home is fast and reliable access to the Internet and this can be an issue in rural areas and in care homes. Damant and Knapp (2015) reported that approximately 25 per cent of registered care homes in the United Kingdom provide Internet access to residents, which can exclude older adults and lead to increased isolation. This is unfortunate given the potential impact noted by Tsai et al. (2010), who showed a significant drop in depressive symptoms three months after using a videoconferencing service in residential care. This is supported by Morris et al. (2014), who report on a systematic review showing how smart technology can positively impact social connectedness, social support and networks, feelings of empowerment, stress, self-efficacy, self-esteem, loneliness, depression, and quality of life. Selwyn (2004) also showed that IT had positively impacted work, leisure, and information-seeking activities of older adults. It should be noted that mobility and transport have been "found to be key to older adults' quality of life as well as their experience of autonomy and participation" (Fahim et al., 2012).

With regard to telecare services, a balance in their use needs to be found. Many older adults resist remote services, as adopting these can result in a loss of contact from healthcare visitors with whom they have developed a stable relationship and who are often seen as part of their extra-familial relationships (Sanders et al., 2012). Whilst telecare services and other monitoring devices can provide considerable reassurance and emotional relief to all stakeholders involved – relatives, physicians and nurses, administrators, the ambulance service, and indeed the resident themselves (Flandorfer, 2012) – it is important to many older adults that IT systems are seen not to be taking over. This is not just due to a loss of control but there are also concerns that an over-reliance on IT may, in time, result in a more lazy lifestyle which could cause their health to deteriorate faster (Portet et al., 2013). Also, many feel that they do not need monitoring and naturally resist admitting they may need help and are perhaps no longer in full control (Mort, Roberts and Callen, 2013). It is however possible that smart technologies linked to healthcare professionals could help older adults gain an enhanced understanding of their health conditions, which may ultimately result in an improvement in conditions associated with being socially connected, such as depression (Morris et al., 2014).

The cost of smart homes and other IT services for the elderly is an issue (Haux et al., 2014) and going forward it is unclear what the balance between consumer spend and government spend should be. Businesses may target the more affluent in the older adult population and of course cost is a significant driver in human behaviour. Insurers may also drive behaviour; for example, the use of smart technology could be seen to reduce the risk of fire, flood, private medical bills, and crime in an elderly person's home. Given the trend to reduce reliance on fossil fuels, governments may subsidise or regulate smart home energy to encourage appropriate behaviour, and they should also not underestimate their power to steer the adoption of technology through campaigns and subsidies (Ehrenhard et al., 2014). However, for the health services, it may be in their interests to fund some of the telecare initiatives, as they may be considerably cheaper in the longer term than continuing to provide traditional visit-based services. As a result, the aging population may be under social, economic, and political pressure to engage with IT technologies and services more (Mort, Roberts and Callen, 2013).

Whilst there are obvious substantial benefits of the use of IT by older adults, the vast majority of IT uses, particularly in smart homes, bring with them significant privacy, ethical, and social issues and these should not be underestimated, as they can become significant barriers to adoption. Research into smart homes technology must be coupled with the appropriate development of frameworks, not only for their design and implementation but also to address the social, ethical, and legal issues that widespread adoption brings. As more data is gathered, it brings with it the potential to aggregate data in ways not previously possible, such as the integration of smart homes data with an electronic patient records, to provide increased levels of intelligence for monitoring older adults. Access to and retention of data is a significant issue that tends to lag behind the technology in an industry that is dominated by a technology push from suppliers as opposed to a demand-pull (Frisardi and Imbimbo, 2011). Quite rightly, people have expressed concerns about technology replacing personal interaction and, whilst in the case of telecare this can be true, it may also intrude on confidentiality and privacy resulting in a sense of autonomy loss (Piau et al., 2014). However, taking an alternative view, to quote from De Silva, Morikawa and Petra (2012), "The house will look at us from many directions to protect us from potential dangers due to our forgetfulness or due to other physical disabilities. Then we will always have a friend to live in with us".

Assistive technologies for specific conditions

Any consideration of assistive technologies has to be contextualised in terms of the purpose and perspective of the use of such technologies. For many years the focus was on the medical perspective of disabilities and assistive technologies were focused on overcoming the disabling effects of various medical conditions. More recently, the focus has moved to a social inclusion perspective, with the focus being on technologies that assist in overcoming the social exclusion occasioned by the impact of various forms of impairment. As Hersh and Johnson (2008) put it, "it is the widespread acceptance of the social model of disability that is driving these changes and it is the tools of assistive technology that are the physical enablers of social inclusiveness". This is particularly important in the context of positive aging, since the medical perspective remains a significant driver for many of the technologies developed to deal with issues and problems associated with aging, but a social inclusion perspective is potentially much more positive. As we said in the introduction to this chapter, the concept of the elderly population now reflects quite as diverse a population as the general adult population (Fozard and Wahl, 2012) and, whilst there are issues associated with aging, considering all forms of assistive technology in terms of social inclusion is beneficial to all. However, as Warschauer (2004) makes clear in his work, it is not simply the provision of technology that enables social inclusion, but the acceptance and integration of that technology into everyday social interaction.

As the Internet has become almost universally pervasive, with more and more information and services readily available from home computers, smartphones, and tablets, Don Norman's vision of "the invisible computer" (Norman, 1999) becomes ever more real. In Norman's vision, computers are replaced by software and hardware technologies within our immediate environments, acting as "information assistants" to help us to live our lives more effectively. This gels entirely with the growth of the Internet of Things (IoT) and, as described earlier, the growth of the Smart Homes/Environments/Cities initiatives (Alam, Reaz and Ali, 2012). In this massively connected world, many of the existing software and hardware tools developed as assistive technologies will be enhanced, realised, or replaced by "apps" running on our chosen information assistants (which can include physical and virtual robots). This process is already well established and represents a significant commercial marketplace for software and hardware developers, moderated by national public bodies, national legislation, and charity organisations representing groups suffering different types of impairment.

So, the combination of the widespread growth of the use and acceptance of IT in everyday social interactions, the ease of use of information assistants embedded into our living environments, and the acceptance of a social model of disability enables assistive technologies to act as agents for social inclusion. From a positive aging perspective, this goes some way to destigmatising the acceptance of assistive technologies by users and, if they are more willing to accept the use of these technologies in the early stages of impairment, then they can have prolonged positive effects on social engagement and inclusion.

In the rest of this section we look at assistive technologies in terms of types of impairment and identify the software and hardware technologies that are currently available to support them. Obviously, technology change in this area is rapid, so the technologies identified are intended as exemplars and we recommend readers to research further before purchasing. To that end, we have also identified some key support bodies in the United Kingdom and United States (please note that exhaustive lists can be found online) who provide advice and support online in these areas. There are similar organisations in many other countries throughout the world, which will provide linguistically and culturally relevant information for those suffering from impairment, and we do encourage all our readers to become familiar and engaged with their local and national support organisations, either as a volunteer, supporter, or user.

Software and hardware for the hearing impaired

In terms of hearing impairment, there is a range of tools available to support users, ranging from those simply requiring some level of audio boost through to the profoundly deaf, who require alternative representations of audio information. In public buildings, legislation in many countries requires the provision of induction loop technology to support members of the public using hearing aids, and some public performance venues provide subtitling/surtitling to help their customers follow the action on stage (Daily Telegraph, 2005). There are many long-standing national support organisations for the hearing impaired around the world, such as Action on Hearing Loss in the United Kingdom (2016) and the National Association of the Deaf in the United States (2016). These organisations offer advice and reviews on assistive technologies for the hearing impaired, offering approved products for sale through their own online site and recommending suppliers or services offering more complex or expensive technologies.

The relevant software and hardware technologies include:

- Digital hearing aids – these offer over-ear or in-ear amplification and have now replaced the older analog hearing aids. They are becoming smaller and lighter, with longer battery life and recharge capability. The latest versions are wifi-linked to software applications that allow users to configure them from their chosen computing device.
- Amplifiers, headphones, portable loops – a wide range of devices providing required levels of amplification to support watching TV, listening to music, and conversations through to hearing-aid support for public events.
- Speech-to-text translators – offering SMS/MMS support for mobile phone communication. In-language translation using tools such as Dragon (Nuance, 2016) and between-language translation using tools such as Google Translate (Google, 2016).
- Alerter systems – ranging from vibrating alarm clocks, flashing light systems for phone calls, doorbells, etc. through to sophisticated computing apps that can be programmed to provide a range of bespoke alerts for chosen conditions, such as Braci (2016) and My Ear Droid (Tecnalia, 2016).
- Subtitling tools – to support watching film or TV, or listening to music, these tools use speech-to-text translation to create subtitles; examples are iSubtitle (Bitfield, 2016) and Subtitles (2016).
- Cochlear implants – serious surgical intervention for the profoundly deaf; unlike hearing aids, which amplify sound, these implants feed signals direct to the brain, replacing the function of damaged parts of the ear (Arndt et al., 1999). The latest versions of these implants are now wirelessly connected and programmable.

Software and hardware for the visually impaired

As with hearing impairment, there are a wide range of tools available to support users with needs ranging from simple vision correction through to alternative representations of visual information for the blind. In many countries, legislation requires the provision of both audio and visual representations of warning information, such as at traffic crossings, to support both visually impaired and hearing impaired citizens. Likewise, the visually impaired community offers many local and national support organisations, such as the Royal National Institute for the Blind (RNIB) in the United Kingdom (2016) and the National Federation of the Blind (NFB) in the United States (2016). These organisations also offer advice and reviews on assistive technologies for the visually impaired, offering approved products for sale through their own online site and recommending suppliers or services offering more complex or expensive technologies.

The relevant software and hardware technologies include:

- Video magnifiers – there are a wide range of these tools, for handheld and desktop use, offering varying levels of magnification depending on the needs of the users. Better quality digital screens and focusing software characterise the developments of this technology, although it is also now embedded as software in many devices, using tools such as MAGic (2016).
- Braille technology – Braille has been in use for the visually impaired for nearly 200 years, and the basic alphabet construction of raised dots remains unchanged and also used for music notation. In many countries there are legal requirements to provide Braille notation on public signage to enable the visually impaired to read signs. Digital technology offers refreshable Braille displays, Braille translators, and text-to-speech synthesisers, such as the Brailliant range (2016) and the Perkins range (2016).
- Accessible information assistants – On computers, laptops, tablets and smartphones, there are a range of information assistants designed to support the visually impaired, including text-to-speech tools such as JAWS (2016), magnification software such as MAGic (2016), and integrated tool suites such as Synapptic (2016).
- Travel assistants – The issue of supporting travel for the visually impaired has exercised the developers of assistive technologies for many years, developing numerous varieties of cane, Braille maps, audio instructions, and enabling legislation on street signage and road crossings. The advent of GPS systems, especially as their accuracy has improved, combined with speech software, such as JAWS, on smartphones and tablets has provided the visually impaired with greater levels of confidence and independence. Smart Canes have now been developed with sensors mounted on the traditional white cane to detect obstacles up to 3m from the user (Smart Canes, 2015), and there is now work in progress to mount camera technology on the cane to enable it to recognise other pedestrians!

Software and hardware for the physically impaired

There is an enormous range of physical impairments that can affect humans, some of which are more prevalent amongst the aging population, such as stroke and arthritis. However, all of the issues of physical impairment are present in the aging population and the same software and hardware products are relevant for them. There is also a large number of local and national organisations representing the needs of physically impaired citizens, such as the Stroke Association in the United Kingdom (2016) and the National Stroke Association in the United States (2016), Arthritis Care in the United Kingdom (2016) and Arthritis Foundation in the United States (2016), multi-representational organisations such as Disability Rights UK (2016), and international organisations such as the Leonard Cheshire Foundation (2016). Given the huge range of conditions that cause physical impairment, it is not feasible here to consider all the tools relevant to each condition; however we can identify some broad categories of software and hardware and identify the key developments impacting this provision.

Therefore, the relevant software and hardware technologies include:

- Prosthetics – whilst there has long been a mechanical prosthetics industry, modern digital technologies have enabled the development of advanced robotic prosthetics, together with software control technologies (Chen, 2009). The latest developments of these technologies are to develop mind control of the software (Chang, 2015).

- Neural implants – a wide range of neural implants are already possible: wiring electronic technology directly to the relevant area within the brain. The best known of these are cochlear implants, described earlier, but their use for control of prosthetic limbs or to control physical symptoms of diseases such as Parkinson's are currently being supported by new chip technologies (Chen, Yao, and Basu, 2015).
- Wheelchair technology – advanced wheelchair technology uses electronic controls and stepper motors to allow wheelchairs to climb kerbs and stairs, as well as operate from breath control or simple muscle movements. The technology for brain-controlled wheelchairs is now so widespread that DIY instructions using a simple EEG monitor are available online (Emotiv, 2015).
- Assistive rehabilitation apps – many of the apps developed for the Wii and the Kinect involved physical games, exercises, and physiotherapeutic activities, and these have been widely used for assistive rehabilitation. This continues to be true with smartphone apps, using web cams or external devices such as the Kinect, and undertaking physical exercise controlled by such an app can improve recovery and rehabilitation from a number of conditions.
- Environmental control devices – POSSUM have been developing environmental control systems in the United Kingdom for many years, initially using mechanical and electrical motors from electronic control boards. Like similar companies in other countries, they have moved to integrated digital control systems, combining hardware and software components, still with the view of enabling physically impaired customers to retain control of their environment. They are now offering Smart Room and Smart Home technologies (POSSUM, 2016).

Software and hardware for the mentally impaired

Whilst the range and variety of physical impairment has become more socially accepted, the picture for those suffering from mental health or mental impairment issues is less positive. Although the World Health Report in 2001 (WHR, 2001) estimated there were 400 million people worldwide living with mental health issues, it was still an area of suspicion, social exclusion, and stigma. More recently, the significant growth in the numbers of the aging population suffering from Alzheimer's and other Dementia conditions, and the attendant publicity, has meant that many more citizens have been directly affected and some progress has been made in terms of social acceptance. However, it is still a major issue, as evidenced by MIND (2016), the UK Mental Health Charity, whose tag-line reads "We won't give up until everyone experiencing a mental health problem gets both support and respect". Another major support organisation in the United Kingdom is the Alzheimer's Society (2016), whilst in the United States there are a large number of organisations in this area such as the National Alliance for Mental Illness (NAMI, 2016) and the Alzheimer's Association (2016).

The relevant software and hardware technologies include:

- Diary and reminder systems – almost any of the standard diary software available on computers today can be used to capture events and provide reminder notifications to help those needing support in planning or memory management. For those who need greater levels of support to maintain memory and recall events, particularly those with dementia, reminiscence software can be extremely beneficial (My Life, 2016).
- Social media and group support software – clearly there is no reason why the mentally impaired should not use standard social media tools, not least since Facebook, Linked-in, WhatsApp, etc. all provide the opportunity to interact in either open or closed groups.

Specialist group support tools, such as Ava (2016), support interactions between users with a variety of impairments, whilst still offering the same range of social media services.

- Medication control and self-reporting systems – medical dosage control and administration systems combine physical controlled-dosage containers with management control and prescription software (MCS, 2016). A variety of self-reporting systems have been developed, predominantly based on the work in the diabetes community (Charron-Prochownik et al., 2007), and they offer the prospect of far greater levels of patient-controlled monitoring of chronic conditions in independent living.
- Monitoring and alarm systems – there are a huge number of monitoring and alarm systems developed for the elderly and those with chronic conditions, ranging from simple alarm siren triggers to fully monitored alerting systems. Many of the services offered by such systems are now available as smartphone apps, such as the Man Down app originally developed for fire-fighters (Man Down, 2016).
- Neural implants – a range of direct neural implants for pain control and to address a number of the symptoms of mental illness, particularly in areas such as post-traumatic syndromes, are currently under development (Thomas, 2015).

Future directions for IT for positive aging

While the discussions on IT technology in this chapter paint a picture of widely connected, developed, and integrated services, there is still a considerable body of work to be undertaken to make this vision a reality. As Damant and Knapp say:

> There is a lot of anticipation that ICT-based services such as telecare and telehealth will develop to provide timely, personalised services to individuals, while providing reassurance to family members and carers and also remaining socially affordable. Robust evidence to date does not support that anticipation.
>
> *(2015)*

However, there are good reasons for optimism that the necessary work will take place:

- The growing size of the aging population, and others who require assistive technologies, make this a significant commercial marketplace. So, competition is growing, and will continue to grow, and with the bulk of these IT technologies being web-enabled and widespread, the days of variable-quality, limited-service provision at the behest of specialist suppliers are numbered.
- As discussed in Section 3, in 2015, 4.8 million people over the age of 64 had never used the Internet (ONS, 2015). However, to set this in context, the Internet turned 21 in 2015, which means that those 4.8 million people were already at least in their mid-40s when the modern era of Internet access and availability began. Over the next 21 years, the user demographic will change significantly, with those who were in their 20s and 30s when the web arrived reaching their 60s. These individuals will be much more tech-savvy, used to receiving services and managing their lives online, with a far higher expectation and demand of online services. The issues associated with training users how to use services will disappear and will be replaced with user demand for higher quality, more efficient, and more effective services and technologies.
- The development of the Internet of Things and the growth of Smart Home technologies will continue apace, linking in to the development of Smart Communities and Smart

Cities. To date most smart home studies have been conducted in artificial environments; very few have been conducted in people's own homes (Portet et al., 2013), so we can expect to see more work reported on the use of these technologies in practice. This will also drive the growth of interconnected services supporting home and community care for citizens, as well as care networks supporting all forms of impairment within a socially inclusive model (Hersh and Johnson, 2008).

- In many countries, interactive online health services already exist, certainly within the private sector and increasingly in the public sector (NHS 24, 2016). We can expect to see continued growth and development of such services, with health authority and government policy support, to enable more chronic front-line services to be provided online. Not only is this approach more cost effective, but the potential to provide new companion-based services, such as the online buddy systems used in games (Vendetta Online, 2016) and the military (defining someday, 2008), could also be linked in to address the needs of isolated patients seeking social contact.
- In many countries, there is already a thriving commercial market for home care, home nursing, and home support services for the aging population and those requiring support due to impairment. Many of these services already have an online presence and this will undoubtedly grow, along with authority and citizen advisory support for regulation, monitoring, and recommendation. The Care Inspectorate in the United Kingdom already provides such a service for Care Homes (2016) and we can expect to see that extended to online care services from a variety of organisations worldwide.
- A substantial percentage of the adult population currently use social media and online gaming (MMORPGs) as social clubs (Blizzard, 2004) to interact regularly with friends and acquaintances, and occasionally to meet up on holidays, at conventions, or more personally. This presents an interesting counterpoint to the range of day care, meal club, and social trip activities organised by local authorities and various care organisations for their clients. All of these activities afford opportunities to counter social isolation, encourage social inclusion, and extend the potential for individuals to find like-minded correspondents and contacts. There are also a range of group apps that have been developed for visually and hearing impaired users to interact online with others in the same impaired community (Ava, 2016). Given the existing well-established and wide-ranging social use of these online services by the community, we can only envisage that this will continue and grow as more of this adult community joins the aging population, significantly changing the dynamics of social isolation and inclusion.

As we said in the introduction, the notion that there is a homogeneous population of elderly people, whether over the age of 55 or 60, is simply nonsensical. Since there is no magical, or otherwise, change that comes over us when we join the aging population, we must assume that they are just as heterogeneous – with as wide a range of wishes, interests, and views – as the rest of the population. They can be better characterised as having more experience of life and potentially suffering greater levels of physical and mental decline, but otherwise no different. As better healthcare, diet, exercise and living conditions enact to enable the population to live longer, and in many countries life expectancy is now over 80, the concept of retirement for 25 years or longer is now commonplace. This seems to be a criminal waste of talent and expertise, and many people are now choosing to continue working well into their 70s and beyond. However, there is also a pool of people who take the opportunity to retire and then take on a new career, often part-time and lower paid or unpaid, in the voluntary and/or social sectors. This has been true for many years and these individuals often form the life-blood of organisations in those sectors. As more digitally aware and IT-capable people reach retirement age, we can anticipate that more online services, run and supported by the aging population themselves, will emerge to support and campaign for the needs of that population. We can also anticipate that the community themselves will begin to distinguish variations in the demographic, whether by age band or other criteria, and develop or specify the services and technologies appropriate to the needs of those variants.

Whether or not this represents a long-term change to the demographic, or whether legislative changes to retirement ages, combined with the financial costs of being retired for that long, will drive people to further prolong their working careers, is a matter for conjecture. However, for an indeterminate period of time we will have a growing community of individuals who are not only aging positively, but have the potential to enable and support the development of ever-better IT services and technologies to support positive aging for all.

References

Action on Hearing Loss. (2016). http://actiononhearingloss.org.uk (accessed March 2016).

Alam, M. R., Reaz, M. B. I., and Ali, M. A. M. (2012). A review of smart homes: Past, present, and future. *IEEE Transactions on Systems, Man, and Cybernetics - Part C: Applications and Reviews*, 42(6), 1190–1203.

Alzheimer's Association. (2016). http://alz.org (accessed March, 2016).

Alzheimer's Society. (2016). www.alzheimers.org.uk (accessed March, 2016).

Amirabdollahian, F., Bedaf, S., Bormann, R., Draper, H., Evers, V., Pérez, J. G., Gelderblom, G. J., Ruiz, C. G., Hewson, D., Hu, N., and Koay, K. L. (2013). Assistive technology design and development for acceptable robotics companions for ageing years. *Paladyn, Journal of Behavioral Robotics*, 4(2), 94–112.

Arndt, P. S., Arcaroli, J., Hines, A., and Ebinger, K. (1999). *Within subject comparison of advanced coding strategies in the nucleus 24 cochlear implant*. Cochlear Corporation.

Arthritis Care. (2016). www.arthritiscare.org.uk (accessed March, 2016).

Arthritis Foundation. (2016). www.arthritis.org (accessed March, 2016).

Ava. (2016). www.indiegogo.com/projects/ava-group-conversations-made-accessible#/ (accessed March, 2016).

Barlow, J., Bayer, S., and Curry, R. (2006). Implementing complex innovations in fluid multi-stakeholder environments: Experiences of 'telecare'. *Technovation*, 26, 396–406.

Bitfield. (2016). www.bitfield.se/isubtitle/ (accessed March, 2016).

Blizzard. (2004). http://us.battle.net/wow/en/ (accessed March, 2016).

Bouchard, K., Giroux, S., Bouchard, B., and Bouzouane, A. (2014). Regression analysis for gesture recognition using passive RFID technology in smart home environments. *International Journal of Smart Home*, 8(5), 245–260.

Braci. (2016). http://braci.co (accessed March, 2016).

Brailliant. (2016). www.humanware.com (accessed March, 2016).

Care Inspectorate. (2016). www.careinspectorate.com (accessed March, 2016).

Chan, M., Estève, D., Fourniols, J. Y., Escriba, C., and Campo, E. (2012). Smart wearable systems: Current status and future challenges. *Artificial Intelligence in Medicine*, 56(3), 137–156.

Chang, L. (2015). *Digital trends*. www.digitaltrends.com/cool-tech/mind-controlled-bionic-prosthetics-announced/ (accessed March, 2016).

Charron-Prochownik, D., Zgibor, J. C., Peyrot, M., Peeples, M., McWilliams, J., Koshinsky, J., Noullet, W., and Siminerio, L. M. (2007). The Diabetes Self-Management Assessment Report Tool (D-SMART): Process evaluation and patient satisfaction. *Diabetes Educator*, 33(5), 833–838, September–October.

Chen, D. (2009). *Medical design technology*. www.mdtmag.com/article/2009/05/orthotics-and-prosthetics-go-digital (accessed March, 2016).

Chen, Y., Yao, E., and Basu, A. (2015). A 128-channel extreme learning machine-based neural decoder for brain machine interfaces. *IEEE Transactions on Biomedical Circuits and Systems*, 2015, 1. doi:10.1109/TBCAS.2015.2483618

Czaja, S. J., Charness, N., Fisk, A. D., Hertzog, C., Nair, S. N., Rogers, W. A., and Sharit, J. (2006). Factors predicting the use of technology: Findings from the Center for Research and Education on Aging and Technology Enhancement (CREATE). *Psychology and Aging*, 21(2), 333.

Daily Telegraph. (2005). www.telegraph.co.uk/culture/3643750/The-arts-column-why-we-have-to-learn-to-love-surtitles.html (accessed March, 2016).

Damant, J., and Knapp, M. (2015). *What are the likely changes in society and technology which will impact upon the ability of older adults to maintain social (extra-familial) networks of support now, in 2025 and in 2040?* London: Future of ageing: Evidence review, Government Office for Science. www.gov.uk/government/organisations/government-office-for-science (accessed May 4, 2017).

defining someday. (2008). www.definingsomeday.com/2008/10/24/a-buddy-system-for-goals/ (accessed March, 2016).

Demeris, G., Doorenbos, A., and Towle, C. (2009). Ethical considerations regarding the use of technology for older adults. *Research in Gerontological Nursing*, 2(2), 128–136.

De Silva, L. C., Morikawa, C., and Petra, I. M. (2012). State of the art of smart homes. *Engineering Applications of Artificial Intelligence*, 25(7), 1313–1321.

Disability Rights UK. (2016). www.disabilityrightsuk.org (accessed March, 2016).

Dutton, W. H., and Blank, G. (2011). *Next generation users: The Internet in Britain*. Oxford Internet Survey 2011 Report. www.oii.ox.ac.uk/publications/oxis2011_report.pdf (accessed January 1, 2016).

Ehrenhard, M., Kijl, B., and Nieuwenhuis, L. (2014). Market adoption barriers of multi-stakeholder technology: Smart homes for the aging population. *Technological Forecasting and Social Change*, 89, 306–315.

Emotiv. (2015). https://emotiv.com/blog/brain-controlled-wheelchair/ (accessed March, 2016).

Fahim, M., Fatima, I., Lee, S., and Lee, Y. K. (2012). Daily life activity tracking application for smart homes using android smartphone. In *Advanced Communication Technology (ICACT), 2012 14th International Conference on IEEE* (pp. 241–245).

Flandorfer, P. (2012). Population ageing and socially assistive robots for elderly persons: The importance of sociodemographic factors for user acceptance. *International Journal of Population Research*, Article ID 829835, 13 pages.

Fozard, J. L., and Wahl, H. W. (2012). Age and cohort effects in gerontechnology: A reconsideration. *Gerontechnology*, 11(1), 10–21.

Frisardi, V., and Imbimbo, B. P. (2011). Gerontechnology for demented patients: Smart homes for smart aging. *Journal of Alzheimer's Disease*, 23(1), 143.

Google. (2016). https://translate.google.co.uk/m/translate (accessed March, 2016).

Gudur, R. R., Blackler, A., Popovic, V., and Mahar, D. (2013). Ageing, technology anxiety and intuitive use of complex interfaces. In *IFIP Conference on Human-computer interaction* (pp. 564–581). Berlin, Heidelberg: Springer.

Hardhill, I., and Olphert, C. W. (2012). Staying connected: Exploring mobile phone use amongst older adults in the UK. *Geoforum*, 43(6), 1306–1312.

Haux, R., Hein, A., Kolb, G., Künemund, H., Eichelberg, M., Appell, J. E., Appelrath, H. J., Bartsch, C., Bauer, J. M., Becker, M., and Bente, P. (2014). Information and communication technologies for promoting and sustaining quality of life, health and self-sufficiency in ageing societies-outcomes of the Lower Saxony Research Network Design of Environments for Ageing (GAL). *Informatics for Health and Social Care*, 39(3–4), 166–187.

Hersh, M. A., and Johnson, M. A. (2008). *Assistive technology for visually impaired and blind people*. London: Springer.

Intosalmi, H., Nykänen, J., and Stenberg, L. (2013). *The use of technology and attitudes of 75–89 years of age – Report of the survey (in Finnish)*. Helsinki: KÄKÄTE Project.

JAWS. (2016). http://freedomscientific.com (accessed March, 2016).

Jia, P., Lu, Y., and Wajda, B. (2015). Designing for technology acceptance in an ageing society through multi-stakeholder collaboration. In *6th International Conference on Applied Human Factors and Ergonomics (AHFE 2015) and the Affiliated Conferences, AHFE 2015*.

Lai, C. K.Y., Chung, J. C. C., Leung, N. K. L., Wong, J. C. T., and Mak, D. P. S. (2010). A survey of older Hong Kong people's perceptions of telecommunication technologies and telecare devices. *Journal of Telemedicine and Telecare*, 16(8), 441–446.
Lee, B., Chen, Y., and Hewitt, L. (2011). Age differences in constraints encountered by seniors in their use of computers and the internet. *Computers in Human Behavior*, 27(3), 1231–1237.
Leonard Cheshire Foundation. (2016). www.leonardcheshire.org (accessed March, 2016).
MAGic. (2016). http://freedomscientific.com (accessed March, 2016).
Man Down. (2016). www.mandownapp.com (accessed March, 2016).
MCS. (2016). http://medicationcontrolsystems.com (accessed March, 2016).
Mertens, A., Hurtmanns, J., Wacharamanotham, C., Kronenbueger, M., Borchers, J., and Schliek, C. M. (2012). Swabbing: Touchscreen-based input technique for people with hand tremor. *Work*, 41(Suppl. 1), 2405–2411.
Milligan, C., Roberts, C., and Mort, M. (2011). Telecare and older people: Who cares where? *Social Science & Medicine*, 72(3), 347–354.
MIND. (2016). www.mind.org.uk (accessed March, 2016).
Morris, M. E., Adair, B., Miller, K., Ozanne, E., Hansen, R., Pearce, A. J., Santamaria, N., Viega, L., Long, M., and Said, C. M. (2013). Smart-home technologies to assist older people to live well at home. *Journal of Aging Science*, 1(1), 1–9.
Morris, M. E., Adair, B., Ozanne, E., Kurowski, W., Miller, K. J., Pearce, A. J., Santamaria, N., Long, M., Ventura, C., and Said, C. M. (2014). Smart technologies to enhance social connectedness in older people who live at home. *Australasian Journal on Ageing*, 33(3), 142–152.
Mort, M., Roberts, C., and Callen, B. (2013). Ageing with telecare: Care or coercion in austerity? *Sociology of Health & Illness*, 35(6), 799–812.
My Life. (2016). http://mylifesoftware.com (accessed March, 2016).
Mynatt, E. D., and Rogers, W. A. (2001). Developing technology to support the functional independence of older adults. *Ageing International*, 27(1), 24–41.
NAMI. (2016). www.nami.org/About-NAMI (accessed March, 2016).
National Association of the Deaf (NAD). (2016). https://nad.org (accessed March, 2016).
National Federation of the Blind (NFB). (2016). http://nfb.org (accessed March, 2016).
National Stroke Association. (2016). www.stroke.org (accessed March, 2016).
NHS 24. (2016). www.nhs24.com (accessed March, 2016).
Norman, D. A. (1999). *The invisible computer: Why good products fail, the personal computer is so complex, and information appliances are the solution*. Cambridge, MA: MIT Press.
Nuance. (2016). http://shop.nuance.co.uk/store/nuanceeu/en_GB/Content/pbPage.dragon-anywhere?utm_source=google&utm_medium=emea-cpc&utm_campaign=DBU+%7C+Dragon+Anywhere+%7C+Product+%7C+UK+-+EN&keyword=dragon+dictation+app-e (accessed March, 2016).
Nugent, C. D., Finlay, D. D., Fiorini, P., Tsumaki, Y., and Prassler, E. (2008). Editorial: Home automation as a means of independent living. *IEEE Transactions on Automation Science and Engineering*, 5(1), 1–9.
Parra, C., Silveira, P., Far, I. K., Daniel, F., De Bruin, E. D., Cernuzzi, L., D'Andrea, V., and Casati, F. (2013). Information technology for active ageing: A review of theory and practice. *Interaction*, 7(4), 351–448.
Peine, A. (2008). Technological paradigms and complex technical systems: The case of Smart Homes. *Research Policy*, 37, 508–529.
Peine, A., Rollwagen, I., and Neven, L. (2014). The rise of the 'innosumer': Rethinking older technology users. *Technological Forecasting and Social Change*, 82, 199–214.
Perkins Braillers. (2016). www.perkinsproducts.org (accessed March, 2016).
Piau, A., Campo, E., Rumeau, P., Vellas, B., and Nourhashémi, F. (2014). Aging society and gerontechnology: A solution for an independent living? *The Journal of Nutrition, Health & Aging*, 18(1), 97–112.
Portet, F., Vacher, M., Golanski, C., Roux, C., and Meillon, B. (2013). Design and evaluation of a smart home voice interface for the elderly: Acceptability and objection aspects. *Personal and Ubiquitous Computing*, 17(1), 127–144.
Possum. (2016). www.possum.co.uk/products-and-services/environmental-control (accessed March, 2016).

Renaud, K., and Biljon, J. van. (2008). Predicting technology acceptance and adoption by the elderly: A qualitative study. *Proceedings of the 2008 Annual Research Conference of the South African Institute of Computer Scientists and Information Technologists on IT Research in Developing Countries: Riding the Wave of Technology (SAICSIT '08)*, ACM, New York (pp. 210–219).

RNIB. (2016). www.rnib.org.uk (accessed March, 2016).

Sanders, C., Rogers, A., Bowen, R., Bower, P., Hirani, S., Cartwright, M., Fitzpatrick, R., Knapp, M., Barlow, J., Hendy, J., Chrysanthaki, T., Bardsley, M., and Newman, S. P. (2012). Exploring barriers to participation and adoption of telehealth and telecare within the Whole Systems Demonstrator trial: A qualitative study. *BMC Health Services Research*, 12, 220–231.

Selwyn, N. (2004). The information aged: A qualitative study of older adults' use of information and communications technology. *Journal of Ageing Studies*, 18(4), 369–384.

Smart Canes. (2015). www.phoenixmedicalsystems.com (accessed March, 2016).

Soliman, M., Abiodun, T., Hamouda, T., Zhou, J., and Lung, C. H. (2013). Smart home: Integrating internet of things with web services and cloud computing. In *Cloud Computing Technology and Science (CloudCom), 2013 IEEE 5th International Conference on IEEE* (Vol. 2, pp. 317–320).

Stroke Association. (2016). www.stroke.org.uk/ (accessed March, 2016).

Subtitles App. (2016). http://subtitlesapp.com (accessed March, 2016).

Synapptic. (2016). www.visionaid.co.uk (accessed March, 2016).

Taipale, V. T. (2014). Preventive policies, politics, profit and gerontechnology. *Gerontechnology*, 13(2), 139.

Tecnalia. (2016). www.tecnalia.com/es/myeardroid/que-es-myeardroid.htm (accessed March, 2016).

Thomas, J. (2015). *San Jose Mercury News*. www.mercurynews.com/health/ci_26185135/future-is-now-neural-implants-may-hold-key (accessed March, 2016).

Tsai, H., Tsai, Y., Wang, H., Chang, Y., and Hua, H. (2010). Videoconference program enhances social support, loneliness, and depressive status of elderly nursing home residents. *Ageing and Mental Health*, 14(8), 947–954.

Valero, M. Á., Bravo, J., Chamizo, J. M. G., and López-de-Ipiña, D. (2014). Integration of multisensor hybrid reasoners to support personal autonomy in the smart home. *Sensors*, 14(9), 17313–17330.

Van de Kaa, G., Den Hartog, F., and De Vries, H. J. (2009). Mapping standards for home networking. *Computer Standards & Interfaces*, 31, 1175–1181.

Väyrynen, R. (2012). *Count of regular home-care clients on 30 November 2012*. Helsinki: THL Statistical report.

Vendetta Online. (2016). www.vendetta-online.com/manual/mul_buddy.html (accessed March, 2016).

Wagner, N., Hassanein, K., and Head, M. (2010). Computer use by older adults: A multidisciplinary review. *Computers in Human Behavior*, 26, 870–882.

Walsh, K., and Callan, A. (2011). Perceptions, preferences and acceptance of information and communication technologies in older-adult community care settings in Ireland: A care-study and ranked-care program analysis. *Ageing International*, 36(1), 102–122.

Walsh, L., Kealy, A., Loane, J., Doyle, J., and Bond, R. (2014). Inferring health metrics from ambient smart home data. In *Bioinformatics and Biomedicine (BIBM), 2014 IEEE International Conference on IEEE* (pp. 27–32).

Warschauer, M. (2004). *Technology and social inclusion – Rethinking the digital divide*. Cambridge, MA: MIT Press.

World Health Organization. (2001). The World Health Report 2001: Mental health: new understanding, new hope. World Health Organization.

Xie, B. (2003). Older adults, computers, and the internet: Future directions. *Gerontechnology*, 2(4), 289–305.

PART IV

Care delivery

17

QUALITY OF LIFE OF ELDERLY RESIDENTS OF UK CARE HOMES

A systematic review

Elizabeth West, Pauline McGovern, Val Chandler, Jane Banaszak-Holl and David Barron

This chapter discusses:

- Residents in care homes
- Quality of life in care homes
- Towards the development of a model of quality of life in care homes
- Approaches to improving the quality of life in UK care homes

Introduction

Many people will spend time, often close to the end of their lives, in residential care or nursing care homes. The decision to move into a care home is often taken after several years of living at home with the support of informal carers (either families, friends or domiciliary carers) whose services are purchased privately or provided by the local authority. Moving to a care home may be experienced as a loss of independence and relatives may feel a sense of inadequacy or failure at their inability to provide enough care to enable their relative to remain in their home. Consequently, care home services are routinely viewed negatively and considered only when all other alternatives are exhausted. In this chapter we argue that the concept of positive aging must be extended to the care home sector and, as an initial step, we describe what is known about the quality of life in care homes and consider some of the policy initiatives that seek to improve older people's experiences.

This chapter will, after giving some demographic information about the residents of care homes, report the results of a systematic review of the literature identifying empirical research on the factors most relevant to quality of life in residential and nursing care homes in the United Kingdom. To anticipate the conclusions, this will show that whilst there is scant United Kingdom -based empirical research in this area, especially in comparison to the extensive literature produced in other European and North American countries, there is a pattern of findings that is consistent enough to justify its immediate influence on how care is delivered. This literature review emphasises the central importance of choice and autonomy, social connectedness, characteristics of the care environment and the residents' own health, particularly whether or not they have dementia. We use these themes to develop a heuristic model of the factors contributing to the quality of life in care homes. Finally, in this chapter we describe how the United Kingdom has responded to the challenges of improving quality of life in care homes by deploying agencies including the National Institute for Health and Care Excellence (NICE), the Care Quality Commission (CQC), the National Institute for Health Research (NIHR), and the Social Care Institute for Excellence (SCIE).

Residents in care homes

The Office of National Statistics (ONS) estimates that there are 352,727 residents of care homes in England and Wales (2011 data, ONS, 2014, p. 1). Of these, 291,000 are aged 65 or over in 2011, representing 3.2 per cent of the population of this age in England and Wales. The number of elderly residents in care has remained almost stable since 2001, increasing only by 0.3 per cent, but on average, they are older than they were in the 2001 census. In 2011 people aged 85 years and older represented 59.2 per cent of the older care home population compared to 56.5 per cent in 2001. The proportions of men and women is also changing. Whereas in 2001, there were around 3.3 women for each man aged 65 and older living in care homes, by 2011, this had reduced to 2.8. Whilst there are still many more women than men living in care homes, the gender gap has narrowed.

ONS suggests that one explanation for the stability of the size of the elderly population in care homes is that the health of the population in England and Wales has improved. Many more people can stay at home longer. However, over the last decade, the number of unpaid carers has increased by 600,000 and ONS suggest that more relatives or friends may have chosen to relieve the financial burden of care home costs by providing care themselves. An additional reason for the stability in the number of people living in care homes may be that more services are now provided at home under the provision of the *National Health Service and Community Care Act 1990*, thus enabling more people who need help with activities of daily living to remain at home.

The demand for care home placements for older people is likely to rise in the future. The NHS Confederation website which has key statistics on the NHS states:

> the number of people aged 65 and over is projected to increase from 10.84m in 2012 to 17.79m by 2037. As part of this growth, the number of over-85's is estimated to more than double from 1.44 million in 2012 to 3.64 million by 2037.
>
> *(www.nhsconfed.org/resources/key-statistics-on-the-nhs accessed 17 July 2015)*

Indeed, over the last 30 years, the number of people aged 90 or over in the United Kingdom has nearly tripled (CQC, 2015). With a rising population of older people, many will have years of coping with multiple health problems and, whilst many may benefit from care in the community, some will inevitably need supported care in residential or nursing homes. However, funding for social care, which includes the provision of residential and nursing care homes, has been cut over the last few years in England. In the run-up to the elections in 2015, the Kings Fund Review of Social Care stated that government spending on social care has been falling since 2009, which leads to concerns about the impact on individuals, families, the NHS, the quality of care that is provided in care homes and the quality of life that residents experience there.

Quality of life in care homes

Quality of life has been defined and measured in many ways. A systematic review of research on quality of life concluded that: "the choice of Quality of Life measures tends to reflect the conceptual bias of the researcher" (Courtney et al., 2003, p. 3). They suggest that measures be assigned to three broad categories: those that focus on objective indices (such as economic circumstances or health outcomes), those that measure purely subjective aspects of well-being (such as happiness) and those containing both objective and subjective components (see also Gabriel & Bowling, 2004; Murphy, O'Shea & Cooney, 2007).

The World Health Organisation's definition of quality of life encompasses every aspect of social life: "Individuals' perceptions of their position in life in the context of the culture and value systems in which they live and in relation to their goals, expectations, standards and concerns" (WHO, 1998, p. 8). A tighter definition is provided by MedLine in its Medical Subject (main) Heading that emphasises the possibility of enhancing quality of life: "A generic concept reflecting concern with the modification and enhancement of life attributes, e.g., physical, political, moral and social environment; the overall condition of a human life".

Quality of life is a significant predictor of mortality, physical dependence and service utilization amongst older people (Ho et al., 2002; Dorr et al., 2006). Elderly residents of care homes are more likely to have a reduced quality of life because of deteriorating health, changes in their mode of living and social environment (Kane et al., 2003; Wong et al., 2004).

We found one international systematic review of quality of life of elderly people in residential care. Lee et al. (2009) identified 18 studies published between 1994 and 2008, but only one study was conducted in the United Kingdom. This systematic review identified the perceived autonomy of residents and their capacity to make choices about their day-to-day life as the one factor of overriding importance to quality of life.

Lee, Yu and Kwong (2009) also identified a number of individual characteristics affecting the quality of life for older adults, including physical functioning and residents' capacity to perform activities of daily living (ADL) as well as the amount and quality of social interaction that residents have with family members and staff. This systematic review also identified different approaches used in studies to improve quality of life for care home residents, including physical interventions, mental stimulation and environmental modification. They found the greatest effect was achieved by modifying the care home environment by removing nursing stations and providing residents with private rooms and accessible outdoor spaces. These authors remark that 'institutionalization is a stressful experience for older people' (Lee, Yu & Kwong, 2009, p. 123).

There were three other systematic reviews relevant to our enquiry, but none of them focused specifically on quality of life in residential care for older people in the United Kingdom or Ireland. Spilsbury et al. (2011) focused on the quality of *nursing* care, as measured using clinical outcomes for older residents of care homes. None of the studies in their review was conducted in the United Kingdom. Bostick et al. (2006) reviewed US empirical research only, focused on staffing and clinical outcomes and was not specific to older residents. The third review, by Bradshaw, Playford and Riazi (2012), focused on quality of life in United Kingdom and Ireland care homes but was not specific to older residents. Finally, we found one systematic review about the quality of life of elderly people at home (Thome, Dykes & Hallberg, 2003). The fact that after a systematic search we could not find a systematic review of quality of life in care homes led us to formulate the following research question: what factors affect the quality of life for older residents in institutional care in the United Kingdom and Ireland?

Search methods

The search strategy for this revised research question is shown in the PRISMA 2009 flow diagram in Figure 17.1 (following the model proposed by Liberati et al., 2009). Eight databases were searched using EBSCOhost, including Academic Search Complete; Academic Search Premier; MEDLINE; CINAHL Plus with Full Text; Psychology and Behavioural Sciences Collection; SPORTDiscus; PsycINFO; eBook Collection and PsycARTICLES. We searched using the keywords: "homes for the aged" OR "nursing home" OR "residential" AND "quality of life" AND "quality". The limiters were: full text; scholarly (peer reviewed) journals; and a published date of 01/01/1960 to 31/03/2015. This yielded 700,503 citations.

When narrowed by age, 65+ years, the citations reduced to 14,010. When narrowed by geography to United Kingdom and Ireland, this reduced to 5,945. In the final delimiter, when

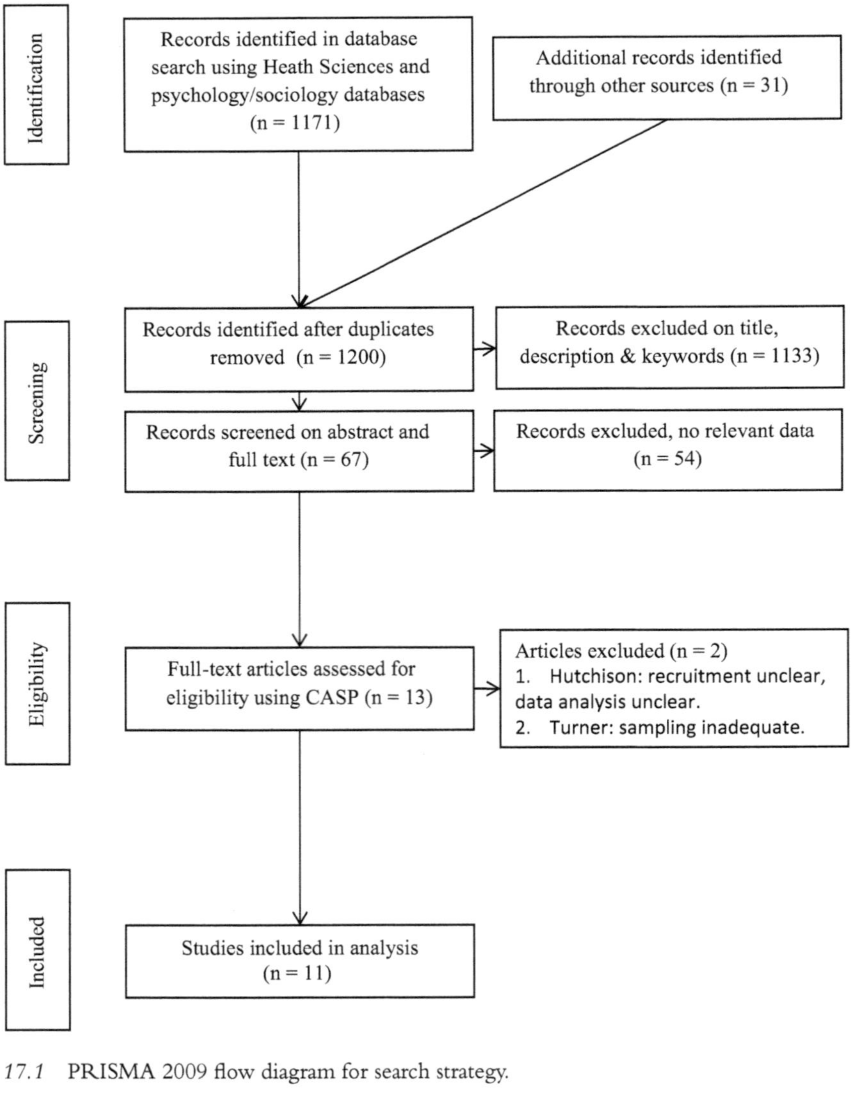

Figure 17.1 PRISMA 2009 flow diagram for search strategy.

reduced by major subject to quality of life, the citations reduced to 1,171. This is noted in the Identification Stage of the PRISMA diagram and summarised in Table 17.1.

When duplicates were removed, the number of citations was further reduced to 1,169. A separate manual search was conducted, using references from the systematic reviews and the identified articles and added a further 31 studies. The title, description and keywords of these citations were then scanned to check whether the studies were within the search terms and delimiters. Citations went forward to the next stage if they either clearly met the search criteria or if it was unclear about the scope of the study. This reduced the number of citations to 67.

The abstracts and full text of these 67 studies were then checked independently by two researchers in order to confirm that they met the search criteria. Studies were included if they reported research conducted in the United Kingdom and Ireland on long-term care in residential and nursing homes and also long-stay hospital wards. We excluded day care, hospices, studies of informal caregivers and of the elderly at home or in the community. We also excluded studies on quality of life after operations, articles that discussed other research and articles that focused on the validation of quality of life tools. The list of inclusions and exclusions is in Table 17.2.

Table 17.1 Search criteria

Research question: What factors affect the quality of life of residents in institutional care for the elderly in the United Kingdom and Ireland?			
Homes for the aged OR nursing home OR residential AND quality of life OR quality	Limiters – full text; scholarly (peer reviewed) journals; pub. 19600101–20150331	Academic Search Premier; MEDLINE; Psychology and Behavioral Sciences Collection; PsychINFO; SPORTDiscus; CINAHL Plus with Full Text; PsychARTICLES; Academic Search Complete; eBook Collection	700,503
	AND narrow by age: aged 65+ years		14,010
	AND narrow by geographic: UK & Ireland		5,945
	AND narrow by subject major: quality of life		1,171

Table 17.2 Inclusion and exclusion criteria

Research question: What factors affect the quality of life of residents in institutional care for the elderly in the United Kingdom and Ireland?	
Include	Studies of institutional care in the UK and/or Ireland
	Care homes, nursing homes and long-stay hospital wards
	Studies that analyse secondary data sets
Exclude	Day care
	Hospices and palliative care
	Studies of informal caregivers
	Studies of the elderly at home or in the community
	Studies of quality of life after operations
	Articles that discuss other studies rather than describe research
	Studies that focus on validation of quality-of-life tools

In total, 13 studies (qualitative, quantitative and mixed methods) went through to the quality appraisal stage. The quality appraisal was conducted by two independent members of the research team using the Critical Appraisal Skills Programme (CASP) checklists for qualitative studies and for cohort studies. They assessed studies independently and reached a consensus on which studies to review, based on their quality. Where the reviewers differed in their views on whether a study should be included, there was a negotiated agreement. This resulted in 11 studies for review.

As a final note on systematic review, it is telling that when this search was repeated adding the keywords for third-sector organisations (TSO), this initially returned 750,116 citations, this being 49,613 citations more than the search without TSO keywords. However, when the search criteria in Table 17.1, rows 3 to 5 were added, the final result was the same – 1,171 citations. This suggests that including TSOs as search terms adds nothing to this review and that there is, indeed, a gap in research on the links between TSOs and the quality of life of residents in institutional care for the elderly in the United Kingdom and Ireland.

Results

The qualitative studies are summarised in Table 17.3. The details of the quantitative studies are in Table 17.4. Of the 11 studies of quality of life of older people in United Kingdom and Ireland care homes, 10 focused either on the resident perspective or on both resident and nurse/staff perspectives. One focused solely on nurse/staff perspectives.

Choice

Seven studies indicated that, from the residents' point of view, autonomy and expressing self-identity through making choices in relation to day-to-day living was the most important aspect of quality of life for residents. This matches the global finding of Lee, Yu and Kwong (2009). The United Kingdom and Ireland studies that mentioned resident autonomy went further in suggesting that residents valued autonomy regardless of the degree of their cognitive impairment. Even those with severe dementia wanted some choices in day-to-day living. For example, in their qualitative study of elders in Irish care homes, Cooney, Murphy and O'Shea (2009) found that residents were more likely to 'feel at home' if they had choices in relation to: personal appearance; personal possessions; spirituality; and preferences for private space. They comment that: 'These are the very things that can be neglected in busy facilities' (Cooney, Murphy & O'Shea, 2009, p. 1036). This is a dominant theme that runs from the oldest to the most recent study. In Hoe et al.'s (2009) study of the quality of life of elders with dementia, they conclude that:

> Increased frailty does not necessarily diminish the strength of self, thus supporting the concept of personhood, in that individuality is maintained throughout the dementia process. An individual's sense of control is also core to QoL and this incorporates feelings of self-efficacy, perceived control, and learned helplessness, which relate to people's personal beliefs and expectations.
>
> *(Hoe et al., 2009, p. 288)*

Although mobility issues and problems with activities of daily living make a difference to the quality of life of older adults, the studies show that residents can be provided with

Table 17.3 Qualitative studies

Summary of qualitative studies (quality of life findings)			
Authors & coverage	*Methods*	*Sample/participants*	*Findings*
Cahill & Diaz-Ponce (2011) **Dublin**	Semi-structured interviews	61 people with cognitive impairment in 3 sites	People with CI can still communicate preferences. Factors associated with QoL include positive social relationships; pleasurable activities; feeling at home; attachment to the home; positive affect. (residents' perspectives)
Clark & Bowling (1989) **London**	Non-participant observation	RCT, 106 patients assessed for 1 year	Patient preferences are most important. Routines and organisation were not crucial determinants of the QoL of residents. Recommends staff training: activities; restructuring leisure areas; more flexibility. (residents' perspectives)
Cooney, Murphy & O'Shea (2009) **Northern Ireland**	Grounded theory	101 interviews at 12 sites	Themes connected to QoL of residents: ethos of care; sense of self & identity; connectedness; activities & therapies. (residents' perspectives)
Draper (1996) **Single NHS trust**	Ethnographic interviewing	14 residents, 11 nurses (long-stay), 3 other nurses at 5 sites	Nurses said that residents should be treated as individuals with freedom of choice in their lives but some engaged in tactics by which choice was denied – using compromise; massive encouragement; forcing. (nurses' perspectives)
Oleson, Heading et al. (1994) **SW England**	Semi-structured interviews	10 residents, 65+ years; 9 nurses (long-stay) at 3 sites	Themes connected to QoL of residents: individuality; professionalism; connectedness; physical function. Residents' perspective: having a meaningful social environment with own choices supported by nurses. Nurses' perspective: external factors important – more intervention-based view of QoL of residents.
Stathi & Simey (2007) **SE England**	Phenomenological, exercise intervention	14 residents at baseline 86–99 years, 7 at follow-up	Exercise improved QoL: better mobility; decreased fear of falling; feelings of achievement. Residents viewed exercise as opportunity to do something for themselves, add to routine, meet other people, be more active. (residents' perspectives)

Table 17.4 Quantitative studies

Summary of quantitative/mixed studies (quality of life findings)			
Authors & coverage	*Methods*	*Sample/participants*	*Findings*
Ballard et al. (2001) **Newcastle**	Dementia Care Mapping & other scales	209/112 residents (6 sites)	Reduced QoL of residents linked to lower performance on ADLs, more social withdrawal, less engagement in activities & taking psychotropics. (residents with dementia focus)
Hoe et al. (2006, 2009) **UK**	QoL-AD scales & other, follow-up at 20 weeks	238 residents at 24 sites, 192 at follow-up, staff	For residents: high QoL scores correlated with lower scores for depression & anxiety. For staff: high QoL of residents correlated negatively with increased dependency & behaviour problems. (both residents with dementia & staff perspectives)
Innes & Surr (2001) **England**	Dementia Care Mapping	76 residents with dementia (6 sites) 269 hours observation	Homes are meeting the physical needs but not the broader psycho-social care needs of residents. More understanding is required of a resident's likes & dislikes, hopes & fears, personality, habits, achievements & successes. (residents' perspectives)
Murphy, O'Shea & Cooney (2007) **Ireland**	Postal survey, qualitative interviewing	Survey (526 sites) qual interviews (101 residents; 48 staff)	Themes connected to QoL of residents: care environment & ethos of care; personal identity; connectedness to family & community; activities & therapies. There must be clear identification of what is important to residents in service delivery. (both residents' & staff perspectives)
O'Shea, Devane et al. (2014) **Ireland**	RCT, QoL-AD scale, reminiscence intervention	304 residents (18 sites): 153 intervention group; 151 control group	Intervention fieldwork by site staff. Intention-to-treat analysis: non-sig. for QoL. Per-protocol analysis (site staff followed protocol): sig. Reminiscence exercise may have positive effects on QoL in some long-stay settings. (residents with dementia focus)

choices with the support of staff as necessary. For example, Oleson et al. (1994) conclude that:

> Residents tended to perceive their QOL more as a meaningful internal environment that might best be created by themselves alone via coping strategies and/or within a therapeutic relationship with a compassionate nurse.
>
> *(Oleson et al., 1994, p. 31)*

This was true even of the most elderly residents. Stathi and Simey (2007) conducted a six-month exercise intervention with care home residents aged 86–99 years (14 at baseline, 7 at follow-up). They concluded that exercise enhanced the elders' quality of life, not simply by improving their physical health but by offering them "the opportunity to self-reflect and self-regulate. Most important, participants realised that they were still capable of actively shaping their environment, allowing them to reconnect with their human potential" (2007, p. 281).

In the four studies that explored the perspectives of both residents and staff in care homes, studies revealed staff felt differently about residents' choice. Even whilst expressing the view that resident behavioural choices were important, staff remained interventionist. Methods of restricting resident choices include: forcing, with or without physical restraint; encouragement within restricted choices; and suggesting compromises from a limited range of options (Draper, 1996). Draper concludes that the mechanisms of control in care homes ensure that the institutions operate without substantial disruption by residents of the established status quo. Although some may see this as overstated and indeed as minimising the extent to which all organisations exert their influence over individuals, it is especially important to consider the constraints to autonomy exerted in care homes as the residents have very limited ability to alter or remove themselves from their living situation, whereas younger adults may be able to move from a work setting or living situation that is overly restrictive or controlling.

Social connectedness

The link between membership of social networks (social capital) and health is well established (see McGovern & Nazroo, 2015). In this review, social connectedness has proved to be the other important factor in the quality of life of elders in care homes. Six studies found that opportunities to interact with staff and other residents made a difference to the level of resident quality of life. For example, Stathi and Simey found that exercise, as well as improving mobility, gave participants the opportunity for personal achievement and to meet other people:

> Being together with other people gave residents a new, more optimistic perspective. This is manifested in their comments at the end of the program regarding the need for social interaction, the increased opportunities to meet and talk with other residents, the need to reward the nursing home staff for their efforts, the interest in aspects of their social well-being, and the increased need to "escape" the monotony and restriction of living in one room.
>
> *(2007, p. 282)*

The need for social connectedness persists even in the presence of severe cognitive impairment. Cahill and Diaz-Ponce, who interviewed 61 adults with mild, moderate or severe cognitive impairment living in nursing homes in the Dublin area, state:

> The narratives of those with a severe cognitive impairment reflected an absence of social contact, a quest for human contact and a lack of awareness of structured

> pleasurable activities. A large majority also reported feelings of loneliness, isolation and a search for home.
>
> *(2011)*

The care environment

The care environment also emerged as an important factor with three studies concluding that the care environment is important in resident quality of life. This includes the physical layout as a spur to attachment to the care home (Clark & Bowling, 1989; Cahill & Diaz-Ponce, 2011), but goes beyond the physical arrangement of the rooms and the placement of furniture. Murphy et al. identify the management style as a key component of the care environment, stating that: "an open visiting policy, a feeling of welcome, a homely atmosphere and strong links with the community were the main enhancing factors" (2007, p. 2172). Clark and Bowling (1989) suggest that staff need training to increase morale and level of activities for residents, leading to more positive interactions and better communication.

Cognitive impairment and affect

Dementia rates are rising in the United Kingdom, and we found an increasing focus on dementia in more recent studies. Described by the Alzheimer's Society as the "hidden voice of loneliness", dementia is defined as: "a set of symptoms including memory loss, mood changes and problems with communication and reasoning" (www.alzheimers.org/site/scripts/download_info.php?fileID=1409). There is increasing interest in developing research methods for gathering information from groups that would hitherto be considered unable to reveal their thoughts and feelings due to cognitive deficits. In this review, two studies (reported in three articles) of residents with dementia found that affect was of importance to their quality of life (Cahill & Diaz-Ponce, 2011; Hoe et al., 2006, 2009). Cahill and Diaz-Ponce (2011, p. 569) found that loneliness was a "striking subtheme" in their qualitative data, collected from residents with a severe cognitive impairment. A small minority of residents with moderate to severe cognitive impairment revealed feelings of hopelessness.

The studies suggest that those with advanced dementia have a poorer quality of life and feel isolated in care homes, whilst staff have inadequate understanding of the needs of residents with cognitive impairment. Cahill and Diaz-Ponce argue that care home staff need more training to understand the multiple and unique needs of these residents and that more resources are required to promote their quality of life. They suggest that:

> In particular, for those with a severe CI, momentary pleasures that are sensory stimulating may have an important role to play in promoting QoL.
>
> *(Cahill & Diaz-Ponce, 2011, p. 570)*

In their quantitative study, Hoe et al. (2006, p. 462) compared staff and resident ratings on the QoL-AD scale (with 13 items relevant to physical and mental health, personal relationships, finances and overall life quality) and found differences in their perceptions of factors relevant to resident quality of life. The inter-item correlation was low ($r<0.4$), indicating a discrepancy between staff and resident ratings of each item within the scale.

Ballard et al. suggest that care home staff rely too heavily on using psychotropic drugs to make residents compliant:

> Within the current cohort, more than 40% of people were taking a neuroleptic agent, many of whom did not have clinically significant behavioural and psychological symptoms of dementia, implying that either the treatment was initiated inappropriately or that the treatment had not been reviewed following resolution of the target symptom.
>
> *(2001, p. 103)*

Our review focuses on quality of life and does not necessarily identify many of the studies of the impact of psychotropic drugs, which may be more likely to appear in the quality of care literature. Suffice to say though that psychotropic drug use is the focus of much of the literature on quality of care in nursing homes and the recognition of potentially deadly side effects of these drugs, particularly in patients with dementia, has led to many changes in standard practice.

Two studies (Innes & Surr, 2001; Ballard, 2001) use Dementia Care Mapping, a tool developed in the United Kingdom but now used worldwide to measure aspects of both dementia and quality of life. Dementia Care Mapping is not just a research instrument. The findings can be fed back to staff and used in a repeated cycle of improvement and can be used to identify staff training and development needs.

Towards the development of a model of quality of life in care homes

The findings of the systematic review identify factors important to the quality of life of care home residents. These include, from the residents' point of view, regardless of their level of cognitive impairment, the ability to have autonomy and express self-identity through making choices related to day-to-day living and the ability to form and maintain social connections. The care environment, particularly the attitudes and actions of carers, their training and management were also found to be important factors affecting the quality of life experienced by care home residents. These findings are supported by the reports "My Home Life, Quality of life in care homes", a review of the literature prepared for Help the Aged by The National Care Homes Research and Development Forum in 2007 and "A Place to Call Home? A Review into the Quality of Life and Care of Older People living in Care Homes in Wales" in 2014.

In the reviewed studies there was a marked difference between the views of residents and staff on the important elements of residents' quality of life. In their systematic reviews, both Courtney et al. (2003) and Xu, Kane and Shamliyan (2013) argue that, because quality of life is inherently subjective, residents are the best reporters of their own quality of life. Xu et al. in their review of quantitative studies, found that:

> Proxy measures (from staff or family members) are weak reflections of resident perceptions. Proxy measures tend to be associated with each other, and least well with resident measures.
>
> *(2013, p. 133)*

Although care home residents and people with dementia more generally have been seen in the past as difficult to access as research participants because they lack the ability to articulate

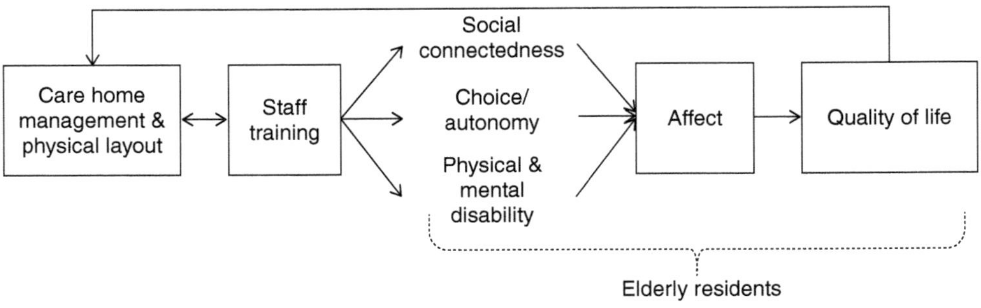

Figure 17.2 Factors that affect the quality of life of elderly residents of UK and Ireland care homes.

their thoughts and feelings, this has been challenged by researchers, and a number of new and innovative approaches have been developed to gather information about their experiences and attitudes. It is important that future research focuses on the residents' views of care they receive as well as the quality of care, just as research in the acute healthcare sector surveys patients about their subjective evaluation of care as well as gathering data about how effective the care was in terms of objective measures.

In this systematic review, we find that staff are the connecting link between the care home and the residents and are key to quality of life for older adults. Staff provide daily support for residents especially those with cognitive and physical impairments. Staff set boundaries within which residents have autonomy and can make choices about how they live. They are also an important source of social interaction and it is through staff that residents are enabled to interact with other residents and visitors.

This suggests that staff training contributes in an important way to the quality of life of care home residents. The studies show that elders in residential care have as much desire for autonomy and control in their lives as do other people who live independently. They also benefit from diverse activities that break up the monotony of institutionalised life and that allow residents to interact with other residents, staff and visitors. The studies suggest that staff require training in the personalised care of residents and in providing a livelier and more varied environment for residents. Effective training has the potential to create a positive feedback loop that can improve care home management generally. This is summarised in Figure 17.2.

There are a number of initiatives and policy instruments that have been developed in the United Kingdom to improve the quality of life of older adults in care homes. These are briefly reviewed in the next section.

Approaches to improving the quality of life in UK care homes

Through the specification of improvements

Over the last few years, there have been changes in UK legislation and regulatory regimes that have facilitated discussion about what good care in UK and Ireland residential homes for the elderly might be. There is now acknowledgement from the top that providing a reasonable quality of life for older people in care homes is more than just about having adequate care.

In the review of quality of life and care of older people in care homes in Wales, by the Older Peoples Commissioner for Wales, changes to be made, actions to be taken and evidenced by commissioners, regulators, providers and staff are all stipulated (Older Peoples Commissioner for Wales, 2014). There is a moral imperative from the champion of older people to make things better for those who deserve more and an exhortation that a

> simple concept needs to be reclaimed across residential care: that it is not just about being safe or having basic physical needs met, essential as these are, it is also about having the best quality of life, in whatever way that is defined by an individual older person.
>
> *(Older Peoples Commissioner for Wales, 2014, p. 3)*

Through registration, regulation and inspection

In England, care homes are registered, regulated and inspected by the Care Quality Commission CQC. In the devolved administrations, the Care Inspectorate in Scotland, Care and Social Services Inspectorate Wales and the Regulation and Quality Improvement Authority Northern Ireland, perform a similar function. Regulatory regimes facilitate a more holistic approach to quality of life in care homes rather than focussing solely on quality of care. Care homes are assessed on five criteria – whether they are safe, effective, caring, responsive and well-led. Inspection may identify improvements required and actions and deadlines are set.

Through guidance, standards and pathways

The National Institute for Health and Care Excellence (NICE) provides guidance, quality standards and pathways for the health and care of older people in care homes for local authorities, health and well-being boards, scrutiny panels, councillors and adult social care commissioners in England (NICE, 2015). To support caregiving staff, NICE recommends the report "Older people's vision for long term care" (Bowers et al., 2009), which focuses on the voice, choice and control of older people with high support needs as well as providing practical guidance, such as a pathway for managing medicines in care homes (NICE, 2014) and quality standards for the mental well-being of older people in care homes (NICE, 2013).

Through research and development

Part of the increasing focus on the quality of life are recent health and social care research initiatives to enhance the life experience of elders in care homes. For example, My Home Life is a UK-wide initiative from the National Care Homes Research and Development Forum supported by the Henry Smith Charity. The website provides resources for care home managers and staff, including examples of evidence-based best practice which use a relationship-centred approach.

The National Institute for Health Research has a Department of Health Policy Research programme which includes research projects in care homes in areas such as strategies to enhance physical activity in care homes and a randomised controlled trial to evaluate a falls prevention intervention.

Through organisational culture, training and development of care home managers and staff

Shifting the focus toward quality of life has resulted in positive changes to the organisational culture of care homes. Promoting a positive culture is one of the eight evidence-based themes that Age Cymru published in 2014 and is key to improving care home residents' quality of life. Good leadership with an aspirational vision of care home life is an integral part of promoting positive culture and nurturing and developing leaders is as important as training of front-line staff. The Social Care Institute for Excellence provides resources to stimulate learning for workforce training and development, such as short films for front-line staff about promoting independence whilst balancing choice, control and risk (Carr & Robbins, 2009). There is an educational framework ranging from an introductory care certificate through occupational competence to continuous professional development supported by Skills for Care and Health Education England as well as professional development for registered care managers.

Limitations of this study

This systematic review has descriptive findings from a mixture of qualitative and quantitative studies. It was not possible to conduct a meta-analysis. The scope of studies makes a descriptive account appropriate. It is notable that there was only one RCT (O'Shea et al., 2014) and this was not successful. This review of the literature explores the factors that promote the "overall condition of a human life" (MedLine) in care homes. This is a wide-ranging and holistic concept. The variety of ways of measuring quality of life that we found mean that the conclusions from these studies vary considerably. This, and the large number of qualitative studies included, indicates that quality of life in care homes is about *constitutive* relations as well as the technical aspects of care. The challenge, in future research, will be to integrate research on quality of care and quality of life; that is, research that attends both to residents' subjective experience of care as well as the objective clinical outcomes that different services deliver.

Summary and conclusions

The motivation for this paper was the desire to extend the concept of positive aging to the time of life when independent living is no longer possible. To that end, we conducted a systematic review of studies that have investigated the factors that are related to the quality of life in UK care homes. The main findings are that there are currently few studies available that meet the standard quality criteria for inclusion in a systematic review. However, the findings of those that do are of great interest. They show that the residents of care homes can be included in studies about their quality of life, even in the presence of mild to moderate cognitive impairment, and that they can, with the appropriate research methods, communicate their experiences. This is important because the few studies that have gathered data from residents and staff have found that they have very different perspectives and evaluations of quality. It could therefore be misleading to treat the observations of staff or visitors to the care home as adequate proxies for the provision of data about residents' experiences, although they have value in and of themselves.

Our synthesis of the existing literature suggests that the most important factors related to the quality of life in care homes includes the ability of residents to exercise choice, whether or not the environment is homelike and welcoming and the resident's own health status, particularly whether or not they have any cognitive impairment. These findings mirror those of reviews of the international literature (e.g. Lee, Yu & Kwong (2009)), suggesting that there are some commonalities across the different care settings.

In this study we also devised a simple model of how the factors that affect quality of life might relate to each other, and we described some of the policy initiatives and other mechanisms that have been employed in the United Kingdom to improve residents' quality of life. These include the specification of improvements required; registration, regulation and inspection of care homes; provision of guidance, standards and pathways; and the training and development of care home managers and staff to change the organisational culture in care homes. Finally, we see great potential for research to further the goal of extending the concept of positive aging to this population. This would involve devising innovative ways of gathering data about residents' evaluation of their living situation, investigating the different perspectives of residents and staff and finally, linking the large and growing international literature on quality of care in care homes, to further studies of quality of life.

References

Age Cymru. (2014). *Promoting a positive culture.* http://myhomelife.org.uk/wp-content/uploads/2014/11/MHL-CYMRU-PROMOTING-A-POSITIVE-CULTURE.pdf (accessed February 3, 2016).

Ballard, C., O'Brien, J., James, I., Mynt, P., Lana, M., Potkins, D., Reichelt, L. L., Swann, A., & Fossey, J. (2001). Quality of life for people with dementia living in residential and nursing home care: The impact of performance on activities of daily living, behavioural and psychological symptoms, language skills, and psychotropic drugs. *International Psychogeriatrics*, 13(1), 93–106.

Bostick, J. E., Rantz, M. J., Flesner, M. K., & Riggs, C. J. (2006). Systematic review of studies of staffing and quality in nursing homes. *Jamda*, 366–376, July.

Bowers, H., Clark, A., Crosby, G., Easterbrook, L., Macadam, A., MacDonald, R., Macfarlane, A., Maclean, M., Patel, M., Runnicles, D., Oshinaike, T. & Smith, C. (2009). *Older people's vision for long term care. Commissioned by the Joseph Rowntree Foundation.* www.jrf.org.uk/report/older-peoples-vision-long-term-care (accessed February 2, 2016).

Bradshaw, S. A., Playford, E. D., & Riazi, A. (2012). Living well in care homes: A systematic review of qualitative studies. *Age & Ageing*, 41, 429–440.

Cahill, S., & Diaz-Ponce, A. M. (2011). 'I hate having nobody here. I'd like to know where they all are': Can qualitative research detect differences in quality of life among nursing home residents with different levels of cognitive impairment? *Aging & Mental Health*, 15(5), 562–572.

Care Quality Commission. (2015). *The state of health care and adult social care in England 2014/15.* HMSO. www.gov.uk/government/publications/health-and-adult-social-care-in-england-2014-to-2015 (accessed May 4, 2017).

Carr, S., & Robbins, D. (2009). *The implementation of individual budget schemes in adult social care.* Social Care Institute for Excellence, Research Briefing 20, London.

Clark, P., & Bowling, A. (1989). Observational study of quality of life in NHS nursing homes and a long-stay ward for the elderly. *Ageing & Society*, 9(2), 123–148.

Cooney, A., Murphy, K., & O'Shea, E. (2009). Resident perspectives of the determinants of quality of life in residential care in Ireland. *Journal of Advanced Nursing*, 65(5), 1029–1038.

Courtney, M. D., Edwards, H., Stephan, J., O'Reilly, M. T., & Duggan, C. (2003). Quality of life measures for residents of aged care facilities: A literature review. *Australasian Journal on Ageing*, 22(2), 58–64.

Dorr, D. A., Jones, S. S., Burns, L., Donnelly, S. M., Brunker, C. P., Wilcox, A., & Claton, P. D. (2006). Use of health-related quality of life metrics to predict mortality and hospitalizations in community-dwelling seniors. *Journal of American Geriatrics Society*, 54, 667–673.

Draper, P. (1996). Compromise, massive encouragement and forcing: A discussion of mechanisms used to limit the choices available to the older adult in hospital. *Journal of Clinical Nursing*, 5(5), 325–531.

Gabriel, Z., & Bowling, A. (2004). Quality of life from the perspective of older people. *Ageing & Society*, 24, 675–691.

Help the Aged. (2007). *My home life: Quality of life in care homes. A review of the literature.* Prepared for Help the Aged by the National Care Homes Research and Development Forum. www.scie.org.uk/publications/guides/guide15/files/myhomelife-litreview.pdf?res=true (accessed January 29, 2016).

Ho, H. K., Matsubayashi, K., Wade, T., Kimura, M., Kita, T., & Saijoh, K. (2002). Factors associated with ADL dependence: A comparative study of residential care home and community-dwelling elderly in Japan. *Geriatrics & Gerontology International*, 2, 80–86.

Hoe, J., Hancock, G., Livingston, G., & Orrell, M. (2006). Quality of life of people with dementia in residential care homes. *British Journal of Psychiatry*, 188, 460–464.

Hoe, J., Hancock, G., Livingston, G., Woods, B., Challis, D., & Orrell, M. (2009). Changes in the quality of life of people with dementia living in care homes. *Alzheimer Disorders & Associated Disorders*, 23(3), 285–290.

Innes, A., & Surr, C. (2001). Measuring the well-being of people with dementia living in formal care settings: The use of Dementia Care Mapping. *Aging & Mental Health*, 5(3), 258–268.

Kane, R. A., Kling, K. C., Bershadsky, B., Kane, R. L., Giles, K., Degennoltz, H. B., Liu, J., & Cutler, L. J. (2003). Quality of life measures for nursing home residents. *Journal of Gerontology: Medical Sciences*, 58A, 240–248.

Lee, D. T. F., Yu, D. S. F., & Kwong, A. N. L. (2009). Quality of life of older people in residential care home: A literature review. *Journal of Nursing and Healthcare of Chronic Illness*, 1(2), 116–125.

Liberati, A., Altman, D. G., Tetzlaff, J., Mulrow, C., Gotzsche, P. C., Loannidis, J. P. A., Clarke, M., Devereaux, P. J., Kleijnen, J., & Moher, D. (2009). The PRISMA statement for reporting systematic reviews and meta-analyses of studies that evaluate healthcare interventions: Explanation and elaboration. *British Medical Journal*, 339, b2700.

McGovern, P., & Nazroo, J. Y. (2015). Patterns and causes of health inequalities in later life: A Bourdieusian analysis. *Sociology of Health & Illness*, 37(1), 143–160.

Murphy, K., O'Shea, E., & Cooney, A. (2007). Quality of life for older people living in long-stay settings in Ireland. *Journal of Clinical Nursing*, 16(11), 2167–2177.

National Care Homes Research and Development Forum. (2007). *My home life: Quality of life in care homes – a review of the literature*. London: Help the Aged. www.scie.org.uk/almost-there (accessed May 4, 2017).

NICE. (2013). *Mental wellbeing of older people in care homes*. www.nice.org.uk/guidance/qs50 (accessed February 1, 2016).

NICE. (2014). *Managing medicines in care homes overview*. www.nice.org.uk/guidance/SC1/chapter/1-Recommendations (accessed February 2, 2016).

NICE. (2015). *Older people in care homes*. www.nice.org.uk/advice/lgb25/chapter/Introduction (accessed February 1, 2016).

NHS Confederation. (2015). *Key statistics on the NHS*. www.nhsconfed.org/resources/key-statistics-on-the-nhs (accessed July 17, 2015).

Office for National Statistics. (2014). *Changes in the older resident care home population between 2001 and 2011*. www.ons.gov.uk (accessed August 1, 2014), Crown Copyright.

The Older People's Commissioner for Wales. (2014). *A place to call home: A review into the quality of life and care of older people living in care homes in Wales*. Cambrian Buildings, Mount Stuart Square, Cardiff. www.olderpeoplewales.com/en/Reviews/Residential_Care_Review/ReviewReport.aspx (accessed May 4, 2017).

Oleson, M., Heading, C., McGlynn Shadick, K., & Bistodeau, J. A. (1994). Quality of life in long-stay institutions in England: Nurse and resident perceptions. *Journal Advanced Nursing*, 20, 23–32.

O'Shea, E., Devane, D., Cooney, A., Casey, D., Jordan, F., Hunter, A., Murphy, E., Newell, J., Connolly, S., & Murphy, K. (2014). The impact of reminiscence on the quality of life of residents with dementia in long-stay care. *Geriatric Psychiatry*, 29, 1062–1070.

Spilsbury, K., Hewitt, C., Stirk, L., & Bowman, C. (2011). The relationship between nurse staffing and quality of care in nursing homes: A systematic review. *International Journal of Nursing Studies*, 48, 732–750.

Stathi, A., & Simey, P. (2007). Quality of life in the fourth age: Exercise experiences of nursing home residents. *Journal of Aging & Physical Activity*, 15(3), 272–286.

Thome, B., Dykes, A.-K., & Hallberg, I. R. (2003). Home care with regard to definition, care recipients, content and outcome: Systematic literature review. *Journal of Nursing Care*, 12, 860–872.

Wong, E. W., Woo, J., Hui, E., & Ho, S. C. (2004). Examination of the Philadelphia geriatric morale scale as a subject quality-of-life measure in elderly Hong Kong Chinese. *The Gerontologist*, 44, 408–417.

World Health Organization. (1998). *WHOQOL user manual*. Geneva, Switzerland: Division of Mental Health and Prevention of Substance Abuse.

Xu, D., Kane, R. L., & Shamliyan, T. A. (2013). Effect of nursing home characteristics on residents' quality of life: A systematic review. *Archives of Gerontology & Geriatrics*, 57, 127–142.

18

ADVANCE CARE PLANNING FOR OLDER ADULTS AT THE END OF LIFE

Gary Bellamy

Learning outcomes

- An understanding of advance care planning as a means of achieving a 'good' death
- The benefits and risks associated with advance care planning
- Cultural influences and their impact on the uptake of advance care planning discussions
- An awareness of how technology might be used to underpin the interoperability of advance care planning documentation to ensure care provision between health and social care providers is in line with patient preferences

Introduction and chapter overview

Meeting the needs of older people as they approach the end of their lives is now a key public health challenge as changes in demography and epidemiology transform trends in longevity, morbidity and mortality. These changes mean that death and chronic illness are now largely concentrated in older age groups. Nonetheless, Seymour et al. (2005) observe that, historically, health and social care services have been slow to respond to the needs of older adults in their last year of life. Current policy direction reflects an increasing recognition that palliative and end-of-life care is not only about the management of the last days of life but is also about supporting people with long-term health conditions to live as well and as comfortably as possible until they die. A key emphasis is on enabling participation in care planning both during and in advance of any illness, as well as on taking into account the individual's values and preferences as well as the views of family members and healthcare professionals to achieve a 'good' death.

Older people who are nearing the end of life should receive timely help if they want or need it to discuss and plan for the end of life. End-of-life care services should provide high-quality care, support, choice and control, and should avoid 'over-medicalising' what is a natural phase of the aging life course in order to achieve a 'good death'. Whilst the concept itself might appear something of an oxymoron – how could anything about dying be good? – you only need to watch someone, or listen to the experiences of others who have witnessed someone die badly to recognise that dying well is not only a valid goal but also hard to achieve. Overall, older people receive poorer quality care towards the end of life compared to younger people. They are less likely to be involved in discussions about their future care and treatment options, less likely to die where they choose and less likely to receive specialist palliative services care or access hospice beds (Seymour et al., 2005; Gott and Ingleton, 2011).

Advances in medical technology have made it possible to treat conditions that even a decade ago would have been considered almost futile. Whilst these advances are important, the seemingly miraculous power of technology to transform healthcare provision has also encouraged the attitude that it should always be used. As a result, patients or their families indulge the nearly irresistible urge to 'Do something!' when faced with a life-threatening medical problem, even when that something is far more likely to prolong the dying process than halt it. In this way, people have become complicit in reducing the likelihood of experiencing a good death.

Generally speaking, however, death and dying still remain taboo subjects: most people find them embarrassing, uncomfortable and potentially distressing to talk about. Yet there is increasing consensus in the public sphere including both the United Kingdom and internationally that talking explicitly about death and dying is necessary in order to make death as positive an experience as possible, both for the person who is dying and for those close to them. Good and timely advance care planning (ACP) is widely regarded as fundamental to avoiding futile, costly and invasive treatment to enable death in the preferred place of care (Higginson and Sen-Gupta, 2000) and, in doing so, avoid 'over-medicalising' what is a natural phase of the aging life course.

What is ACP and why is it important?

ACP has been defined by Henry and Seymour as:

> a voluntary process of discussion about future care and treatment preferences between an individual and their care providers, irrespective of discipline. This might include a discussion of the individual's concerns and wishes, their important values or personal goals for care; their understanding of their illness and prognosis, and their preferences and wishes for the type of care or treatment that may be beneficial in the future and the availability of these.
>
> *(2008, p. 5)*

There is an increasing body of research and guidance, nationally and internationally, on the best use of ACP for people nearing the end of life (Thomas and Lobo, 2010; International Society of Advance Care Planning and End-of-life Care, 2011). ACP helps to meet patient preferences (Abel et al., 2013) and must be handled sensitively. A major international study found that no fewer than three-quarters of people wanted to be fully informed if they had less than a year to live (Harding et al., 2013). It is also vitally important that care planning is not seen as a one-off event; communication with patients and their families should be a continuous process.

ACP has become increasingly important as a means of improving care for people with a life-limiting illness and a key component of end-of-life care policy in many countries of the developed world. In 2008, the first 'End-of-Life Care Strategy' for England and Wales was published by the United Kingdom's Department of Health which outlined a 10-year strategy for improving care at the end of life in all care settings in England. One of the key aims of the strategy is to ensure, as far as possible, that services meet the needs of people and that their end-of-life care is in keeping with any expressed preferences. According to Henry and Joseph (2011), the common factors in attaining a 'good death' include the following:

1 Being treated as an individual, with dignity and respect
2 Being without pain and other symptoms

3 Being in familiar surroundings
4 Being in the company of close friends and family

Studies of dying in hospitals conducted internationally, most notably the SUPPORT study in the United States (Freeborne, Lynn and Desbiens, 2000) and the later APROPRICUS study in nine European countries and Israel (Piers et al., 2011), identified that the use of invasive medical technology was prolonging dying for many patients at the expense of optimising the remaining quality of life experienced by those individuals. There is also evidence to suggest that facilitating ACP with patients and their families can increase the likelihood that preferences for end-of-life care are known and respected (Detering et al., 2010) and is therefore a fundamental part of the end-of-life process.

ACP differs from general care planning based on its use primarily in the context of progressive illness and anticipated deterioration. This has implications for its acceptability to patients as well as any informal or family caregivers who may have involvement. The process may result in a written record of that person's wishes which can subsequently be referred to by carers and healthcare professionals in the future. If the individual concerned loses capacity, health and social care professionals should make use of the information gathered to guide them in their decision-making when needed.

The Royal College of Physicians (2009) underscores the importance of the process of ACP not being document driven or a 'tick box' exercise – an issue that has been corroborated by other research (Barnes et al., 2007; Billings, 2012; Mahon, 2011). In a similar manner, other authors focus on the importance of good communication and that the success of advance care planning should not be measured on the completion of ACP documentation alone (Fried and O'Leary, 2008).

What are the benefits and risks associated with ACP?

Despite an original focus on the completion of written documents such as advance directives (including living wills and durable powers of attorney for healthcare) and do not attempt to resuscitate (DNAR) orders, there has been a move to a more informal process of discussion and reflection about goals of care (Thomas and Lobo, 2010; Horne, Seymour and Payne, 2009; Davison, Holley and Seymour, 2010). The process of ACP can facilitate patients' future wishes regarding care and treatment to be carried out in the event that they lose mental capacity (Hayhoe and Howe, 2011). The Mental Capacity Act 2005 enables people to appoint a family member, carer or professional as a welfare attorney to make decisions on their behalf should the need arise. At the same time, ACP can also serve as a basis for decision-making for those who retain capacity.

The particularly poor end-of-life care experienced by older adults with dementia can be the result of either overly interventionist care (such as tube feeding and the use of restraints) or sub-optimal care (inadequate pain control, malnutrition and dehydration and inadequate emotional and social support) (Hughes et al., 2007). Reasons for this include the difficulty of identifying when people with dementia enter the end-of-life phase and difficulties in communication. These make it difficult to accurately assess and treat pain, as well as to ascertain the patient's wishes and preferences. As a consequence, it is vital that ACP discussions occur at an early stage of dementia so that the patient's preferences can be expressed before their condition deteriorates (Shega et al., 2003).

For those individuals with dementia and cognitive impairment, the benefits of ACP can lead to less aggressive forms of medical care and better quality of life near death, decreased rates of hospital admission (especially those admitted from care homes) and increased rates of hospice admission. There is also evidence to suggest that those with an advance care plan are more likely to receive care in line with their wishes. At the same time, advance care planning can enable family members and partners to prepare for their death, resolve family conflict and deal with the subsequent bereavement whilst knowing that any of the patients' wishes have been carried out accordingly (Rhee, Zwar and Kemp, 2013; Detering et al., 2010).

Evidence from two systematic reviews in relation to ACP (Lorenz et al., 2008; Brinkman-Stoppelenburg, Rietjens and Heide, 2014) examined the evidence for improving palliative care at the end of life. The first, conducted in 2008, included 41 articles associated with ACP and found moderate evidence supporting multicomponent interventions to increase patient uptake of advance directives; however, these studies seldom measured clinically important outcomes. The 41 studies included in the systematic review highlighted the value placed on care planning that respects the patients' individual values, involvement of skilled facilitators and focus on key decision makers such as patients, caregivers and providers (Lorenz et al., 2008). Patients themselves also find the discussion process helpful. Rather than focusing upon particular treatments and interventions alone, there is evidence to suggest patients find the opportunity to focus upon their goals, values and beliefs more beneficial (Detering et al., 2010; Lorenz et al., 2008; Pautex, Hermann and Zulian, 2008; Kaldjian et al., 2009). A second systematic review by Stoppelenburg, Rietjens and Heide (2014) included 113 relevant papers. In a similar way to the first, there was evidence that ACP positively impacts on the quality of end-of-life care. Moreover, rather than focusing on the completion of written documents alone, more complex ACP interventions may be more effective in meeting patients' preferences.

As older people are a diverse group, so too are their attitudes towards ACP. Healthcare professionals planning to engage in these conversations need to be cognisant of the risks and barriers that this group have highlighted. Individual preferences are paramount and research has demonstrated that some may find the topic distressing and actively choose not to engage in discussions about future care on the basis that it involves thinking about deterioration in their condition (Barnes et al., 2007; Billings, 2012; Horne, Symour and Shepherd, 2006). There is evidence to suggest that some older people with chronic conditions such as heart failure or chronic obstructive pulmonary disease may not think of their condition as life limiting in such a way that warrants the need for discussions about future care and treatment preferences (Janssen et al., 2012; Gott et al., 2008). Moreover, opting not to engage in ACP discussions may be the preferred coping strategy of some older adults wanting to live 'in the here and now', and should therefore be seen as a positive coping strategy and not counterproductive (Horne, Seymour and Payne, 2012). Furthermore, other studies have found that asking patients to anticipate their future experiences of illness and the treatments they would opt for can often prove too difficult (Halpern, 2012; Dening, Jones and Sampson, 2013).

There are a number of barriers that healthcare professionals have highlighted for not initiating ACP discussions with older adults with a life-limiting illness. Previous research findings have emphasised how holding these discussions brings death to the fore and, in doing so, destroys any hope that the patient may have had prior to the discussion (Curtis et al., 2008). Difficulties associated with prognostication can be a particular barrier for healthcare professionals looking to engage in ACP discussions with older people. Unlike a patient receiving a terminal diagnosis, for many older people nearing the end of life, there is no sentinel event that presents itself an opportunity for a clinician to 'break bad news'. Talking about dying is difficult and a survey of GPs conducted in 2012 revealed that 35 per cent had never initiated a conversation about end-of-life care with one of their patients (Royal College of General Practitioners and Royal College of Nursing, 2012). Indeed, those conditions characterized by a pervasive deterioration such as chronic obstructive pulmonary disease (COPD) and heart failure (Momen and Barclay, 2011) can be particularly challenging in terms of knowing the 'right' time to hold ACP discussions. As a result, there is sometimes reluctance on the part of healthcare professionals who fear destroying hope or being proved wrong (Christakis, 1999).

Whilst professionals cite the fear of jeopardising their relationship with patients as one reason for not engaging in ACP-related discussions (Seymour, Almack and Kennedy, 2010), being in a trusting relationship with the individual or being able to develop such a relationship is considered fundamental (Prendergast, 2001). Another factor is the skilled communication required of healthcare professionals to facilitate these discussions, which is crucial to the success of ACP (Janssen et al., 2012). Evidence of poor communication about end-of-life care is widespread (Gott et al., 2011; Healthcare Commission, 2007) and this has, in part, led to the provision of increased workforce training and support to deliver good care at the end of life. The National Gold Standards Framework Centre (GSF) in End-of-Life Care provides comprehensive training programmes for staff combined with strategic support and tools that aim to ensure that end-of-life care services provide 'the right care, for the right person in the right place at the right time, every time' (www.goldstandardsframework.org.uk/).

Cultural influences and their impact on the uptake of advance care planning discussions

ACP has developed within a particular cultural and professional ideology. According to Pollock and Seymour (2013) it is one which stresses the importance of individual autonomy, personal choice and a culture of practice promoting a particular vision of a 'good death'. This paradigm does not accommodate for cultural diversity and it is clear that ACP poses challenges for older patients and professionals from diverse cultural backgrounds. Non-Western cultures may not necessarily share Western preoccupations associated with autonomy. For example, international studies have identified the involvement of family in decision-making and place of care as central to good end-of-life care; a preference for family members to make decisions about the patient's care has been reported (Bellamy and Gott, 2013; Bowman and Singer, 2001; McGrath, Vu and McLeod, 2001; Frey et al., 2014), as well as a tendency to withhold prognostic information on the basis that it might cause a loss of hope (Bowman and Singer, 2001; McGrath, Vu, McLeod, 2001; Chan and Kayser-Jones, 2005; Hathaway, 2009). The concept of individual autonomy has only recently begun to take influence amongst Asian populations; commentators have noted a preference for a concept of self, enmeshed within family networks. This has been deemed a particularly important aspect of end-of-life care for Chinese elders (Ho, 1995; Fan, 1997).

In the context in which family decision-making is integral, current formulations of ACP may be seen as unhelpful and at worst as harmful to the caring relationship between family and patient (Candib, 2002; Bito et al., 2007). However, caution must also be exercised by healthcare professionals and policymakers in judgements relating to an individual's level of interest in ACP based on cultural background alone. As Koffmann (2011) has pointed out, when applied to palliative and end-of-life care, 'culture' may serve only to restrict the dialogue to 'an interpretive list of end-of-life care beliefs and practices from a range of so-called "cultural" groups' (p. 117). Others have raised concerns about the deterministic links between cultural, ethnic or religious factors and end-of-life care preferences (often referred to as the 'cookbook' approach) (Jones, 2005). Adopting this approach is one solution to caring for individuals from different cultural backgrounds; however, this may serve to foster new myths or stereotypes (Johnson and Jones, 2002). As Kagawa-Singer and Blackhall (2001) note, there can be a wide variation in the beliefs and behaviours within any given population. Rather, a twofold approach to end-of-life care that acknowledges cultural values – but at the same time focuses on the individual, their care preferences and those of their family and significant others – is key.

Using technology to underpin the delivery of advance care planning and achieve a 'good death'

According to Frey et al. (2014), technology-supported information concerning ACP delivery is a fundamental requisite to facilitate shared decision-making and information sharing. Moreover, in a world of increasing technology, patients have grown accustomed to a wealth of health-related information via high-speed Internet access (Jeannot et al., 2004; Schwartz et al., 2006). This improved access to health-related information has also changed the interpersonal dynamics between patients and their clinicians and has led to more patient involvement in the decision-making process, rather than simply acting as a passive recipient (Weiner and Bondich, 2006). Healthcare providers continue to indicate that patient volume, increasing patient complexity, the need to share information with multiple providers and an increasing paperwork burden have adversely affected quality ACP delivery. However, an increasing and ubiquitous use of health information technology, such as electronic health records and electronic health record-tethered patient portals, affords opportunities to streamline communication methods between various providers and their patients to help provide seamless end-of-life care (Bose-Brill and Pressler, 2012).

Despite these communication methods afforded by new technologies, sharing advance care plans so that the appropriate services (hospitals, GP services and care homes) remain aware of updated plans remains a considerable challenge and service provision is variable. Other than lasting powers of attorney, the United Kingdom has no central register for advance care plans. Nonetheless, the 2008 UK National End-of-Life Care Strategy (Department of Health, 2008) recommended locality registers as a means to enable effective communication amongst professionals. Initiatives in information technology systems, most notably the Electronic Palliative Care Coordination System (EPaCCS) tool, grew from this recommendation and are helping to support better care planning and co-ordination between health and social care providers (www.nhsiq.nhs.uk/improvement-programmes/long-term-conditions-and-integrated-care/end-of-life-care/coordination-of-care.aspx). EPaCCS are designed to improve communication and simplify access to up-to-date information, which enables a consistent approach to care management at the end of life by creating a shared locality record for health and social care professionals. They allow rapid access across care boundaries to key information about an individual approaching the end of life, including their expressed preferences for care. Another such example is Coordinate My Care (http://coordinatemycare.co.uk/). This has been developed to give people the opportunity to create a personalised urgent care plan where they can express their wishes and preferences for how and where they are treated and cared for. In some areas, this has led to an increase in patients dying in their preferred place of care (Smith and Riley, 2011). However, in its present form, as a platform for sharing information, it is only available as a pan-London initiative and not currently available across the United Kingdom.

Given that older adults in their last year of life are likely to be admitted to hospital an average of 3.5 times (Lyons and Verne, 2011), a multidisciplinary model of care with good communication between primary and secondary care providers is essential in end-of-life care to avoid unnecessary admissions and manage discharge from hospital effectively. Individuals and their families must be able to rely on safe, appropriate care consistent with their expressed wishes, at any time of day or night and no matter the care provider.

Conclusion

Populations around the world are rapidly aging and, whilst this is a cause for celebration, it brings its own unique set of challenges. It signals the rise in chronic, often co-morbid health conditions and an increased demand for both acute and primary healthcare, as well as the need for a larger and better trained health workforce. Since death is now most likely to occur at the end of a long life, ACP is a useful tool to promote discussion to explore the views and values which older adults express in relation to their future care and treatment preferences and act upon them accordingly. For some older adults with a life-limiting condition, the opportunity to talk about, and realise their personal goals for living and dying 'well', is fundamental for enabling them to have a say in their own end-of-life care. However, in spite of ACP being promoted as a means of improving healthcare and helping to facilitate patient autonomy, evidence for its effectiveness remains limited and haphazard. It has developed within a dominant Western cultural and professional ideology with little or no input from those non-Western cultures who may not share those prevailing beliefs.

Meeting individual 'cultural' needs forms only part of the picture but can, nonetheless, inform the delivery of end-of-life care. Whilst the Western moral imperative of autonomy, informed consent and truth telling is often at odds with the beliefs of cultural groups who place a much greater emphasis on the role of family in decision-making, determining how much information to give patients from different groups with a life-limiting illness is not straightforward and 'one size does not fit all'. Seymour and Gott note similar discrepancies when they argue that:

> older people tend to take heterogeneous stances towards decision-making and that their abilities (and indeed wishes) to be autonomous often depend on the context in which they find themselves.
>
> *(2011, p. 48)*

ACP is now well established on the professional agenda in developed countries such as the United States, Canada, Australia and New Zealand and much of Europe. In recent years, as a potential outcome of ACP, there has been a move away from the use of legally authorised written advance directives to a more informal process of discussion that may involve family members and significant others. In turn, these discussions can impact positively on the bereavement experiences of family members and significant others safe in the knowledge that any express wishes they may have had have been carried out in accordance with the patients' own preferences.

Whilst these conversations require courage and determination on both the part of the older person, their family members and healthcare providers alike, they should not be seen as a panacea. A substantial minority may not wish to engage in future planning and may instead prefer to live in the 'here and now', thereby corroborating with professional anxieties associated with engaging in these potentially sensitive conversations in the first place. At the very least, ACP requires healthcare staff with excellent communication skills to facilitate these conversations should they arise as a means of achieving a 'good death'. At the same time, in an increasing age of information technology, it should be underpinned by a platform capable of sharing up-to-date plans between different agencies to avoid potentially inappropriate hospital admissions and unwanted life-prolonging treatments.

Ascertaining the wishes of both the individual older person with a life-limiting illness and their family members is important to ensure that preferences are met through individualised assessment that may involve advance care planning discussions and is seen as a hallmark of good practice.

References

Abel, J., Pring, A., Rich, A., Malik, T., and Verne, J. (2013). The impact of advance care planning of place of death, a hospice retrospective cohort study. *BMJ Supportive & Palliative Care*, 3(2), 168–173.

Barnes, K., Jones, L., Tookman, A., and King, M. (2007). Acceptability of a care planning interview schedule: A focus group study. *Palliative Medicine*, 21, 23–28.

Bellamy, G., and Gott, M. (2013). What are the priorities for developing culturally appropriate palliative and end-of-life care for older people? The views of healthcare staff working in New Zealand. *Health and Social Care in the Community*, 21(30), 26–34.

Billings, J. A. (2012). The need for safeguards in advance care planning. *Journal of General Internal Medicine*, 27, 595–600.

Bito, S., Matsumura, S., Kagawa-Singer, M., Meredith, L., Fukuhara, S., and Wenger, N. S. (2007). Acculturation and end-of-life decision making: Comparison of Japanese and Japanese-American focus groups. *Bioethics*, 21, 251–262.

Bose-Brill, S., and Pressler, T. R. (2012). Commentary: Opportunities for innovation and improvement in advance care planning using a tethered patient portal in the electronic health record. *Journal of Primary Care and Community Health*, 3(4), 285–288.

Bowman, K., and Singer, P. (2001). Chinese seniors' perspectives on end-of-life decisions. *Social Science and Medicine*, 53(4), 455–464.

Brinkman-Stoppelenburg, A., Rietjens, A. C., and Heide, A. (2014). The effects of advance care planning on end-of-life care: A systematic review. *Palliative Medicine*, 28(8), 1000–1025.

Candib, L. (2002). Truth telling and advance planning at the end-of-life: Problems with autonomy in a multicultural world. *Family Systems and Health*, 20, 213–228.

Chan, J., and Kayser-Jones, J. (2005). The experience of dying for Chinese nursing home residents. *Journal of Gerontological Nursing*, 31(8), 26–32.

Christakis, N. A. (1999). *Death foretold, prophecy and prognosis in medical care*. Chicago: University of Chicago Press.

Curtis, J. R., Engelberg, R., Young, J. P., Vig, L. K., Reinke, L. F., Wenrich, M. D., et al. (2008). An approach to understanding the interaction of hope and desire for explicit prognostic information among individuals with severe chronic obstructive pulmonary disease or advanced cancer. *Journal of Palliative Medicine*, 11, 610–620.

Davison, S. N., Holley, J. L., and Seymour, J. (2010). ACP in patients with end-stage renal disease. In E. J. Chambers, E. Brown, and M. Germain (Eds.), *Supportive care for the renal patient* (pp. 49–74). Oxford: Oxford University Press.

Department of Health. (2008). *End-of-life care strategy: Promoting high quality care for all adults at the end-of-life*. London: Department of Health.

Dening, K. H., Jones, L., and Sampson, E. L. (2013). Preferences for end-of-life care: A nominal group study of people with dementia and their family carers. *Palliative Medicine*, 27, 409–417.

Detering, K. M., Hancock, A. D., Reade, M. C., and Silvester, W. (2010). The impact of advance care planning on end-of-life care in elderly patients: Randomised controlled trial. *British Medical Journal*, 340, c1345.

Fan, R. P. (1997). Self-determination versus family determination: Two incommensurable principles of autonomy. *Bioethics*, 11, 309–322.

Freeborne, N., Lynn, J., and Desbiens, N. A. (2000). Insights about dying from the support project. *Journal of the American Geriatric Society*, 48, S199–S205.

Frey, R., Raphael, D., Bellamy, G., and Gott, M. (2014). Advance care planning for Māori, Pacific and Asian people: The views of New Zealand healthcare professionals. *Health and Social Care in the Community*, 22(3), 290–299.

Fried, T. R., and O'Leary, J. R. (2008). Using the experiences of bereaved caregivers to inform patient and caregiver-centred advance care planning. *Journal of General Internal Medicine*, 23, 1602–1607.

Gott, M., and Ingleton, C. (2011). *Living with ageing and dying: Palliative end-of-life care for older people*. Oxford: Oxford University Press.

Gott, M., Ingleton, C., Bennett, M. I., and Gardiner, C. (2011). Transitions to palliative care in acute hospitals in England. *BMJ*, 342, d1773.

Gott, M., Small, N., Barnes, S., Payne, S., and Seamark, D. (2008). Older people's views of a good death in heart failure: Implications for palliative care provision. *Social Science and Medicine*, 67, 1113–1121.

Halpern, S. (2012). Shaping end-of-life care: Behavioural economics and advance directives. *Seminars in Respiratory and Critical Care Medicine*, 33, 393–400.

Harding, R., Simms, V., Calanzani, N., Higginson, I. J., Hall, S., Gysels, M., Meñaca, A., Bausewein, C., Deliens, L., Ferreira, P., Toscani, F., Daveson, B. A., Ceulemans, L., and Gomes, B. (2013). If you had less than a year to live, would you want to know? A seven-country European population survey of public preferences for disclosure of poor prognosis. *Psycho-Oncology*, 22(10), 2298–2305.

Hathaway, J. (2009). *Over the great wall: A qualitative descriptive study of the experiences and preferences of Chinese Immigrant families when receiving hospice services in New Zealand*. Unpublished Master's Thesis, Victoria University, Wellington, New Zealand.

Hayhoe, B., and Howe, A. (2011). Advance care planning under the Mental Capacity Act 2005 in primary care. *British Journal of General Practice*, 61, e537–e541.

Healthcare Commission. (2007). *Spotlight on complaints: A report on second stage complaints about the NHS in England*. London: Commission for Health care Audit and Inspection.

Henry, C., and Joseph, S. (2011). Advance care planning for the end-of-life. In B. Lobo and K. Thomas (Eds.), *Advance care planning in end-of-life care* (pp. 73–82). Oxford: Oxford University Press.

Henry, C., and Seymour, J. (2008). *Advance care planning: A guide for health and social care staff*. London: Department of Health.

Higginson, I. J., and Sen-Gupta, G. J. A. (2000). Place of care in advanced cancer: A qualitative systematic literature review of patient preferences. *Journal of Palliative Medicine*, 3(3), 287–300.

Ho, D. Y. F. (1995). Selfhood and Identity in Confucianism, Taoism, Buddhism and Hinduism: Contrasts with the West. *Journal for the Theory of Social Behaviour*, 25, 115–138.

Horne, G., Seymour, J., and Payne, S. (2009). ACP: Evidence and implications for practice. *End-of-Life Care*, 3(1), 58–64.

Horne, G., Seymour, J., and Payne, S. (2012). Maintaining integrity in the face of death: A grounded theory to explain the perspectives of people affected by lung cancer about the expression of wishes for end-of-life care. *International Journal of Nursing Studies*, 49, 718–726.

Horne, G., Seymour, J., and Shepherd, K. (2006). ACP for patients with inoperable lung cancer. *International Journal of Palliative Nursing*, 12(14), 172–179.

Hughes, J., Jolley, D., Jordan, A., and Sampson, E. (2007). Palliative care in dementia: Issues and evidence. *Advances in Psychiatric Treatment*, 13, 251–260.

International Society of Advance Care Planning & End-of-Life Care. (2011). *International society of advance care planning & end-of-life care website*. http://acpelsociety.com/ (accessed April 4, 2016).

Janssen, D. J. A., Engelberg, R. A., Wouters, E. F. M., and Curtis, J. R. (2012). ACP for patients with COPD: Past, present and future. *Patient Education and Counselling*, 86, 19–24.

Jeannot, J. G., Froehlich, F., Wietlisbach, V., Burnand, B., Terraz, O., and Vader, J. P. (2004). Patient use of the internet for health care information in Switzerland. *Swiss Medical Weekly*, 134, 307–312.

Johnson, M., and Jones, K. (2002). *Faith and health: A critical review*. Leicester: The Leicester Faith Forum.

Jones, J. (2005). Diversities in approach to end-of-life care: A view from Britain of the qualitative literature. *Journal of Research in Nursing*, 10 (4), 431.

Kagawa-Singer, M., and Blackhall, L. (2001). Negotiating cross cultural issues at end-of-life: You got to go where he lives. *Journal of the American Medical Association*, 286(23), 2993–3001.

Kaldjian, L. C., Curtis, A. E., Shinkunas, L. A., and Cannon, K. T. (2009). Goals of care toward the end-of-life: A structured literature review. *The American Journal of Hospice and Palliative Care*, 25(6), 501–511.

Koffmann, J. (2011). New public health approaches to address diversity and end-of-life issues for older people. In M. Gott and C. Ingleton (Eds.), *Living with ageing and dying: Palliative and end-of-life care for older people* (pp. 116–131). Oxford: Oxford University Press.

Lorenz, K. A., Lynn, J., Dy, S. M., Shugarman, L. R., Wilkinson, A., Mularski, R. A., et al. (2008). Evidence for improving palliative care at the end-of-life: A systematic review. *Annals of Internal Medicine*, 148, 147–159.

Lyons, P., and Verne, J. (2011). Pattern of hospital admission in the final year of life. *BMJ Supportive and Palliative Care*, 1, 81–82.

McGrath, P., Vu, M., and McLeod, L. (2001). Needs and experiences of non-English speaking hospice patients and families in an English Speaking country. *American Journal of Hospice and Palliative Care*, 18(5), 305–312.

Mahon, M. M. (2011). An advance directive in two questions. *Journal of Pain and Symptom Management*, 41, 801–807.

Momen, N., and Barclay, S. (2011). Addressing 'the elephant on the table': Barriers to end-of-life care conversations- a literature review and narrative synthesis. *Current Opinion in Palliative and Supportive Care*, 5(4), 312–316.

Pautex, S., Hermann, F. R., and Zulian, G. B. (2008). Role of advance directives in palliative care units: A prospective study. *Palliative Medicine*, 22, 835–841.

Piers, R., Azoulay, E., Ricou, B., et al. (2011). Perceptions of appropriateness of care among European and Israeli intensive care unit nurses and physicians. *Journal of the American Medical Association*, 306, 2694–2703.

Pollock, K., and Seymour, J. (2013). Communication and advance care planning for older people. In L. Van den Block, G. Albers, S. Martins Pereira, B. Onwuteaka-Philipsen, R. Pasman, and L. Deliens (Eds.), *Palliative care for older people: A public health perspective* (pp. 236–248). Oxford: Oxford University Press.

Prendergast, T. J. (2001). Advance care planning: Pitfalls, progress, promise. *Critical Care Medicine*, 29, N34–N39.

Royal College of General Practitioners and Royal College of Nursing. (2012). *Matters of life and death: Helping people to live well until they die*. London: Royal College of General Practitioners Clinical Innovation and Research Centre. www.rcgp.org.uk/~/media/Files/CIRC/Matters%20of%20Life%20and%20Death%20FINAL.ashx (accessed April 4, 2016).

Rhee, J. J., Zwar, N. A., and Kemp, L. A. (2013). Advance care planning and interpersonal relationships: A two way street. *Family Practice*, 30, 219–226.

Seymour, J., Almack, K., and Kennedy, S. (2010). Implementing ACP: A qualitative study of community nurses' views and experiences. *BMC Palliative Care*, 9(4), 1–29.

Seymour, J., Witherspoon, R., Gott, M., Ross, H., and Payne, S., with Owen, T., Help the Aged. (2005). *End-of-life care: Promoting comfort, choice and well-being for older people*. Bristol: Policy Press, in association with Help the Aged.

Schwartz, K., Roe, T., Northrup, J., Meza, J., Seifeldin, R., and Neale, A.V. (2006). Family medicine patients' use of the internet for health information: A MetroNet study. *Journal of the American Board of Family Medicine*, 19, 39–45.

Seymour, J., and Gott, M. (2011). The challenges of health technology for ageing and dying. In M. Gott and C. Ingleton (Eds.), *Living with ageing and dying: Palliative and end-of-life care for older people* (pp. 42–51). Oxford: Oxford University Press.

Shega, J., Levin, A., Hougham, G., Cox-Hayley, D., Luchins, D., Hanrahan, P., Stocking, C., and Sachs, G. (2003). Palliative excellence in Alzheimer care efforts (PEACE): A program description. *Journal of Palliative Medicine*, 6(2), 315–320.

Smith, C., Hough, L., Cheung, C-C., et al. (2012). Coordinate My Care: a clinical service that coordinates care, giving patients choice and improving quality of life. *BMJ Support Palliat Care*, 2, 301–7.

Thomas, K., and Lobo, B. (2010). *Advance care planning in end-of-life care*. Oxford: Oxford University Press.

Weiner, M., and Bondich, P. (2006). The influence of information technology on patient-physician relationships. *Journal of General Internal Medicine*, 21(Suppl. 1), S35–S39.

PART V

Conclusion

19
CONCLUSION

Rachael E. Docking and Jennifer Stock

In this *International Handbook of Positive Aging* we have discussed the national and international evidence across a range of topics related to aging. Whilst we aimed to consider the challenges that come with an aging population on a societal level and the challenges faced in later life on an individual level, the key aim was to recognise and identify the opportunity provided to us, as a society, to accept it with both hands and start to rethink how we do things to enable older adults to age more positively.

We have learnt that the population trends seen over the last decade are predominantly due to improvements in health services, environment and overall prosperity, which enable people to live longer. However, we are also experiencing an increase in long-term, often co-morbid health conditions, including diabetes and cardiovascular disease. With this comes an increased demand for acute and primary healthcare services. As more pressure is put on resources, to ensure we promote positive aging, it is time we start shifting responsibility from the state on to the individual, for instance in terms of maximising capacity for prevention and self-management.

To ensure that living with long-term conditions becomes a more positive aging experience, there needs to be a 'whole-system approach' incorporating person-centred and relationship-centred care which have been cited as important concepts with the field of dementia and other long-term conditions. This 'whole-system approach' involves encouraging healthcare professionals to establish relationships with patients and carers that are reliable and dependable; improving training and education both to staff and to older adults themselves; supporting people in their socio-contextual resources and building on their existing social support; taking into consideration individuals' ability to self-manage and the level of support required; and providing clearly identified pathways to access resources. Research outlined in this book demonstrates that those who have access to the support of extended family and friends tend to cope better. Additionally, patients and carers who have a good understanding of their health conditions display lower levels of anxiety and better emotional well-being.

There are aspects of aging that are currently thought of as 'normal'. Pain is becoming an increasingly common problem for our aging population. Increasing numbers of older adults will have to deal with threats to basic day-to-day functioning, mood, sleep and overall quality of life that can result from living with persistent pain, which in older adults is poorly assessed and poorly managed. It is necessary for us to challenge ageist and discriminatory attitudes to challenge those who see pain as a normal part of aging. Similarly, falling is something that people often overlook or do not fully understand in relation to its long-term consequences. Experiencing a fall and the often serious consequences of a fall can have a major impact on an individual's life, and it is therefore imperative that professionals work closely with individuals to assess risk and work on multifactorial and individualised approaches to falls prevention to allow people to live positively.

There are proactive things that we can all look to include in our lives to ensure a positive later life. For example, the role physical activity and healthy eating have to play in promoting positive aging is invaluable; through publicising the importance of engaging in physical activity and following a healthy diet, we can improve our population's health and well-being. These are simple things that we can all do to have a greater sense of control over our own health. Furthermore, we are now experiencing a growing population of older adults who have the potential to enable and support the development of digital technology, to help live independently for longer, potentially offset some of the effects of age-related cognitive decline and use these services to promote positive aging for themselves and others.

Further to enabling individuals to live independently for longer, it is time we were proactive in considering the diversity of future housing options for the changing population's needs and wants. We often underestimate the importance of the place in which we live, the possible changes that environment might need through the different stages of later life, how small changes can make a huge difference to allowing people to live in the comfort of their own homes and the impact that can then have on their well-being. We are at the start of a changing world where individuals will not only want to, but have to, remain in their own homes for as long as possible – residential care will increasingly not be a feasible or favoured choice for most, although one that will remain a necessity for some. Where we live makes a huge difference to our quality of life. By building and sharing evidence, and supporting people in accessing and understanding what options are available, later life can be spent in an environment chosen and designed by the person, ensuring more of us are in control and aging well in place.

There is a growing body of evidence which demonstrates the positive relationship of social engagement with health and well-being in later life. However, this relationship is complex and varies based on gender and cultural differences and the quality, type and number of social connections. Cultural differences are prominent, in particular the traditional family structures and attitudes towards aging in Asia, whereby younger generations traditionally cared for their older relatives within the same household. However, the frequency of this has decreased due to societal changes. Occupation can be considered an integral component of socialisation especially for older people, because of the significant role of positive aspects of work such as providing financial and social support. However, a circular relationship was suggested, as evidence suggests that social engagement is likely to increase the opportunities for working and volunteering in older adults. Therefore, social engagement is an important aspect for promoting positive aging.

Alongside positive aging, it is also essential we consider positive dying. We keep talking about individuals starting to take control of their lives; it is also time that we encourage everyone to take control of the end of their lives too. Having the opportunity to talk about what dying 'well' means for the individual, and indeed those around them, is essential to ensure preferences are met. With increasingly diverse populations in nations around the world and the increasing prevalence of dementia, it is essential that compassionate care at the end of life is flexible and can be delivered to everyone. Starting discussions early are paramount to allowing an individual's thoughts, wishes and preferences to be taken into account to allow for a more positive experience at the end of life.

It is important to note that decline in various aspects of social, physical and mental functioning is not inevitable as we age. For instance, it is commonly believed that sexual desires diminish with age and is also less frequently discussed compared to other aspects of aging. However, pleasure and interest do not diminish with age. Sexual health in older adults has received less research attention in recent years despite the statistics which show that the rate of sexually transmitted diseases has doubled in the last decade. Sexual health care policy and education needs to be improved to include older adult sexual health behaviour to the same level as they address the sexual health needs of adolescents. Safe sexual activity is a fundamental human desire and can continue as long as one chooses and regardless of age, gender or sexual orientation. Additionally, not all cognitive abilities decline inevitably in later life. As we age we continue to maintain, and even grow, our knowledge about the world, which may help us manage declines in other areas of cognition. This highlights our capacity to maintain good functioning into later life and also to adapt to manage decline. Evidence discussed demonstrates that aging is not solely a biological process, but also a psychosocial process whereby attitudes, self-perceptions and stereotypes of aging can affect cognitive and physical health outcomes. This demonstrates the importance of having positive attitudes towards aging.

It is time we moved away from negative and harmful language, which does nothing but entrench ageist and negative views, and instead start to see our changing society as an opportunity rather than seeing the aging population as a 'burden' on health and social care services. This will not happen overnight but by starting to challenge negative thinking, it is hoped that individuals will feel empowered to take control of their lives and reshape the way society views older adults. This seed change will require new thinking about aging and health and well-being which must come from employers, health services and older adults themselves. We need to capitalise on the vast knowledge, wisdom and experience of those older than us to help problem-solve the challenges we are facing. One important way of doing this is to increase the involvement of older adults as people with lived experience in research, agenda setting and decision-making at a policy and wider level. Their input is also valuable because we often have pre-conceived ideas regarding what the aging population 'need' or 'think'.

Amongst all of this, we have to remember that older adults are not a homogenous group. We already know that the definition of 'older adults' varies between nations (50 or 65 years) and between philosophical perspectives (for example, sociological, psychological or biological). Furthermore, strategies put into place today may not be appropriate for the older population of tomorrow. The only way that this can happen is to empower individuals to take control and influence the socio-political agenda which in turn will shape the health and social care agenda and provide services that can be fit for purpose and reactive to the changing needs of society to enable us all to age more positively.

INDEX

Note: Page numbers in *italics* indicate figures and tables.

For Product Safety Concerns and Information please contact our EU
representative GPSR@taylorandfrancis.com
Taylor & Francis Verlag GmbH, Kaufingerstraße 24, 80331 München, Germany

www.ingramcontent.com/pod-product-compliance
Ingram Content Group UK Ltd.
Pitfield, Milton Keynes, MK11 3LW, UK
UKHW050054200926
475702UK00019B/2829
* 9 7 8 0 3 6 7 8 7 3 4 9 3 *